CHROMOSOMES AND CANCER
From Molecules to Man

BRISTOL-MYERS CANCER SYMPOSIA

Series Editor
MAXWELL GORDON
Science and Technology Division
Bristol-Myers Company

1. Harris Busch, Stanley T. Crooke, and Yerach Daskal (Editors).
   Effects of Drugs on the Cell Nucleus, 1979.

2. Alan C. Sartorelli, John S. Lazo, and Joseph R. Bertino (Editors).
   Molecular Actions and Targets for Cancer Chemotherapeutic Agents, 1981.

3. Saul A. Rosenberg and Henry S. Kaplan (Editors).
   Malignant Lymphomas:
   Etiology, Immunology, Pathology, Treatment, 1982.

4. Albert H. Owens, Jr., Donald S. Coffey, and Stephen B. Baylin (Editors).
   Tumor Cell Heterogeneity: Origins and Implications, 1982.

5. Janet D. Rowley and John E. Ultmann (Editors).
   Chromosomes and Cancer: From Molecules to Man, 1983.

In preparation

6. G. Bonadonna and U. Veronesi (Editors).
   Clinical Trials and Cancer Medicine, 1984.

CHROMOSOMES AND CANCER

From Molecules to Man

Edited by

JANET D. ROWLEY
Section of Hematology/Oncology
The University of Chicago
Chicago, Illinois

JOHN E. ULTMANN
Section of Hematology/Oncology
and the Cancer Research Center
The University of Chicago
Chicago, Illinois

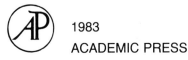

1983
ACADEMIC PRESS

A Subsidiary of Harcourt Brace Jovanovich, Publishers
New York   London
Paris   San Diego   San Francisco   São Paulo   Sydney   Tokyo   Toronto

ACADEMIC PRESS, INC.
111 Fifth Avenue, New York, New York 10003

United Kingdom Edition published by
ACADEMIC PRESS, INC. (LONDON) LTD.
24/28 Oval Road, London NW1 7DX

Library of Congress Cataloging in Publication Data
Main entry under title:

Chromosomes and cancer: from molecules to man.

(Bristol-Myers cancer symposia series; v. 5)
Includes index.
1. Cancer--Genetic aspects--Congresses. 2. Chromo-
some abnormalities--Congresses. I. Rowley, Janet.
II. Ultmann, J. E. (John E.) III. Series. [DNLM:
1. Neoplasms--Familial and genetic--Congresses.
2. Chromosome abnormalities--Congresses. W3 BR429 v.5
/ QZ 200 C557 1982]
RC268.4.C49 1983 616.99'4042   83-11872
ISBN 0-12-600250-9

PRINTED IN THE UNITED STATES OF AMERICA

83 84 85 86 9 8 7 6 5 4 3 2 1

Contents

Introduction to Symposium
JANET D. ROWLEY

PART I   CHROMOSOME STRUCTURE AND FUNCTION

Introduction
HEWSON SWIFT

Long-Range Order Folding of the Chromatin Fibers in Metaphase Chromosomes and Nuclei
U. K. LAEMMLI, C. D. LEWIS, and W. C. EARNSHAW

v

PART II   CHROMOSOME PATTERN IN ANIMAL AND HUMAN TUMORS

Specific Chromosome Changes in the Human Heritable Tumors Retinoblastoma and Nephroblastoma
UTA FRANCKE

Chromosome Abnormalities and Gene Amplification: Comparison of Antifolate-Resistant and Human Neuroblastoma Cell Systems
JUNE L. BIEDLER, PETER W. MELERA, and BARBARA A. SPENGLER

Chromosome Changes in Leukemic Cells as Indicators of Mutagenic Exposure
JANET D. ROWLEY

PART III NEW APPROACHES TO CORRELATING LOCATION OF CHROMOSOME ABNORMALITIES WITH SPECIFIC GENES

Construction and Characterization of Chromosomal DNA Libraries

BRYAN D. YOUNG, MARC JEANPIERRE, MALCOLM H. GOYNS, GORDON D. STEWART, THERESA ELLIOT, and ROBERT KRUMLAUF

States of Differentiation in Leukemias: A Two-Dimensional Gel Analysis of Genetic Expression

ERIC P. LESTER, PETER F. LEMKIN, and LEWIS E. LIPKIN

Localization of Viral-Specific DNA in the Mammalian Chromosome Complement by Cytological Hybridization

ANN S. HENDERSON

A Sensitive Colorimetric Method for Visualizing Biotin-Labeled Probes Hybridized to DNA or RNA on Nitrocellulose Filters

JEFFRY J. LEARY, DAVID J. BRIGATI, and DAVID C. WARD

PART IV   RELATIONSHIP OF CHROMOSOME CHANGES TO NEOPLASTIC TRANSFORMATION

Introduction

JOHN E. ULTMANN

Contributors

Numbers in parentheses indicate the pages on which the authors' contributions begin.

JUNE L. BIEDLER (117), Laboratory of Cellular and Biochemical Genetics, Memorial Sloan-Kettering Cancer Center, New York, New York 10021

DAVID J. BRIGATI[1] (273), Laboratory of Medicine, Yale University School of Medicine, New Haven, Connecticut 06510

A. V. CARRANO (195), Biomedical Sciences Division, Lawrence Livermore National Laboratory, Livermore, California 94550

P. CHAMBON (29), Institut de Chimie Biologique—Faculté de Médecine, Laboratoire de Génétique Moléculaire des Eucaryotes du CNRS et Unité 184 de Biologie Moléculaire et de Génie Génétique de l'INSERM, 67085 Strasbourg, France

GEOFFREY M. COOPER (45), Dana–Farber Cancer Institute, and Department of Pathology, Harvard Medical School, Boston, Massachusetts 02115

J. CORDEN[2] (29), Institute de Chimie Biologique—Faculté de Médecine, Laboratoire de Génétique Moléculaire des Eucaryotes du CNRS et Unité 184 de Biologie Moléculaire et de Génie Génétique de l'INSERM, 67085 Strasbourg, France

C. CROCE (165), The Wistar Institute, Philadelphia, Pennsylvania 19104

R. DALLA-FAVERA[3] (165), Laboratory of Tumor Cell Biology, National Cancer Institute, Bethesda, Maryland 20205

---

[1]Present address: Department of Pathology, The Milton S. Hershey Medical Center, Pennsylvania State University, Hershey, Pennsylvania 17033.

[2]Present address: Department of Molecular Biology, Johns Hopkins University School of Medicine, Baltimore, Maryland 21205.

[3]Present address: Department of Pathology, New York University School of Medicine, New York, New York 10016.

W. C. EARNSHAW[4] (15), Departments of Molecular Biology and Biochemistry, University of Geneva, Geneva 12, Switzerland

THERESA ELLIOT (211), Duncan Guthrie Institute of Medical Genetics, Yorkhill Hospital, Glasgow, Scotland

J. ERIKSON (165), The Wistar Institute, Philadelphia, Pennsylvania 19104

H. JOHN EVANS (333), Clinical and Population Cytogenetics Unit, Medical Research Council, Western General Hospital, Edinburgh, Scotland

J. FINAN (165), Department of Pathology and Laboratory Medicine, University of Pennsylvania School of Medicine, Philadelphia, Pennsylvania 19104

UTA FRANCKE (99), Department of Human Genetics, Yale University School of Medicine, New Haven, Connecticut 06510

M. P. GAUB (29), Institut de Chimie Biologique—Faculté de Médecine, Laboratoire de Génétique Moléculaire des Eucaryotes du CNRS and Unité 184 de Biologie Moléculaire et de Génie Génétique de l'INSERM, 67085 Strasbourg, France

HARVEY M. GOLOMB (311), Section of Hematology/Oncology, The University of Chicago, Chicago, Illinois 60637

PETER N. GOODFELLOW (183), Imperial Cancer Research Fund, London WC2A 3PX, England

MALCOLM H. GOYNS (211), Beatson Institute for Cancer Research, Glasgow G61 1BD, Scotland

J. W. GRAY (195), Biomedical Sciences Division, Lawrence Livermore National Laboratory, Livermore, California 94550

JOHN GROFFEN (183), Laboratory of Viral Carcinogenesis, National Cancer Institute—Frederick Cancer Research Facility, Frederick, Maryland 21701

NORA HEISTERKAMP (183), Laboratory of Viral Carcinogenesis, National Cancer Institute—Frederick Cancer Research Facility, Frederick, Maryland 21701

R. HEN (29), Institut de Chimie Biologique—Faculté de Médecine, Laboratoire de Génétique Moléculaire des Eucaryotes du CNRS et Unité 184 de Biologie Moléculaire et de Génie Génétique de l'INSERM, 67085 Strasbourg, France

ANN S. HENDERSON[5] (247), Department of Human Genetics and Development, Columbia University School of Health Sciences, New York, New York 10032

LYNNE R. HIORNS (183), Imperial Cancer Research Fund, London WC2A 3PX, England

[4]Present address: Department of Cell Biology and Anatomy, Johns Hopkins University School of Medicine, Baltimore, Maryland 21205.

[5]Present address: Department of Biological Sciences, Hunter College, New York, New York 10021.

MARC JEANPIERRE[6] (211), Beatson Institute for Cancer Research, Glasgow G61 1BD, Scotland

C. KÉDINGER (29), Institut de Chimie Biologique—Faculté de Médecine, Laboratoire de Génétique Moléculaire des Eucaryotes du CNRS et Unité 184 de Biologie Moléculaire et de Génie Génétique de l'INSERM, 67085 Strasbourg, France

ROBERT KRUMLAUF[7] (211), Beatson Institute for Cancer Research, Glasgow G61 1BD, Scotland

U. K. LAEMMLI (15), Departments of Molecular Biology and Biochemistry, University of Geneva, Geneva 12, Switzerland

MARY-ANN LANE (45), Dana–Farber Cancer Institute, and Department of Pathology, Harvard Medical School, Boston, Massachusetts 02115

R. G. LANGLOIS (195), Biomedical Sciences Division, Lawrence Livermore National Laboratory, Livermore, California 94550

RICHARD A. LARSON (311), Section of Hematology/Oncology, The University of Chicago, Chicago, Illinois 60637

JEFFRY J. LEARY (273), Department of Human Genetics, Yale University School of Medicine, New Haven, Connecticut 06510

PETER F. LEMKIN (225), Image Processing Section, National Cancer Institute, Bethesda, Maryland 20205

ERIC P. LESTER (225), Section of Hematology/Oncology and the Cancer Research Center, The University of Chicago, Chicago, Illinois 60637

C. D. LEWIS (15), Departments of Molecular Biology and Biochemistry, University of Geneva, Geneva 12, Switzerland

LEWIS E. LIPKIN (225), Image Processing Section, National Cancer Institute, Bethesda, Maryland 20205

PAUL A. MARKS (291), DeWitt Wallace Research Laboratory, Memorial Sloan-Kettering Cancer Center, New York, New York 10021

PETER W. MELERA (117), Laboratory of RNA Synthesis and Regulation, Memorial Sloan-Kettering Cancer Center, New York, New York 10021

FELIX MITELMAN (61), Department of Clinical Genetics, University of Lund, Lund S-22185, Sweden

P. NOWELL (165), Department of Pathology and Laboratory Medicine, University of Pennsylvania School of Medicine, Philadelphia, Pennsylvania 19104

MARILYN G. PEARSON (311), Section of Hematology/Oncology, The University of Chicago, Chicago, Illinois 60637

SUSAN POVEY (183), MRC Human Biochemical Genetics Unit, The Galton Laboratory, University College, London NW1 2HE, England

[6]Present address: Institut de Pathologie Moleculaire, 24 rue du Faubourg Saint Jacques, Paris, France.
[7]Present address: Fox Chase Institute for Cancer Research, Philadelphia, Pennsylvania 19111.

RICHARD A. RIFKIND (291), DeWitt Wallace Research Laboratory, Memorial Sloan-Kettering Cancer Center, New York, New York 10021

JANET D. ROWLEY (1, 57, 139, 163), Section of Hematology/Oncology, The University of Chicago, Chicago, Illinois 60637

P. SASSONE-CORSI (29), Institut de Chimie Biologique—Faculté de Médecine, Laboratoire de Génétique Moléculaire des Eucaryotes du CNRS et Unité 184 de Biologie Moléculaire et de Génie Génétique de l'INSERM, 67085 Strasbourg, France

DENISE SHEER (183), Imperial Cancer Research Fund, London WC2A 3PX, England

MICHAEL SHEFFERY (291), DeWitt Wallace Research Laboratory, Memorial Sloan-Kettering Cancer Center, New York, New York 10021

ELLEN SOLOMON (183), Imperial Cancer Research Fund, London WC2A 3PX, England

BARBARA A. SPENGLER (117), Laboratory of Cellular and Biochemical Genetics, Memorial Sloan-Kettering Cancer Center, New York, New York 10021

JACK SPIRA (85), Department of Tumor Biology, Karolinska Institute, Stockholm S-10401, Sweden

JOHN R. STEPHENSON (183), Laboratory of Viral Carcinogenesis, National Cancer Institute—Frederick Cancer Research Facility, Frederick, Maryland 21701

GORDON D. STEWART (211), Duncan Guthrie Institute of Medical Genetics, Yorkhill Hospital, Glasgow, Scotland

DALLAS M. SWALLOW (183), MRC Human Biochemical Genetics Unit, The Galton Laboratory, University College, London NW1 2HE, England

HEWSON SWIFT (5), Department of Biology, The University of Chicago, Chicago, Illinois 60637

JOHN E. ULTMANN (309), Section of Hematology/Oncology and the Cancer Research Center, The University of Chicago, Chicago, Illinois 60637

DAVID C. WARD (273), Departments of Human Genetics and Molecular Biophysics–Biochemistry, Yale University School of Medicine, New Haven, Connecticut 06510

BRYAN D. YOUNG (211), Beatson Institute for Cancer Research, Glasgow G61 1BD, Scotland

L.-C. YU (195), Biomedical Sciences Division, Lawrence Livermore National Laboratory, Livermore, California 94550

Editor's Foreword

This fifth volume of the Bristol-Myers Cancer Symposium Series comes at a time of extraordinary ferment in cancer research. The subject of this symposium, namely,"Chromosomes and Cancer:From Molecules to Man,"surveys the newer areas of excitement in cancer research, especially work on oncogenes, gene expression, and translocations.

The process of carcinogenesis appears to be a complex one involving many steps, several of them under genetic control. Until recently it was not possible to identify the genes specifically involved in malignant transformation. However, modern techniques now make it possible to select out transforming genes and to isolate and characterize their protein products. The involvement of viruses in the genetic transformations leading to cancer is receiving increasing attention, and certain sequences present in viruses have been shown to correspond to homologous DNA sequences found in human cells, both normal and cancer cells. In provocative experiments the treatment of cancer cells *in vitro* with interferon caused not only a redifferentiation to normal but also a disappearance of a viral sequence detected in the cancer cell.

In this volume, topics such as chromosome patterns in human cancer, chromosome abnormalities and gene amplification, chromosome changes in mutagenesis, chromosome translocations as they relate to immunoglobulin loci and neoplasia, flow cytogenetics as applied to cancer research, genetic expression in leukemias as related to state of cell differentiation, cytological hybridization for localization of viral-specific DNA, and chromatin structure, are treated in depth. This area of science is moving so rapidly that it is impossible to predict where we will be even a year from now.

The sixth volume of the Bristol-Myers Cancer Symposium Series will relate to the clinical sphere with a review of the impact of research on cancer treatment and how this interaction will grow over the years.

Maxwell Gordon
Series Editor

Foreword

This is a time of ferment and excitement in the world of cancer research and therapy. The authoritative British scientific journal, *Nature,* has said that "1983 may be the year in which carcinogenesis is finally understood" and asserted that "for the first time there is a chance of getting to the bottom of the phenomenon of cancer."

Among the signs of a quickening pace in our knowledge of cancer is the progress being announced each month at laboratories around the world and at scientific meetings, such as the fifth annual Bristol-Myers Cancer Symposium Series, reported in this volume. I am pleased that Bristol-Myers has been able to contribute to this progress. The annual Bristol-Myers Symposium on Cancer Research and the annual Bristol-Myers Award for Distinguished Achievement in Cancer Research are two aspects of Bristol-Myers' support of cancer investigation.

Over the past 6 years, we have also made unrestricted research grants to thirteen medical schools and cancer centers—10 in the United States, 2 in Europe, and 1 in Canada. The grants, which now total $6.34 million, are made with the suggestion that they be used to underwrite cancer research that is promising and potentially significant but for one reason or another unlikely to attract public funding. Each grant carries a firm understanding, however, that the recipient institution alone will determine how the grant is used—with no strings attached.

The success of this program has led us to use it as a model for support by our company of research in two other fields of medicine: human nutrition, where we initiated a program in 1980, and orthopaedics, where we announced a program earlier in 1983.

As a result, Bristol-Myers' commitment to unrestricted medical research now exceeds 8 million dollars. We expect the figure to rise even higher in the years ahead.

Many new pieces of the cancer puzzle are being found, and many cancer patients are surviving longer. In basic research, there are exciting developments taking place which also raise our hopes. To turn that hope into reality is the purpose that unites all of us. Bristol-Myers is proud to be playing a role in today's progress in cancer research.

Richard L. Gelb
Chairman of the Board
Bristol-Myers Company

Preface

The Fifth Annual Bristol-Myers Symposium on Cancer Research was held at The University of Chicago Cancer Research Center in October 1982. The topic "Chromosomes and Cancer: From Molecules to Man" was chosen to highlight the progress which has occurred in the past decade in this area.

Nonrandom chromosome changes have been detected in a variety of human tumors. Many of them are specifically associated with particular types of tumors. The challenge for the 1980s is to determine which genes carried by the aberrant chromosomes are affected and how the chromosome changes modify the function of these genes that in turn affect cell proliferation and malignant transformation.

This Symposium included presentations on our present understanding of chromosome structure, gene organization, and the control of gene function. The current status of our knowledge about chromosome changes in a variety of human and animal malignant tumors and leukemias was reviewed.

With these reviews of the chromosome and chromosome abnormalities as background, a major focus of the Symposium was on the techniques that are currently available to bridge the gaps between the identification of the aberrant chromosome and our understanding of the function of the affected gene. The papers included discussions of the improved techniques of chromosome banding, chromosome sorting, and the use of somatic cell hybrids to isolate the chromosomes of interest. *In situ* chromosome hybridization and the use of protein maps to analyze gene function were also described. The aim was to highlight the areas that are likely to be productive in our search for the molecular mechanisms of carcinogenesis.

This increased knowledge should result in improved, more targeted therapy because we will be able to classify disease more precisely (i.e., in CML, Ph[1] positive from Ph[1] negative) and to understand the basis for the development of drug resistance in some patients (i.e., gene amplification). Moreover, as we identify the fundamental alterations in gene structure and function in malignant cells, we will be able to institute rational therapy tailored to correct the specific genetic change.

The success of the Symposium was assured by the dedicated work of many individuals. We wish to thank Marie Garza, Marianne Hartzmark, Steven Honingfeld, Marjorie Isaacson, Theresa Kelley, Susan Morin, Nancy Nagel, Patricia Rosner, Jacqueline Samuel, Jennifer Sanders, and Pamela Stokes. We acknowledge with deep gratitude the sponsorship by the Bristol-Myers Company which made this Symposium and the publication of its transactions possible.

Janet D. Rowley
John E. Ultmann

Abbreviations

AA, only chromosomally abnormal metaphase cells
ABR, abnormal banding regions
Ad2ML, adenovirus type 2 major late
Ad2MLP, adenovirus type 2 major late promoter
ALL, acute lymphoblastic leukemia
AML, acute myelogenous leukemia
AMMOL, acute myelomonocytic leukemia
AN, mixture of chromosomally normal and abnormal cells
ANLL, acute nonlymphocytic leukemia
APL, acute promyelocytic leukemia
AWTA, Aniridia-Wilms' tumor association

BACSE, biotinyl-ϵ-aminocaproic acid N-hydroxysuccinimide
bp, base pair
BP, benzo(a)pyrene

CFU-e, colony forming units-erythroid
CHO, Chinese hamster ovary
CHL, Chinese hamster lungs
CLL, chronic lymphocytic leukemia
CML, chronic myelogenous leukemia

DHFR, dihydrofolate reductase
DM, double-minute chromosomes
DMBA, 7,12-dimethylbenz(a)anthracene
DMSO, dimethyl sulfoxide

EBV, Epstein-Barr virus
EL, erythroleukemia

FAB, French/American/British classification
FACS, fluorescence activated cell sorter

HCL, hairy cell leukemia
HD, Hodgkin's disease
HMBA, hexamethylene bisacetamide
HSR, homogeneously staining regions

Kb, kilobase

LTR, long terminal repeat

MD, myelodysplastic diseases
MELC, murine erythroleukemia cells
MM, multiple myeloma
ML, malignant lymphoma

PDL, poorly differentiated lymphocytic lymphoma
PHA, phytohemagglutinin
PV, polycythemia vera

RB, retinoblastoma

SRL, search result list

WCE, whole cell extract
WT, Wilms' tumor

Introduction to Symposium

JANET D. ROWLEY

Section of Hematology/Oncology
The University of Chicago
Chicago, Illinois

The question of the role of consistent chromosome changes in human cancer has been debated for quite some time (see Mitelman, Chapter 4). The veritable explosion of information regarding the chromosome location of the cellular genes that are homologous to the viral oncogenes has awakened an interest in this topic in the entire biomedical community. It is, thus, especially appropriate to have a symposium on chromosomes and cancer at this particular time.

This Symposium has two main goals. The first is to review what we have learned about recurring chromosome abnormalities in various human and animal malignant diseases. The emphasis is on both the specificity of various abnormalities in particular human tumors and on the remarkable concordance of much of the data from human and mouse lymphoid neoplasms. One of the most striking examples of chromosome specificity is the presence of particular translations, usually involving the same pair of chromosomes, in restricted types of tumors. The data of some of these consistent aberrations will be discussed in Part II.

The second goal is to ask about the nature of the genes at the sites of the breakpoints in these translocations and about the changes in the function of these genes as they are moved to a different location as the result of the translocation. The techniques that are appropriate to isolating the DNA of interest and to determining the function of these genes are reviewed in Part III. The strategies presented in this session are of great importance, because our aim as cytogeneticists is not merely to catalog the chromosome abnormalities that we find in a particular tumor, but rather to identify chromosome regions that are clearly of biologic importance in a particular malignant disease because of their recurring nature.

As indicated earlier, there has been a remarkable burst of information regarding the chromosome location of the cellular counterparts of viral transforming

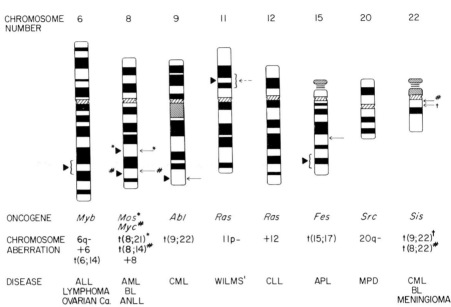

CHROMOSOME NUMBER	6	8	9	11	12	15	20	22
ONCOGENE	Myb	Mos* Myc#	Abl	Ras	Ras	Fes	Src	Sis
CHROMOSOME ABERRATION	6q- +6 t(6;14)	t(8;21)* t(8;14)# +8	t(9;22)	11p-	+12	t(15;17)	20q-	t(9;22)† t(8;22)#
DISEASE	ALL LYMPHOMA OVARIAN Ca.	AML BL ANLL	CML	WILMS'	CLL	APL	MPD	CML BL MENINGIOMA

Fig. 1. Diagram of chromosomes containing known cellular oncogenes; the number is above each chromosome, and the oncogene, karyotypic aberrations, and neoplastic diseases associated with these abnormalities are indicated below the chromosome. The arrowhead (▶) to the left of each chromosome indicates the band carrying the cellular oncogene; the arrow or arrows to the right of a chromosome identify specific bands involved in consistent translocations (←) or deletions (←--) observed in patients having the disorders listed. The asterisk indicates the c-mos and t(8;21), and # indicates the c-myc and t(8;14) or t(8;22). AML, acute myeloblastic leukemia; CML, chronic myelogenous leukemia; APL, acute promyelocytic leukemia; ANLL, acute nonlymphocytic leukemia; CLL; chronic lymphocytic leukemia; and MPD, myeloproliferative disorder. The letter p indicates the short arm, and q, the long arm of the chromosome. Reprinted by permission from *Nature* **301,** 290, Copyright © 1983, Macmillan Journals Limited.

genes called oncogenes. Some of the initial data were presented at this Symposium; events here moved so swiftly that we now know the chromosome location of 9 cellular oncogenes and the band location for 6 of these (Fig. 1). To call these genes "oncogenes" is quite likely a misnomer because their functions, almost certainly, are not as cancer genes, but rather as essential genes in some step of cellular proliferation or differentiation. Whatever their function, and the function of the other genes at the sites of specific translocations or deletions, some of the techniques reviewed in Part III will be useful in our attempts to clarify the nature and the purpose of these remarkable genes.

It is important to relate the chromosome abnormalities that we have detected in various tumors to our current understanding of chromosome structure and function. It is, thus, appropriate that the first part in this Symposium be devoted to these fundamental topics.

PART I

Chromosome Structure and Function

Introduction

HEWSON SWIFT

Department of Biology
The University of Chicago
Chicago, Illinois

In his studies of sea urchin eggs, Theodor Boveri in 1902 reported on the anomalous mitoses produced when fertilization occurred with multiple sperm nuclei. He noted that many cytoplasmic lesions could be repaired by the embryo to provide almost normal development, but nuclear abnormalities produced by polyspermy invariably resulted in distorted cleavage patterns and death of the embryo. He discussed his conviction that cancer cells, like the aneuploid sea urchin cells, involved ''a particular incorrectly combined chromosome array'' in the monograph ''Zur Frage der Entstehung maligner Tumoren'' published in 1914, the year before his death. Our Symposium begins with studies, like those of Boveri, concerned with the basic aspects of cell biology. His conviction that ''the tumor problem is a cell problem'' today requires little further argument.

Several basic questions will be approached in this session: First, how is the genetic material held together in mitotic chromosomes, and in the chromatin of the interphase nucleus? Second, what are the genetic signals that mark the attachment sites for the RNA polymerase molecules, required to initiate specific RNA synthesis? Third, what molecular events may precede or accompany this transcription process, and fourth, what factors may disrupt the usual orderly mechanisms of transcription control, leading to abnormal patterns of cell growth?

The tremendous extent and complexity of the genome confronts the cell biologist working with eukaryote cells. The 3.2 pg of DNA in a human sperm or ovum contains almost 3×10^9 bp, more than 100 times the total number of letters and punctuation marks in a complete set of the ''Encyclopedia Britannica.'' It is of

5

importance to understand the way this tremendously long and complex genome, the cell memory, is arranged within a typical interphase nucleus and partitioned into the 46 chromosomes of a dividing human cell. The DNA molecules that make up the human genetic material, one per chromosome, if arranged end to end would stretch for slightly more than 2 m, or more than 200,000 times the diameter of the lymphocyte nucleus that could contain them. This huge length of double helix must be organized in the nucleus in an untangled array, and like the disk drives in a microcomputer, specific regions must be available for rapid read-out when the proper activitating signals are provided. As mentioned in Chapter 1 by Laemmli *et al.,* spaced every 200 bp along the double helix is a small bead of eight histone molecules. The DNA molecule winds twice around each of these histone octamers to form an ordered string of beads, the nucleosomes. Another kind of histone molecule (H1) bridges the gap between nucleosomes, and ties the beads together into a thicker and more compact chromatin fiber. Each histone molecule is designed to combine with the DNA in a specific way, to neutralize the acid groups with arginine or lysine residues, and at the same time to cross-pair with other histones. The nucleosome pattern of chromatin is fundamental to all eukaryote cells, and in evolutionary terms it is very old, similar in plants and animals and from primitive protozoa to man.

Even though the association with histones shortens the genetic material to 2% of the length of the DNA molecules that it contains, chromatin fibers still have great length. A human lymphocyte encompasses strands of nucleohistone totaling 30 cm. These wind, like Laocoön, through the interphase nucleus, forming densely packed clumps of heterochromatin around the nucleolus and against the nuclear margin, and unraveling into diffuse regions in the interchromatin areas. The chromatin fibers seem to adhere to the inner surface of the nuclear envelope, apparently held in place by their association with the fibrous lamina. This lamina coats the nuclear envelope except in the region of the pores, which are kept open for the exchange of materials between nucleus and cytoplasm. It is formed of three major proteins, 70,000, 67,000, and 60,000 daltons in size, which constitute a peripheral meshwork around the entire nuclear margin (Gerace *et al.,* 1978).

Within the interphase nucleus the specific patterns of the chromosomes have been dissolved into diffuse areas and irregular clumps of chromatin, and yet it is obvious that the continuity of the DNA fibers must be maintained. Again, it was Boveri (1899) who pointed out in his studies on development of the parasitic worm, *Ascaris,* that chromosomes must somehow stay intact in spite of their apparent dissolution in interphase. He showed that the terminal knobs of heterochromatin on the chromosomes formed small projections on the nuclear margin as telophase nuclei proceeded into interphase, and when the next mitosis came around, the same chromosome end could be seen to condense within the projection.

How specific is this arrangement of chromosome fibers? Do individual gene loci possess specific sites of localization within most interphase nuclei? We know already that the distribution of DNA is not random. In many nuclei, heterochromatin occurs in specific clumps at one side of the nucleus, but this is often the result of their location at the centromeres of chromosomes, since the centromeres are concentrated at the spindle pole of the preceding telophase (Woodard *et al.*, 1961). Metaphase chromosomes in some cells tend to have specific sites on the mitotic spindle, the smaller chromosomes inside and the larger more peripheral, but this again seems the result of the kinetics of cell division (Schrader, 1953). Specific metaphase chromosomes have a tangible probability of occurring beside their homologs on the metaphase plate in most flies (e.g., *Drosophila*) and some higher plants (Feldman *et al.*, 1966), but this positioning probably depends on a generalized tendency for homologous association, rather than on a specific ordering of the interphase genome. One finding has repeatedly been made. Most chromosomal inversions or translocations, involving new associations between chromosome regions, are widely tolerated in somatic cells without visible effect, a lesson learned from countless cytogenetic studies with *Drosophila,* maize, and numerous other systems. Specific translocations associated with oncogenicity must do more than disrupt a vague gestalt of the interphase nucleus, and can probably be attributed instead to cis acting events along single chromatin fibers of a much more detailed scope, acting to disrupt control sequences at the molecular level. Chromosome abnormalities can, however, cause specific problems in meiosis where events of chromosome pairing, recombination, and segregation are involved, but the cytogenetics of gamete formation are not the concern of this Symposium.

The interphase nucleus obviously contains much more than just the chromatin fibers and the outer lamina. Nuclei that are synthetically active enlarge and are filled with proteins of the nucleoplasm and the complex array of proteins required for RNA synthesis and processing. Some workers (Berezney and Coffee, 1974; Basler *et al.*, 1981) have described the nuclear matrix, which they feel is specifically involved in holding the chromatin fibers in an ordered array, necessary for the events of transcription, and also to orient and bind the DNA polymerase molecules during DNA replication. The specific proteins involved in the nuclear matrix have proved difficult to characterize and to separate as a fraction distinct from the outer lamina. In Chapter 1, Laemmli *et al.* describes recent evidence for an attachment between the proteins of the lamina and the chromatin fibers. Whether or not this interesting association is sufficient to account for the structural arrangement of chromatin fibers within the interphase nucleus must await better characterization of the presently somewhat enigmatic matrix.

With the onset of mitosis a series of events occurs, leading to the appearance of the 46 chromosomes and their orderly segregation at anaphase. The work of Laemmli and colleagues has brilliantly described the presence of a scaffold protein that must play a major role in this condensation process, including evidence that the chromatin fiber is attached at periodic points to a fibrous scaffold that forms a central chromosome axis from which the nucleohistone fiber loops out and back. As prophase proceeds into metaphase the scaffold proteins somehow shorten, bringing the chromatin fiber more and more tightly into the metaphase chromosome. Such "cores" have long been known in meiotic chromosomes (Moses, 1968) where paired homologs provide a thicker and more rigid structure, but the delicate axes of somatic chromosomes suspected earlier are difficult to demonstrate (Wray and Stubblefield, 1970), needing sophisticated protein chemistry to make them clearly evident.

As prophase proceeds into metaphase the nuclear envelope breaks down, and with it the nuclear lamina proteins are depolymerized, as clearly shown by Gerace and Blobel (1980). Just before the nuclear envelope falls apart, in many cells the condensing chromosomes can be seen to move to the nuclear margin. Such a localization is nicely explained if the chromatin fiber is attached both to the central scaffold to form loops, and each loop near its apex is also attached to the lamina. It seems possible that cyclic changes in two attachment systems for the chromatin fiber, lamina in interphase and scaffold in mitosis, may go far toward providing an understanding of the complex changes in chromatin condensation and decondensation during the mitotic cycle. Whether other structural elements, such as the more elusive matrix proteins, are also involved, remains to be seen.

Tablets engraved with languages long dead may be difficult if not impossible to translate. To be able to read the genetic code, with all the subtleties required for an understanding of the mechanisms for gene control, we must somehow change the dead language of base sequences to a living one. The process of extricating specific coding regions and their flanking sequences, altering them by deletion or base substitution, and then reinserting them into living cells to study the effects on transcription, has been called "reverse genetics" by C. Weissmann, inverting as it does the usual procedure of the classic geneticist, who glimpsed the gene only through the effects of mutation on the organism. The new methods provide powerful tools in the understanding of gene function. In some of the most sophisticated "reverse genetics" yet accomplished, Hen and colleagues (see Chapter 2) have demonstrated the importance of DNA base sequences far removed from the coding region for the T antigen of SV40. It seems particularly significant that the findings from intact HeLa cells, made to synthesize the new protein by microinjection or with calcium phosphate precipitated DNA transfection, have also been duplicated in studies on cell homogenates, where the transcription of specific RNAs has been quantified with S_1 nuclease. One further gap in our understanding of gene action has thus been breached, where *in vitro* systems have been made to mirror the complexities of eukaryote gene action in intact cells. Indications have been provided that an active promoter region for the T antigen protein requires not only the TATA sequence, shown to be a necessary code for RNA polymerase attachment about 30 bases up stream of many gene loci, but also regions almost 100 bp away from the beginning cap site for the gene. In addition, the *in vitro* system provides an indication of more subtle aspects of chromatin structure that may also influence the relative strength or efficiency of the promoter region, since under conditions where the homogenate was partially fractionated, covalently closed circular templates showed the upstream effect whereas linear DNA did not. The importance of the three-dimensional configuration of DNA templates, or the presence of free ends, can thus be evaluated.

Gene transcription begins when a promoter region complexes with a molecule of RNA polymerase. A prevalent model for oncogenic transformation supposes that a locus important in the control of cell proliferation is inappropriately activated. Two major classes of theories suppose that activation occurs either by alterations in the DNA structure itself (genetic theories) or by induced configurational changes in the promoter region akin to the events of differentiation (epigenetic theories). The two mechanisms are not mutually exclusive. In this age of molecular biology our ignorance of molecular events in cell differentiation is rather appalling, but one fact seems reasonably clear. Although more and more cases of developmentally directed alterations in the DNA are being described, involving genome amplification, diminution, and changes induced by transposable elements (see Schimke, 1982, and *Cold Spring Harbor Symp. Quant. Biol.* **45,** 1981, for reviews), most cell differentiation is clearly based on the epigenetic pattern. The research of Weintraub and collaborators has been specifically directed to an understanding of epigenetic changes in normal differentiation. When a gene for hemoglobin is turned on in embryonic chick blood cells in the normal course of differentiation, specific sites in the chromatin fiber upstream from the gene locus become sensitive to pancreatic DNase digestion (an indication of shifts in DNA–histone relationships), and also sensitive to S_1 nuclease (an indication that the double helix is locally separated into two strands). Most recently, Groudine and Weintraub (1982) have shown that similar changes occur in chick fibroblasts induced to abnormal synthesis of hemoglobin by infection with Rous sarcoma virus. There is no indication that the viral infection alters the DNA, but only that it produces an abnormal activation of the hemoglobin promoter. It has also been shown that the same effect can even be produced in the total absence of virus, if the cells are shocked with hypertonic saline. This treatment, like the virus, apparently alters the relationship between DNA and surrounding protein molecules, since these chromatin fibers, like those in normal development, show similar changes upstream of the globin locus in DNase and S_1 sensitivity. Most remarkable, these viral- or saline-induced changes persist through many cell divisions, after the initial activating stimulus has been withdrawn. This experimental system comes as close as any to mirror the events of gene activation in normal cell differentiation. It should be possible to apply precisely the same approach to cell systems involving oncogenic transformation.

Recent studies on the effects of transposable elements in eukaryotic cells have served to blur the distinction between infective and endogenous alterations in the genome. Retroviruses are clearly extracellular infective agents, and yet the provirus DNA that they synthesize readily integrates into the host cell genome. In addition, the provirus DNA can induce its own excision from the chromosome, and may take along a piece of covalently linked normal host genome as it does so. This produces a highly variable class of DNA fragments, both extrachromosomal and inserted at a variety of places in the genome of eukaryote cells. Some fragments maintain intact viral RNA genomes and synthesize core and capsid proteins to continue the infection cycle. Others are defective, and unable to propagate, except in the presence of helper virus (see Varmus, 1982, for review).

A major discovery of modern genetic biology is that a profusion of retrovirus-like DNA sequences contribute a large portion of the DNA of many, if not most, eukaryote genomes (see *Cold Spring Harbor Symp. Quant. Biol.* **45,** 1981, for review). These moderately repetitive DNA sequences are dispersed throughout the genome of *Drosophila melanogaster,* and constitute some 10% of the total genome. They exist as families of very similar sequences, 500 to 13,000 bp long. They are variable in position when different strains of *D. melanogaster* are compared, and there is evidence that like retroviruses at least some sequences are infective (Engels, 1981; Spradling and Rubin, 1981). These sequences in almost all cases also carry terminal redundancies of 250 to 500 bp, much like the long terminal repeats (LTRs) of retroviruses. Certain of these repetitive sequences have even been used in experimental transformation studies, where microinjection of specific infective DNA into developing *Drosophila* eggs has been shown genetically to transform the resulting insect (Rubin and Spradling, 1982). The presence of infective middle repetitive DNA sequences, or transposable elements, has been suspected for many years. It is clear that insertion of such a sequence, near the TATA promoter region, or within the structural gene itself, can result in gene inactivation, as in the inactivation of a cuticle protein gene by the insertion of a ''Beagle'' sequence in the TATA box of *Drosophila* (Snyder *et al.,* 1982). In some cases, as in the insertion of the TY-1 sequence upstream from the *leucine-2* gene of yeast, the inserted element can result in a marked stimulation of gene activity (Elder *et al.,* 1981). The effects of these variable genetic elements in the pigment and starch patterns of developing maize kernels has been carefully investigated by McClintock (1965, 1967, 1978) in studies bridging many years. Thus the distribution of amylose in the endosperm and anthocyanin pigmentation of the aleurone were shown to be affected by either the supressor–mutator or activator system of control elements. Like transposable elements in *Drosophila,* these elements were variable in position in the genome and were able to act either as supressors or activators of gene activity, presumably in relation to the positions for insertion that they established within the genome. By analysis of sectors of pigment cells, or of starch accumulation within the developing endosperm, it was possible to determine the time in development at which specific genes were activated or suppressed. Some control elements acted early in development, producing large clones of altered cells. Others acted late, involving pigment or starch changes in a small clone of only a few cells.

Transposable elements follow different patterns of insertion and inactivity in different organisms. For example, sequence length is much longer in *Drosophila* elements than the apparently comparable elements in mammalian cells. We have much to learn of their probable role in mutagenesis and in understanding the extent to which they provide genetic variability in natural populations, and thus generate the raw materials of evolution. It is also of great importance to determine the evolutionary origins of transposable elements themselves, whether or not they represent a degenerate class of molecules derived from a retrovirus-like ancestor. Finally, the complex relationships between retroviruses and host cell oncogenes in vertebrate cells are obviously of primary importance, as discussed elsewhere in this Symposium. The retrovirus terminal repeat regions (LTRs) may themselves contain powerful promoters (Varmus, 1982; Temin, 1982). A translocation event that brings a new promoter adjacent to an important control element can clearly play a major role in the alteration of cell growth. There are indications that the oncogenes associated with retrovirus LTRs, at least in some instances, are purely normal gene loci associated with cell growth (Goyette *et al.*, 1983).

The transfection studies of G. M. Cooper and collaborators leave little doubt that some oncogenic transformation, as studied in mouse 3T3 cells, involves alteration in host genomic DNA. Calcium phosphate-treated DNA is readily taken up by cultured cells. When the donor cells are normal, transformation is rare and inefficient. When DNA is from most donor tumor cells the oncogenic transformation is more efficient by several orders of magnitude, though DNA from some carcinoma cell lines lacks transforming ability. Transformation tends to be specific for tissue type, indicating that the same dominant "transforming gene" is activated by tumor DNA from the same cell type, regardless of whether the donor tumor was induced by viruses, carcinogens, or was spontaneous. Transforming genes are also stage specific, different transforming genes being activated in prelymphocyte neoplasms, lymphomas, and myelomas.

These impressive results, discussed in detail in Chapter 3 by Cooper and Lane, demonstrate clearly that the activation of a limited number of genes, closely related to normal components of the genome, is associated with transformation. At least in some instances the activated genes produce proteins indistinguishable from normal gene products, e.g., for the P21 proteins from the ras^H transforming gene in EJ bladder carcinoma cells. In other cases, however, gene products were clearly abnormal. The factors in the tumor DNA that turn a normal gene locus into a transforming gene are thus still unclear, and may well be different in different tumors. The transfection system, however, coupled with the repeated testing of cloned restriction fragments, has enabled this laboratory in some instances to localize the region of the transforming gene to a finite part of the genome. For example, the transforming gene activated in a lymphoma cell line was localized to an 1800 bp fragment that produced a translation product 65 amino acids long, partially homologous to transferrin. Analyses of this kind, time consuming as they are, should enable the oncologist ultimately to determine the specific lesion associated with the transformation process. One might predict from the extensive studies of Cooper and other laboratories, that oncogenesis will involve a spectrum of changes, from modified promoters and major DNA insertions and deletions to individual point mutations involving minimal changes in the amino acid sequences of key proteins for gene control.

With the transfection analysis for transforming genes, the investigations into the role of transposable elements in mutagenesis and gene control, the detailed studies on DNase sensitivity associated with normal or induced activity of genes in development, the *in vivo* and *in vitro* systems for the study of promoter structure in the synthesis of specific proteins, and the structural relationships between scaffold and lamina in the mitotic cycle, we can glimpse something of the ingenious and multifaceted approach to cell biology that characterizes today's molecular biologist. The results of this labor will not only be a vital insight into the causal stages in the development of cancer cells, but also what may prove to be even more important in the last analysis, a deeper understanding of the normal developmental process. From the studies of Boveri on the basic cell, the biologist has been aware of the problems of oncology, and the oncologist has also realized that solutions to the problems he considers will provide basic insight into the normal processes of cell growth.

References

Basler, J., Hastie, N. D., Pietras, D., Matsui, S-I, Sandberg, A. A., and Berezney, R. (1981). *Biochem.* **20**, 6921–6929.

Berezney, R., and Coffee, D. (1974). *Biophys. Biochem. Res. Comm.* **60**, 1410–1417.

Boveri, T. (1899). "Fetschr. f.c.V. Kupfler," Fischer, Jena, pp. 383–430; (1902). *Verh. phys.-med. Ges. Würtzburg, N.F.* **35**, 67–90; (1914). "Zur Frage der Entstehung maligner Tumoren." Fischer, Jena, (M. Boveri, transl., 1929, Williams & Wilkins, Baltimore).

Elder, R. T., St. John, T. P., Stinchcomb, D. T., and Davis, R. W. (1981). *Cold Spring Harbor Symp. Quant. Biol.* **45**, 581–583.

Engels, W. R. (1981). *Cold Spring Harbor Symp. Quant. Biol.* **45**, 561–565.

Feldman, M., Mello-Sampayo, T., and Sears, E. R. (1966). *Proc. Nat. Acad. Sci.* **56**, 1192–1199.

Gerace, L., and Blobel, G. (1980). *Cell* **19**, 277–287.

Gerace, L., Blum, A., and Blobel, G. (1978). *J. Cell Biol.* **79,** 546–566.

Goyette, M., Petropoulos, C. J., Shaule, P. R., and Fausto, N. (1983). *Science* **219,** 510–512.

Groudine, M., and Weintraub, H. (1982). *Cell* **30,** 131–139.

McClintock, B. (1965). *Brookhaven Symp. Biol.* **18,** 162–184; (1967). *Dev. Biol. Symp.* **1,** 84–112; (1978). *Symp. Soc. Dev. Biol.* **36,** 217–237.

Moses, M. (1968). *Ann. Rev. Genet.* **2,** 363–412.

Rubin, G., and Spradling, A. (1982). *Science* **218,** 348–352.

Schrader, R. (1953). "Mitosis." Columbia Univ. Press, New York.

Schimke, R. (1982). "Gene Amplification." Cold Spring Harbor Lab., Cold Spring Harbor, New York.

Snyder, M. P., Kimbrell, D., Hunkapillar, M., Hill, R., Fristrom, J., and Davidson, M. (1982). *Proc. Nat. Acad. Sci.* **79,** 7430–7434.

Spradling, A., and Rubin, G. (1981). *Ann. Rev. Gen.* **15,** 219–264.

Varmus, H. E. (1982). *Science* **216,** 812–820.

Temin, H. M. (1982). *Cell* **28,** 3–5.

Woodard, J., Rasch, E., and Swift, H. (1961). *J. Biophys. Biochem. Cytol.* **9,** 445–462.

Wray, W., and Stubblefield, E. (1970). *Exp. Cell Res.* **59,** 469–478.

1

Long-Range Order Folding of the Chromatin Fibers in Metaphase Chromosomes and Nuclei

U. K. LAEMMLI, C. D. LEWIS, AND W. C. EARNSHAW*

Departments of Molecular Biology and Biochemistry
University of Geneva
Geneva, Switzerland

I. Introduction

At mitosis the entire eukaryotic genome is compacted into the metaphase chromosome by histones and nonhistone proteins for ready distribution to daughter cells. Chromosomes not only deliver the DNA sequences in an orderly fash-

*Present address: Department of Cell Biology and Anatomy, Johns Hopkins University School of Medicine, Baltimore, Maryland 21205.

ion to the daughter cells, but they must also bear epigenetic information that maintains the transcriptional repertoire. Epigenetic information is defined as the structural information in chromatin that will permit or forbid transcription of a given gene or cluster of genes. In this view, cell reproduction involves both replication of genetic information, in terms of DNA sequences, and replication of epigenetic information, in terms of chromatin structure. The epigenetic information must be preserved and maintained during chromosome condensation prior to delivery to the daughter cells.

The DNA of the eukaryotic cell is organized on several distinguishable levels; the basic chromatin fiber encompasses the first two levels of organization. The nucleosome is the fundamental structural subunit of the basic chromatin fiber, and a wealth of data have accumulated that describe this subunit in detail (for recent review see Igo-Kemenes et al., 1982). The nucleosome is composed of the four core histones H2A, H2B, H3, H4 (two each), and it determines, together with the H1 histone, the structure of the basic chromatin fiber. Early electron microscopy (reviewed by Ris and Kubai, 1970) reported different dimensions for the chromatin fiber, but it is now generally accepted that the chromatin fiber has, under physiological conditions, an irregular diameter of about 250 Å (e.g., Thoma et al., 1979). The arrangement of the nucleosomes in the basic fiber is not entirely understood despite intensive study. Three possibilities have been suggested: (a) a helical packing of the nucleosome into a coiled structure (Finch and Klug, 1976), (b) an assembly of the nucleosomes into particles called "superbeads" (Hozier et al., 1977, Jorcano et al., 1980), and (c) a "zig-zag" packing of the nucleosomes (Worcel et al., 1981).

The basic chromatin fiber appears to be the same in both interphase and metaphase chromosomes. Morphological studies in the electron microscope by surface spreading or thin sectioning show the "thick" 250 Å fiber in both cases (Dupraw, 1966; Ris, 1978; Marsden and Laemmli, 1979). Moreover, nucleosomes have been observed in both structures to be packed into the thick fiber (Rattner and Hamkalo, 1979, 1978a,b). Thus, common fiber structure has been observed despite the dramatic difference between interphase and metaphase chromosomes. This remarkable feature suggests that the condensation of the chromosome at mitosis is due largely to an altered higher-order packaging of the basic fiber. This higher-order level of organization, or third level, encompasses the folding or coiling of the basic fiber into chromosomes (for a review see Paulson, 1981).

Evidence for order in metaphase chromosomes, on a gross morphological level, comes from chromosome banding phenomena. Chromosomal bands were first observed by Caspersson et al. (1971), who found that certain fluorochromes produce a chromosome-specific pattern of bright and dark bands. Various banding patterns were subsequently developed that greatly stimulated the area of cytogenetic research. The biochemical basis for the banding phenomena is not understood in detail, but this phenomenon might provide two important clues about chromosome structure: (1) It suggests that chromatin of similar biochemical composition is grouped together to form a disk or ring. One might view chromosomes, in this light, as consisting of a series of stacked disks, a given disk containing chromatin of a certain biochemical composition (detected by the fluorochromes) that is different from that of the neighboring disks as to generate differential staining. (2) Also important is the observation that structurally similar chromatin is packed into a disk, while chromatin of different composition is separated along the long axis of the chromatid. Indeed, longitudinally oriented banding is not observed, except for the enhancement of an axial structure by the silver staining technique (Howel and Hsu, 1979). The idea that the banding phenomenon is brought about by a series of stacked disks of chromatin of different biochemical composition suggests that the long axis of the chromatid may have rotational symmetry at least at some low resolution.

II. Order in Metaphase Chromosomes: The Loop

A. Histone-Depleted Chromosomes

Chromosomes are large enough structures so that an understanding of them cannot be achieved by a single approach. Electron micrographs usually display a hopeless entanglement of fibers with no indication of a repeating higher-order subunit organization. A remarkable observation is that it appears to be possible to reversibly swell the volume of chromosomes about 50-fold by decreasing the ionic strength and then reversibly to regain the "normal" compacted form with physiological salt solutions. Such studies (reviewed by Cole, 1967) suggested to us some time ago that the structural integrity of chromosomes might be due to a network of cross ties which stabilize the structure. Such cross ties would be arranged at certain intervals along the chromatin fiber serving as the "nuts and bolts" of the chromosome. This type of organization would convert the chromatin between the cross ties into loops, which could assume various extended or contracted conformations without loss of the overall chromosome morphology.

The first evidence for loops in mitotic chromosomes came from studies of histone-depleted chromosomes (Adolph et al., 1977a,b; Paulson and Laemmli, 1977; Laemmli et al., 1978). We were able to show that it is possible to extract, either by competition with polyanions such as dextran sulfate/heparin or by high salt, virtually all the histones and many nonhistone proteins and to isolate a residual structure that maintains the total DNA in a highly folded form. These histone-depleted chromosomes have the following properties: (1) They can be isolated on sucrose gradients as fast sedimenting structures (4000–7000 S). (2) Their structural integrity is due to nonhistone proteins, since treatment of these structures with SDS, urea, or pronase, but not RNase, unfolds the DNA completely (Adolph et al., 1977a,b). (3) Important metalloprotein interactions stabilize the histone-depleted chromosomes (Lewis and Laemmli, 1982). Dissociation of these interactions by metal chelation completely unfolds the histone-depleted chromosomes. (4) The histone-depleted chromosomes retain the overall morphology of the metaphase chromosome as observed in the fluorescent microscope. (5) Electron micrographs confirm this and show a halo of DNA strands converging on a central skeletal structure referred to as the scaffolding (Paulson and Laemmli, 1977). (6) The DNA strands are clearly attached to the scaffolding, and are organized as loops. The length of the loops vary statistically, the average length corresponding to about 65 kb of DNA. (7) The loops observed are regularly spaced, that is, they start at a point on the scaffolding and return to an adjacent point (Paulson and Laemmli, 1977). The loops are supercoiled if care is taken to avoid the introduction of nicks into the DNA during the process of isolation (Mullinger and Johnson, 1979). (8) The scaffolding retains its structural integrity and metaphase shape despite extensive digestion of the accessible DNA with nucleases or high salt (Adolph et al., 1977b). (9) The scaffolding extends through the entire length of the chromatid and appears to retain a residual kinetochore structure (Earnshaw and Laemmli, 1983).

B. Thin Section through Intact Mitotic Chromosomes

The observations made with histone-depleted chromosome are consistent with a model in which loops of chromatin are stabilized by a scaffolding consisting of proteins that somehow cross-link the bases of the loops (Laemmli et al., 1978). The idea of a backbone or core to help organize the chromatin fiber has been expressed previously (e.g., Taylor, 1958; Stubblefield and Wray, 1971). Independent evidence for a scaffold organizing principle comes from thin sectioning of HeLa chromosomes swollen at low divalent cation concentration or in the presence of EDTA (Marsden and Laemmli, 1979). Such micrographs of swollen chromosomes show a ''star-like'' arrangement of the chromatin fiber, supporting the idea of centrally arranged cross links that anchor the fibers (Fig. 1). Loops of about 3–4 μm can sometmes be traced. Since the DNA is compacted 6- to 7-fold in the string of beads, and 25- to 40-fold in the thick 250 Å fiber, these measurements agree roughly with the length measurements of loops in histone-depleted chromosomes (Paulson and Laemmli, 1977). Similar micrographs have been obtained using HeLa metaphase cells or isolated chromosomes (Adolph, 1980a) and mitotic Chinese hamster cells (Ris, 1978).

C. Examination of Chromosomes by Spreading Procedures

Low magnification micrographs of metaphase chromosomes spread for microscopy by the Miller technique show lateral loops that appear to emanate from the central chromosome axis (Rattner and Hamkalo, 1978a,b). Radially arranged

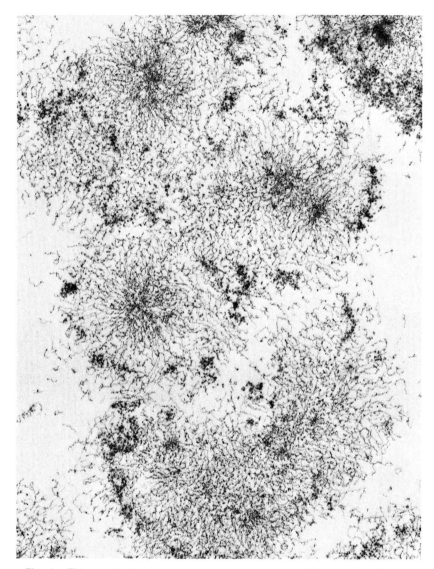

Fig. 1. Thin section through chromosomes swollen with EDTA prior to fixation and embedding showing the radial arrangement of the fibers. The nucleoprotein fiber is in the 10-nm-thick ("string of beads") configuration. Several cross sections of chromatids appear in the lower portion of the micrograph, while a longitudinal section can be seen at the top. From Marsden and Laemmli (1979), with permission.

loops are more convincingly observed in micrographs of chromosomes spread by a similar but modified technique (Fig. 2) (Earnshaw and Laemmli, 1983). A central organizing element cannot always be seen in such micrographs, but in certain cases it is possible to discern an axial element. Such micrographs show kinetochores, apparently as a specialized region of the scaffolding (Earnshaw and Laemmli, 1983). Residual kinetechore material is also associated with isolated scaffolds following extraction of all histones and DNA (Earnshaw and Laemmli, 1983).

Additional evidence for loops in mitotic chromosomes comes from impressive micrographs of Victoria E. Foe (Foe *et al.*, 1982). These chromosomes, prepared from early embryos of the milkweed bug *Oncepeltus fasciatus,* and observed by a modified Miller technique, show peripheral loops that can often be traced to a central structure. This central structure is differentially enhanced with PTA (phosphotungstic acid) stain.

The organization of chromatin into loops is strongly supported by electron microscope (EM) studies from early stages of meiosis. Clear micrographs were obtained by Rattner *et al.* (1980) at early stages of meiosis of *Bombyx mori.* The chromatin appears to be organized in loops; the bases of the loops are thought to become more closely packed as compaction of the chromosomes proceeds during the leptotene to zygotene transition. The bases of the loops seem to form the lateral element of the synaptonemal complex observed later at pachytene (Rattner *et al.,* 1980). Earlier EM studies of pachytene chromosomes have also suggested loops (Comings and Okada, 1970).

Chromatin loops in lampbrush chromosomes of intact amphibian oocyte nuclei at the diplotene stage have been observed directly with the light microscope for many years (Callan and Lloyd, 1960, for a review see Scheer *et al.,* 1979). The lampbrush loops contain a single DNA strand (Gall, 1963) and are made visible by the tightly packed transcriptional complexes. Only the actively transcribing region of these chromosomes are visible as loops (about 5%), the rest being tightly compacted in chromomeres.

In summary, the available evidence clearly supports the notion that chromatin loops are the fundamental organizing unit of both meiotic and mitotic chromosomes.

D. Proteins of the Chromosomal Scaffold: Involvement of Metalloprotein Interactions

The structural stability of the histone-depleted chromosomes is due to a series of high molecular weight proteins, as shown previously (Adolph *et al.,* 1977a,b). Chromosomes isolated by differential centrifugation are usually heavily contaminated with cytoskeletal material, but we have recently developed procedures that permit the isolation of highly purified chromosomes (Lewis and Laemmli, 1982).

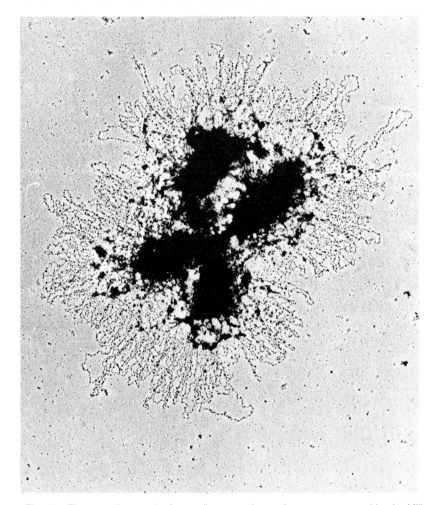

Fig. 2. Electron micrograph of a swollen metaphase chromosome spread by the Miller technique. Note the radial loops of the chromatin in the periphery and the general convergence of the fibers on the chromatid axis. A scaffolding cannot be seen in such a micrograph due to the dense chromatin material that did not expand. From Earnshaw and Laemmli (1983), with permission.

The protein composition of the scaffolding derived from such highly purified chromosomes is less complex then previously reported. It consists largely of two high molecular weight proteins SC_1 and SC_2 (170,000 and 135,000 MWr, respectively), and a series of minor bands. Most interestingly, we discovered that metalloprotein interactions are important in stabilizing the scaffold structure. The evidence is based on sedimentation studies of histone-depleted chromosomes.

These structures have a sedimentation coefficient of 4000–7000 S, but these particles unfold dramatically and lose all aspect of structure if certain metal chelators or thiols are added to the lysis solution (Lewis and Laemmli, 1982). The chelators effective for this dissociation are 1,10-phenanthroline, neocuproine, or thiols such as β-mercaptoethanol and dithiothreitol, but not EDTA or $NaBH_4$. The unfolding of the histone-depleted chromosomes is due to a dissociation of the scaffolding proteins as observed both biochemically and structurally. We have used the following evidence to identify the metal involved. It is possible to generate metal-depleted chromosomes that do not have a stable scaffolding; that is, they unfold if challenged with lysis solutions to extract the histones. Such metal-depleted chromosomes can be specifically and reversibly stabilized by as little as $10^{-8}\ M\ Cu^{2+}$, while addition of as much as $10^{-3}\ M$ of Mn^{2+}, Co^{2+}, Zn^{2+}, or Hg^{2+} has no effect. Metal-depleted chromosomes can also be stabilized under certain conditions by Ca^{2+} (at 37°C), but this effect appears less specific than that of Cu^{2+} (Lewis and Laemmli, 1982). Thus, metal interactions confer stability to the scaffold so as to allow extraction of the histones while maintaining the integrity of the scaffold.

In summary, the scaffolding is composed of a discrete and nonrandom set of proteins. This finding and the specificity of the metal effect inspires additional confidence that the scaffolding represents the genuine structural elements of chromosomes.

III. Chromatin Organization in Nuclei

The chromatin fiber of the interphase nucleus is also organized into domains, possibly loops, which are structurally stabilized by residual nuclear elements. One line of evidence in support of this is based on work by Igo-Kemenes and Zachau (1978) who studied the maximum length of chromatin that can be excised from nuclei by restriction enzymes. An upper size limit is expected if nuclear attachment points exist. The maximum length obtained by this approach is about 75 kb. A different line of evidence comes from sedimentation studies with cells extracted in high salt. Such "nucleoids" exhibit a biphasic alteration in sedimentation rate with an increasing concentration of ethidium bromide, suggesting that the DNA is constrained in closed domains (Benyajati and Worcel, 1976; Cook and Brazell, 1976, 1978). The length of the proposed DNA domains was estimated to be about 85 kb in *Drosophila* tissue culture cells (Benyajati and Worcel, 1976) and about 220 kb in HeLa cells (Cook and Brazell, 1978). These observations suggest that the chromatin is attached to a framework in the nucleus. This framework could be the nuclear matrix, as suggested by various researchers (Berezeney and Buchholtz, 1981; Vogelstein *et al.*, 1980; Adolph, 1980b; Beckers *et al.*, 1981). The nuclear matrix has been described as a residual nuclear structure retaining some of the morphological features of the nucleus. It is isolated from nuclei following digestion of the DNA followed by extraction in high salt to eliminate the histones and many nonhistone proteins.

We have recently elucidated the nuclear elements involved in DNA folding and studied their relationship to the chromosomal scaffolding in some detail (Lebkowski and Laemmli, 1982a,b). We were able to distinguish two different levels of folding of the nuclear DNA which are defined as follows:

Level I: This level of organization is sensitive to metal chelation and is similar to that observed in metaphase chromosomes. It is composed of a complex set of proteins that form a network apparently in the interior of the nucleus (Lebkowski and Laemmli, 1982a,b). Briefly, the evidence is as follows: histone-depleted nuclei maintain the nuclear DNA in a highly folded conformation, sedimenting as a compact structure with a sedimentation coefficient of about 18000 S. This type I scaffold is composed partly of the nuclear lamina proteins that are known to constitute the peripheral structure of the nucleus (Gerace et al., 1978). In addition to the lamina proteins, type I scaffolds contain a complex set of non-histone proteins that arise from the network observed in nuclear matrices.

Level II: Level II is observed following addition of metal chelators during histone depletion. Such treatment leads to a partial unfolding of the nuclear DNA as shown by a dramatic reduction in the sedimentation coefficient from 18000 S to 8000 S for the histone-depleted nuclei. An important difference between chromosomes and nuclei is that metal chelation in the case of the chromosome leads to complete dissociation of the folded structure to "linear" DNA, whereas only a partial unfolding is observed in the nuclear case. The metal implicated in both cases is either Cu^{2+} or Ca^{2+}. The type II nuclear scaffold is much less complex than the type I scaffold. It is composed almost exclusively of the nuclear lamina proteins. The complex set of nonhistone proteins observed in the type I scaffold are solubilized by metal chelation. Morphologically, type II scaffolds show the peripheral lamina structure without the interior network (Lebkowski and Laemmli, in preparation). Thus the complex set of nonhistone proteins observed in type I scaffolds must be localized predominantly in the interior. Several of these proteins as well as the nuclear lamina proteins bind DNA as tested in an *in vitro* assay.

These data suggest a model for the organization of the chromatin in nuclei (Lebkowski and Laemmli, 1982a,b). One level of organization is brought about by a repetitive attachment of the DNA to the peripheral nuclear lamina or a structure closely associated with the lamina. At a second level, the DNA is stabilized by a chelation-sensitive network localized more in the interior of the nucleus. We would like to think that those interactions in the nucleus that are sensitive to chelation represent the interphase equivalent of the metaphase scaf-folding. The nuclear lamina structure is known to dissociate in the late G_2 phase of the cell cycle as chromosome condensation proceeds (Gerace et al., 1978;

Gerace and Blobel, 1980). Thus the level of chromatin organization that is imposed by the nuclear lamina is lost in metaphase. We have speculated elsewhere that the chelation-sensitive elements of the nucleus may rearrange to bring about chromosome condensation (Lewis and Laemmli, 1982).

IV. Conclusion and Outlook

Available data are consistent with a model in which chromatin loops are stabilized by a set of nonhistone proteins that link the bases of the loops. These linkers form a network or scaffold that retains some of the morphological features of the intact chromosomes or nuclei. Two levels of folding can be distinguished in nuclei; one level is imposed by the nuclear lamina, while a second level is brought about by a residual network in the interior of the nuclear matrix. This level of folding appears to share structural components with the chromosomal scaffolding. Both are stabilized by similar metalloprotein interactions, and at least one of the major proteins (SC_1) of the chromosomal scaffold is also associated with the nucleus (Lewis and Laemmli, in preparation). The nuclear matrix is compositionally much more complex. A series of recent papers suggest a possible involvement of the nuclear matrix in DNA replication (e.g., Vogelstein *et al.*, 1980), transcription (e.g., Jackson *et al.*, 1981), and RNA processing (e.g., Ciejek *et al.*, 1982), providing a possible rationale for the compositional complexity of the nuclear matrix.

The scaffold model, although strongly supported by different lines of experimentation, is not entirely proved. The difficulty lies in showing that the scaffold interactions observed in the histone-depleted chromosomes are operative in the intact chromosome. One line of argumentation is based on the specificity observed. The chromosomal scaffold is composed of a specific set of proteins and is not a random aggregate. Additionally, highly specific metalloprotein interactions are operative in the scaffold. These interactions can be reversibly stabilized or dissociated by the addition or chelation of Cu^{2+} or Ca^{2+}. Addition of 10^{-8} M Cu^{2+} to metal-depleted chromosomes is enough to stabilize the scaffold interactions. Such treatment would be unlikely to induce new interactions by rearrangement of proteins, but would be more likely to stabilize preexisting protein–protein and/or protein–DNA interactions. A second line of argumentation is based on the coherent picture that emerges from different EM studies. Loops of chromatin converging on a central organizing element are observed in intact chromosomes both in thin sections and in spread preparations (Fig. 2). Moreover, The DNA loops seen in histone-depleted chromosomes have the length expected, taking into account the packaging ratio of DNA in chromatin. The loops are arranged in an orderly fashion and not in a random tangle.

A scaffolding is not always directly visible in all electron micrographs of chromosomes, an observation that has been taken as an argument against the existence of such a structural element (Okada and Comings, 1982). This is due in part to a misunderstanding concerning the amount of protein in the scaffold and certain assumptions made about its structure. The scaffold retains at most about 3–4% of total chromosomal proteins or about 1–2% of the total mass. Examination of the scaffold shows that it is a diffuse, expanded network at the low ionic strength condition used to expand the chromosome (Earnshaw and Laemmli, 1983). Such a diffuse structure is extremely difficult to observe against a background of chromatin fibers. In contrast, the scaffolding becomes very visible in histone-depleted chromosomes spread by the cytochrome c method. The elimination of the histones and the moderately high ionic strength of the spreading solutions leads to a scaffold with a massive appearance. This visual impression has misled some electron microscopists to assume that a scaffold should be observed easily in intact chromosomes.

Various researchers have tried to answer the question of whether the interaction of the DNA at the bases of the loops is sequence specific and fixed for a given loop, or if it is random. A sequence-specific interaction with the scaffolding would establish that this organizational principle is correct. Unfortunately, the current conclusions on this point are in conflict. Some reports claim that the DNA attached to the scaffold is enriched in middle repetitive sequences (Razin *et al.*, 1979; Mantieva *et al.*, 1980), while other reports support an opposite conclusion (Bowen, 1981; Basler *et al.*, 1981; Kuo, 1982). A partially nonrandom distribution for the globin genes has been observed by Cook and Brazell (1980), who found some enrichment of the α-globin genes, versus the β- or γ-globin genes, in the DNA fraction more closely associated with the nuclear matrix. The question of the sequence organization of the loops is not settled; technical and procedural differences may be the source of the discrepancies. This important question needs to be studied in detail to assess the specificities of the DNA–protein interaction in the scaffolding. A specific interaction would go a long way to establish conclusively this concept of chromosome organization.

Acknowledgments

This work was supported by the Swiss National Science Foundation Grant No. 3.621.80 and by the Canton of Geneva.

References

Adolph, K. W. (1980a). *Exp. Cell Res.* **125**, 95–103.
Adolph, K. W. (1980b). *J. Cell Sci.* **42**, 291–304.
Adolph, K. W., Cheng, S. M., and Laemmli, U. K. (1977a). *Cell* **12**, 805–816.

Adolph, K. W., Cheng, S. M., Paulson, J. R., and Laemmli, U. K. (1977b). *Proc. Natl. Acad. Sci. USA* **74**, 4937–4941.

Basler, J., Hastie, N. D., Pietras, D., Matsai, S. I., Sandberg, A. A., and Berezney, R. (1981). *Biochemistry* **20**, 6921–6929.

Beckers, A. G. M., Gijén, H. J., Taalman, R. D. F. M., and Wanka, F. (1981). *J. Res.* **75**, 352–362.

Benyajati, C., and Worcel, A. (1976). *Cell* **9**, 393–407.

Berezeney, R., and Buchholtz, L. (1981). *Exp. Cell Res.* **132**, 1–13.

Bowen, B. C. (1981). *Nucleic Acids Res.* **9**, 5093–5108.

Callan, H. G., and Lloyd, L. (1960). *Phil. Trans. Roy. Soc. Lond.* **B243**, 135–219.

Caspersson, T., Hulten, M., Lindsten, J., and Zech, L. (1971). *Heriditas* **67**, 147–149.

Ciejek, E. M., Nordstrom, J. L., Tsai, M.-J., and O'Malley, B. W. (1982). *Biochemistry* **21**, 4945–4953.

Cole, A. (1967). *In* "Theoretical and Experimental Biophysics" (A. Cole, ed.), Vol. 1, pp. 305–375. Dekker, New York.

Comings, D. E., and Okada, T. A. (1970). *Chromosoma (Berl.)* **30**, 269–286.

Cook, P. R., and Brazell, I. A. (1976). *J. Cell Sci.* **22**, 287–302.

Cook, P. R., and Brazell, I. A. (1978). *Eur. J. Biochem.* **84**, 465–477.

Cook, P. R., and Brazell, I. A. (1980). *Nucleic Acids Res.* **8**, 2895–2906.

DuPraw, E. J. (1966). *Nature, Lond.* **209**, 577–581.

Earnshaw, W. C., and Laemmli, U. K. (1983). *J. Cell. Biol.* **96**, 84–93.

Finch, J. T., and Klug, A. (1976). *Proc. Natl. Acad. Sci. USA* **73**, 1897–1901.

Foe, V. E., Forrest, H., Wilkinson, L., and Laird, C. (1982). *In* "Insect Ultrastructure" (H. Akai and R. King, eds.), Vol. 1, pp. 222–246. Plenum, New York.

Gall, J. G. (1963). *Nature, Lond.* **198**, 36–38.

Gerace, L., Blum, A., and Blobel, G. (1978). *J. Cell. Biol.* **79**, 546–566.

Gerace, L., and Blobel, G. (1980). *Cell* **19**, 277–287.

Howel, W. M., and Hsu, T. C. (1979). *Chromosoma* **73**, 61–66.

Hozier, J., Renz, M., and Nehls, P. (1977). *Chromosoma (Berl.)* **62**, 301–317.

Igo-Kemenes, T., and Zachau, H. G. (1978). *Cold Spring Harbor Symp. Quant. Biol.* **42**, 109–118.

Igo-Kemenes, T., Hörz, W., and Zachau, H. G. (1982). *Ann. Rev. Biochem.* **51**, 89–121.

Jackson, D. A., McCready, S. J., and Cook, P. R. (1981). *Nature* **292**, 552–555.

Jorcano, J. L., Meyer, G., Day, L. A., and Renz, M. (1980). *Proc. Natl. Acad. Sci. USA* **77**, 6443–6447.

Kuo, M. T. (1982). *Biochemistry* **21**, 321–326.

Laemmli, U. K., Cheng, S. M., Adolph, K. W., Paulson, J. R., Brown, J. A., and Baumbach, W. R. (1978). *Cold Spring Harbor Symp. Quant. Biol.* **42**, 351–360.

Lebkowski, J. S., and Laemmli, U. K. (1982a). *J. Mol. Biol.* **156**, 309–324.

Lebkowski, J. S., and Laemmli, U. K. (1982b). *J. Mol. Biol.* **156**, 325–344.

Lewis, C. D., and Laemmli, U. K. (1982). *Cell* **29**, 171–181.

Mantieva, V. L., Razin, S. V., and Georgiev, G. P. (1980). *Mol. Biol. (U.S.S.R.)* **13**, 1065–1072.

Marsden, M. P. F., and Laemmli, U. K. (1979). *Cell* **17**, 849–858.

Mullinger, A. M., and Johnson, R. T. (1979). *J. Cell Sci.* **38**, 369–389.

Okada, T. D., and Comings, D. E. (1982). *Ann. J. Hum. Genet.* **32**, 814–832.

Paulson, J. R. (1981). *In* "Electron Microscopy of Proteins" (R. Harris, ed.), Vol. 3, pp. 78–127. Academic Press, London.

Paulson, J. R., and Laemmli, U. K. (1977). *Cell* **12**, 817–828.

Rattner, J. B., and Hamkalo, B. A. (1978a). *Chromosoma* **69**, 363–372.

Rattner, J. B., and Hamkalo, B. A. (1978b). *Chromosoma* **69**, 373–379.

Rattner, J. B., and Hamkalo, B. A. (1979). *J. Cell Biol.* **81**, 453–457.

Rattner, J. B., Goldsmith, M., and Hamkalo, B. A. (1980).*Chromosoma (Berl.)* **79,** 215–224.
Razin, S. V., Mantieva, V. L., and Georgiev, G. P. (1979). *Nucleic Acids Res.* **7,** 1713–1735.
Ris, H. (1978). *In* "Electron Microscopy 1978" (J. M. Sturgess, ed.), Vol. 3, pp. 545–556. Microscopical Society of Canada, Toronto.
Scheer, U., Spring, H., and Trendelenburg, M. F. (1979). *In* "The Cell Nucleus" (Harris Busch, ed.), Vol. VII, pp. 1–47. Academic Press, New York.
Stubblefield, E., and Wray, W. (1971). *Chromosoma (Berl.)* **32,** 262–294.
Taylor, J. H. (1958). *Genetics* **43,** 515–529.
Thoma, F., Koller, T., and Klug, A. (1979). *J. Cell. Biol.* **83,** 403–427.
Vogelstein, B., Pardoll, D. M., and Coffey, D. S. (1980). *Cell* **22,** 79–85.
Worcel, A., Strogatz, S., and Riley, D. (1981). *Proc. Natl. Acad. Sci. USA* **78,** 1461–1465.

The Adenovirus Type 2 Major Late Promoter: An *in Vitro* System Which Mimics the TATA Box and Upstream Sequences Requirements for Efficient *in Vivo* Transcription*

R. HEN, P. SASSONE-CORSI, J. CORDEN,[†] M. P. GAUB,
C. KÉDINGER, AND P. CHAMBON

*Laboratoire de Génétique Moléculaire des Eucaryotes du
C N R S et Unité 184 de Biologie Moléculaire et de Génie
Génétique de l'INSERM
Institut de Chimie Biologique–Faculté de Médecine
Strasbourg, France*

Abbreviations: Ad2ML and Ad2MLP, adenovirus type 2 major late and adenovirus type 2 major late promoter, respectively; bp: base pair; WCE: whole cell extract.

†Present address: Department of Molecular Biology, Johns Hopkins University School of Medicine, Baltimore, Maryland 21205.

CHROMOSOMES AND CANCER

I. Introduction

The comparison of DNA sequences in the 5' flanking region of genes coding for proteins has revealed two specific regions of homology. The highly conserved TATA box sequence, located about 30 nucleotides upstream from the cap site is a promoter element required for efficient and selective transcription both *in vitro* and *in vivo* (see for reviews, Corden *et al.*, 1980; Breathnach and Chambon, 1981). A second region of homology, located at a variable position upstream from the TATA box appears to be less conserved (Benoist *et al.*, 1980; Efstratiadis *et al.*, 1980) and is necessary for efficient *in vivo* transcription (Grosschedl and Birnstiel, 1980; Dierks *et al.*, 1981; McKnight *et al.*, 1981; Mellon *et al.*, 1981; Struhl, 1981; Grosveld *et al.*, 1982a). The *in vitro* effect of these further upstream sequences is less clear: in some cases they had no or little effect (Corden *et al.*, 1980; Wasylyk *et al.*, 1980; Grosveld *et al.*, 1981; Hu and Manley, 1981; Mathis and Chambon, 1981; Tsai *et al.*, 1981), while in others they appeared to be important for efficient transcription (Myers *et al.*, 1981; Tsuda and Suzuki, 1981; Grosschedl and Birnstiel, 1982; Lee *et al.*, 1982). We demonstrate here that these upstream sequences are required both *in vivo* and *in vitro* for efficient transcription from the adenovirus type 2 major late promoter.

II. Materials and Methods

HeLa cells (20–40% confluence) were transfected as described (Banerji *et al.*, 1981) with 20 μg of Ad2MLP recombinant DNA per 10 cm petri dish and 2 μg of the β-globin plasmid pβ(244+)β (De Villiers and Schaffner, 1981) as an internal control. After 48 hours cytoplasmic RNA was purified from cells lysed with 0.3% NP40. For S_1 nuclease mapping, RNA from *in vivo* (50 μg, equivalent to about one petri dish) and *in vitro* assays was dissolved in 10 μl of 10 mM Pipes, pH 6.5, 400 mM NaCl containing an excess of the *Hin*dIII–*Xho*I probe (see Figs. 1B and 2) and the internal control probe when indicated, heated 5 minutes at 85°C, and hybridized at 68°C for 12 hours. After digestion with 2000 units of S_1 nuclease (Miles) at 25°C for 2 hours in 100 μl containing 30 mM sodium acetate pH 4.6, 0.3 M NaCl, and 3 mM $ZnCl_2$, the S_1-resistant DNA fragments were extracted with phenol–chloroform, precipitated twice with ethanol, and analyzed on a 8% acrylamide–8.3 M urea gel as described (Maxam and Gilbert, 1980). The differences between the various recombinants were repeatedly found in several independent transfection experiments performed with different preparations of DNA. Figures 2–5 represent typical experiments.

III. Results

1. Microinjection in CV1 cell nuclei of recombinants containing the Ad2ML promoter reveals that sequences upstream from the TATA box are essential for efficient *in vivo* expression. A series of Ad2MLP mutants lacking the sequences upstream from positions −200, −150, −97, −62, −34, −29, and −21 were constructed (see Fig. 1; Corden *et al.,* 1980) and linked to the coding sequence of the SV40 T antigen (the pSVA series, Fig. 1). After microinjection of the recombinants into CV1 cell nuclei, T antigen accumulation was used as a functional test for promoter activity. The same level of expression was obtained, irrespective of the amount of microinjected DNA, with the wild-type recombinant pSVA500 and recombinants pSVA200, 150 and 97 (Table I). In addition no decrease in T antigen expression was observed with a recombinant where the sequences between −500 and −260 were deleted (not shown). However T antigen expression was significantly decreased in pSVA34 and pSVA32 (Table I), both of which have an intact TATA box, but are missing sequences upstream from positions −34 and −32, respectively (see Fig. 1). This effect is more pronounced at the lower DNA concentration which is likely better to reflect the

TABLE I

Microinjection of pSVA Recombinants in CV1 Cell Nuclei[a]

Recombinants	Immunofluorescent CV1 cells (%)	
	100 μg DNA/ml	33 μg DNA/ml
pSVA500	100 (6)	100 (2)
pSVA200	89 (3)	140 (2)
pSVA150	95 (3)	127 (2)
pSVA97	110 (3)	138 (2)
pSVA34	32 (6)	6 (2)
pSVA32	31 (2)	5 (2)
pSVA29	7 (6)	0 (2)
pSVA21	9 (3)	0 (2)
pEMP	0 (6)	0 (2)

[a] About 2.10^{-11} ml of recombinant DNA at 33 or 100 μg/ml was injected per CV1 cell nucleus as described previously (Moreau *et al.,* 1981). pEMP and the pSVA series are described in Fig. 1. The results were expressed as the percent of injected cells that were positive for T antigen, taking as 100% the value obtained with pSVA500. Numbers in parentheses correspond to the number of independent assays carried out for each recombinant. For convenience we microinjected CV1 cells, but similar results (not shown) were obtained with HeLa cells.

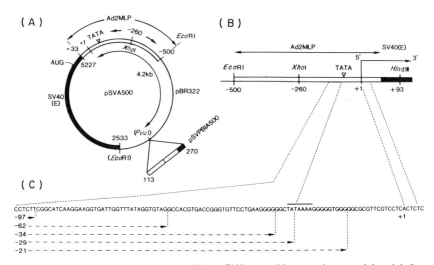

Fig. 1. Construction and structure of the pSVA recombinant series containing deletions in the Ad2ML promoter region. (A) pSVA plasmids were constructed by recombination of parts of the previously described pEMP (Benoist and Chambon, 1980) and pMLA (Corden *et al.*, 1980) plasmids. pEMP contains the entire SV40 T antigen amino acid coding sequence (without the early promoter region) between coordinates 2533 and 5227 (Moreau *et al.*, 1981), inserted between the EcoRI and BamHI sites of pBR322 (restriction sites in parenthesis were lost during the constructions). pMLA contains the Ad2 BalI E fragment inserted into the EcoRI site of pBR322. Deletions in the Ad2MLP region were created (arrows) from the unique −260 XhoI site by limited exonuclease III digestion, followed by S$_1$ nuclease treatment and blunt-end ligation (Corden *et al.*, 1980). The wild type or deletion-containing fragments were excised from the corresponding pMLA recombinants with SalI (position 650 in pBR322) and PvuII (position +33 in the Ad2MLP) and inserted between the repaired BamHI and the nonrepaired SalI sites of pEMP. pSVA500 contains the wild type Ad2MLP region from −500 to +33 (double line) inserted upstream from the SV40 early (E) coding sequences (heavy line). Recombinants pSVA200, 150, 97, 62, 34, 32, 29, and 21 contain 200, 150, 97, 62, 34, 32, 29, and 21 bp upstream from the initiation site (+1), respectively, as determined by sequencing (pSV97, 62, 34, 32, 29, 21) or restriction enzyme mapping (pSVA500, 200, 150). pSVPBIA500, 150, 97, 62, 34, 29, and 21 correspond to the pSVA series in which an SV40 DNA fragment (coordinates 113 to 270; see Moreau *et al.*, 1981), containing the 72 bp repeat, was inserted in the PvuI site of pBR322 in the orientation opposite to that of the SV40 (E) sequence. The direct repeat is represented by the open boxes and a flanking segment by the closed box. (B) Structure of the boundary between the Ad2MLP (double line) and the SV40 early region (heavy line) in pSVA500. The origin and direction of specific transcription from the Ad2MLP is shown by the arrow at +1. (C) Nucleotide sequence of the noncoding strand of the Ad2MLP region (Akusjärvi and Pattersson, 1979) from positions −99 to +3. The TATA box sequence is overlined and the 3' boundary of 5 deletion mutants is indicated by vertical dashed lines.

relative promoter efficiency of the various deletion mutants. Deletion of the first two bases of the TATA box (pSVA29) or of the entire box (pSVA21) resulted in a further decrease, but the values obtained with pSVA29 and pSVA21, at the higher DNA concentration, were still significantly higher than those obtained with pEMP, which has no promoter sequence in front of the T antigen coding region. From these results it appears that at least two sets of sequences are important for the *in vivo* activity of the Ad2MLP. One corresponds to the TATA box region, whereas the other is located further upstream, between positions −97 and −34.

2. Insertion of the SV40 72 bp repeat in the pSVA recombinants allows detection of specific transcription from the Ad2ML promoter after transfection into HeLa cells. To analyze the effect of deletions in the Ad2MLP region at the transcriptional level, we quantitated the amount of specific RNA synthesized in HeLa cells transfected with the various recombinants by S_1 nuclease mapping. We switched to HeLa cells because their transfection efficiency is higher than that of CV1 cells.) With pSVA500 (not shown) or pSVA34 (Fig. 2B, lane 1) a band corresponding to RNA initiated from the Ad2MLP (position MLP+1) could not be detected. This observation prompted us to investigate whether the SV40 72 bp repeat, which is known to enhance gene expression (Banerji *et al.*, 1981; Moreau *et al.*, 1981), could be used to increase the amount of RNA transcribed from the Ad2MLP. We inserted it close to the TATA box into pSVA34 and pSVA29, and the corresponding plasmids pSVBA34 and pSVBA29 (Fig. 2A) were transfected into HeLa cells. Insertion of the 72 bp repeat resulted in a dramatic increase of the amount of Ad2MLP specific RNA (Fig. 2B, lanes 2 and 8). In agreement with our previous results (Moreau *et al.*, 1981), insertion of the 72 bp repeat in the opposite orientation (pSVBIA34 and 29, lanes 3 and 9 of Fig. 2) did not affect the magnitude of its effect, whereas deletions within the 72 bp repeat, known to drastically reduce its effect (Moreau *et al.*, 1981) (see legend to Fig. 2), resulted in a striking decrease in the amount of specific RNA [see Fig. 2; compare pSVBA34 (lane 2) with pTB101A34 (lane 4) and pTB208A34 (lane 5)]. No RNA could be detected with the deletion mutant pTB101A34, which suggested that the sequences deleted in this recombinant are essential for the activity of the 72 bp repeat.

pSVBA29 and pSVBIA29, which have lost the first two bases of the TATA box, were almost as efficient in promoting specific transcription from the Ad2ML cap site as pSVBA34 and pSVBIA34, which possess an intact TATA box (compare in Fig. 2B, lanes 2 and 3 with lanes 8 and 9). This observation, in apparent contradiction with the results shown in Table I for pSVA34 and pSVA29, suggested that insertion of the 72 bp repeat close to the Ad2ML cap site can mask the effect of deletions of promoter elements. Since it is known (Moreau *et al.*, 1981) that the effect of the 72 bp repeat decreases with increasing

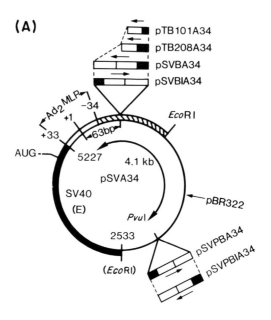

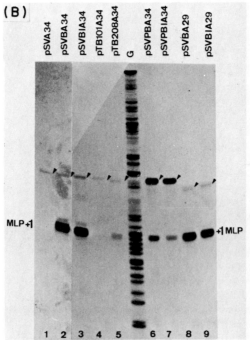

Fig. 2.

length of intervening sequences, we inserted it in the *Pvu*I site of pBR322, more than 4 kb upstream from the Ad2MLP region (pSVPBA34, pSVPBIA34 and pSVPBIA29, see Fig. 1 and 2A), to minimize this masking effect. The amount of specific RNA present in cells transfected with pSVPBA34 and pSVPBIA34 was much lower than that found in cells transfected with the corresponding pSVBA mutants (compare in Fig. 2B lanes 6 and 7 with lanes 2 and 3) and, as expected, a difference could now be seen between the recombinant with an intact TATA box (pSVPBIA34, lane 5, Fig. 3A) and a recombinant with a partially deleted TATA box (pSVPBIA29, lane 6, Fig. 3A). It is striking that by moving the 72 bp repeat 4 kb upstream from the Ad2MLP, a dramatic increase in RNA initiated upstream from the deletion end-point was observed (compare in Fig. 2B, pSVPBA34 and pSVPBIA34 with pSVA34, pSVBA34, and pSVBIA34, arrowheads in lanes 6, 7 and 1–3, respectively. In fact S_1 nuclease mapping experiments have revealed that insertion of the 72 bp repeat in the *Pvu*I site of pBR322 (pSVPBA recombinants) promoted RNA synthesis from several nearby sites (R. Hen, unpublished experiments). This observation supports our previous hypothesis that the 72 bp repeat could act as an entry site for RNA polymerase B (Moreau *et al.*, 1981).

3. S_1 nuclease mapping of RNA synthesized *in vivo* demonstrates that sequences located upstream from the TATA box are essential for efficient transcription from the Ad2ML promoter. The pSVPBIA recombinants (Fig. 1) were transfected into HeLa cells and the RNA accumulated after 48 hours was analyzed by quantitative S_1 nuclease mapping (Fig. 3). Deletions of sequences upstream from −97 had no effect on the amount of RNA initiated from the

---

Fig. 2. The SV40 72 bp repeat enhances specific *in vivo* transcription from the Ad2ML promoter. (A) Construction of derivatives of pSVA34 and pSVA29 containing the wild-type or mutated SV40 72 bp repeat. pSVA34 and pSVA29 were derived from pSVA500 as described in legend to Fig. 1. pSVA34 only is represented and the replacing adenovirus sequences upstream from −34 are hatched. The SV40 DNA segment containing the 72 bp repeat (see Fig. 1A) was then inserted in either orientation [the arrows indicate the natural orientation with respect to the SV40 (E) sequence] at 63 bp (SstI site; see Moreau *et al.*, 1981) (pSVBA34 and pSVBIA34) or at 4.1 kb (pSVPBA34 and pSVPBIA34) from the Ad2ML cap site. Two other recombinants (pTB101A34 and pTB208A34) contain the fraction of the 72 bp repeat sequence present in the two deletion mutants TB101 and TB208, previously described (Moreau *et al.*, 1981). pSVBA29 and pSVBIA29 were constructed as pSVBA34 and pSVBIA34, respectively. (B) S_1 nuclease mapping of the 5′ end of RNA transcripts isolated from HeLa cells transfected with the pSVA34 and pSVA29 series. Total cellular RNA was hybridized to an excess of *Hind*III–*Xho*I single-stranded probe (5′-end labeled at the *Hind*III site, see Fig. 1B) and analyzed as described in Section II of the text. Lane G corresponds to a G sequence ladder (Maxam and Gilbert, 1980) of the probe. The S_1 nuclease-resistant probe fragments corresponding to specific transcription from the Ad2MLP are indicated by MLP + 1. Bands pointed out by the arrowheads correspond to nonspecific transcription initiated upstream from the deletion end-points (see Section III of the text).

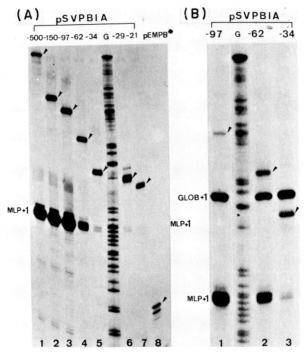

Fig. 3. Effect of deletions in the Ad2ML promoter region on specific *in vivo* transcription. (A) Quantitative S$_1$ nuclease mapping of Ad2MLP transcripts produced in HeLa cells transfected with pSVBIA500 and its deletion mutants pSVPBIA150, 97, 62, 34, 29 and 21 (Fig. 1A) as indicated. The specific transcripts were mapped with the *Hind*III–*Xho*I probe as in Fig. 2B. pEMPB* corresponds to pSVPBIA500 (see Fig. 1A) but lacks all the Ad2MLP sequence. (B) Same as in (A), but the HeLa cells were cotransfected as indicated with the pSVPBIA mutants and a polyoma–β-globin recombinant [pβ(244+)β in De Villiers and Schaffner, 1981] used as an internal transcription control. The probe used to map the specific globin transcripts was a single-stranded BstNI restriction fragment (202 nucleotides), prepared from the globin recombinant. GLOB+1 refers to the position of the S$_1$ nuclease-resistant band that corresponds to RNA initiated at the β-globin cap site. Experimental conditions and other symbols (G and arrowheads) are as in Section II and Fig. 2.

Ad2MLP (compare pSVPBIA500, 150 and 97 in lanes 1–3 of Fig. 3A). Further deletions resulted in a threefold decrease in the amount of specific RNA when sequences were deleted up to −62 and in an additional tenfold reduction when the deletion was extended to −34 (lanes 3–5 in Fig. 3A and Table II). Deletion of the first two bases of the TATA box (pSVPBIA29, lane 6) caused an additional twofold reduction, whereas deletion of the entire TATA box resulted in a further 2.5-fold decrease (pSVPBIA21, lane 7). It is remarkable that even in the absence of the TATA box (pSVPBIA21, lane 7) the only band (excluding the

TABLE II

Comparison of the *in Vivo* and *in Vitro* Efficiency of Adenovirus Type 2 Major Late Promoter Mutants[a]

		In vitro (%)			
		S100 Extract		Whole cell extract	
Recombinants	in vivo (%)	Linear template	Circular template	Linear template	Circular template
pSVPBIA97	100	100	100	100	100
pSVPBIA62	33	100	53	30	33
pSVPBIA34	3	80	20	5	3
pSVPBIA21	0.6	0	0	0	0

[a] *In vivo* and *in vitro* efficiency of the Ad2MLP mutants was determined by quantitative S_1 nuclease mapping as described in Figs. 3–5. The intensity of the specific band corresponding to initiation from the Ad2MLP (MLP+1, in Figs. 3–5) was determined by densitometry of autoradiograms exposed for various periods of time. The values for the pSVPBIA21 recombinant used as a circulate template were taken from unpublished experiments. In all cases the results were expressed in percent of the value obtained with pSVPBIA97.

deletion end-point band) which was seen on the original autoradiogram corresponds to RNA initiated at the Ad2ML cap site. This band was absent in the lane corresponding to pEMPB* which lacks all of the Ad2MLP region (legend to Fig. 3A and lane 8). Two sets of observations indicate that the differences found between the various pSVPBIA recombinants in Fig. 3A are not artifactual. First, in all cases there was very little variation in the amount of RNA initiated upstream from the deletion end-points, as shown by the intensity of the bands pointed out by arrowheads in Fig. 3A. Second, a rabbit β-globin recombinant [pβ(244+)β; De Villers and Schaffner, 1981] was cotransfected as an internal control with pSVPBIA97, 62 or 34. There was little variation in the intensity of the globin band (GLOB+1, in lanes 1, 2, and 3 of Fig. 3B), whereas the differences between the various pSVPBIA recombinants were very similar to those seen in Fig. 3A.

4. The effect of the upstream sequences of the Ad2ML promoter can be faithfully reproduced *in vitro*. Previous *in vitro* studies using an S100 extract and a run-off assay (Weil *et al.*, 1979) did not demonstrate any effect of sequences upstream from the TATA box on specific *in vitro* transcription from the Ad2MLP (Corden *et al.*, 1980). We therefore reinvestigated the promoter sequence requirement for *in vitro* transcription using the quantitative S_1 nuclease assay while varying the type of cellular extract and the form of the template. As expected (Corden *et al.*, 1980), deletions down to position −34 (Fig. 4A, lanes

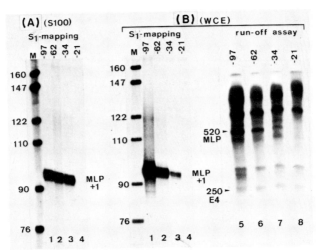

Fig. 4. Effect of deletions in the upstream region of the Ad2ML promoter on specific *in vitro* transcription of linear templates. (A) *In vitro* transcription with an S100 extract. The S100 extract was prepared from HeLa cells as described (Weil *et al.*, 1979). Unlabeled RNA was synthesized in a threefold standard reaction (Sassone-Corsi *et al.*, 1981) in the presence of 10 μg/ml of the pSVPBIA97, 62, 34 and 21 deletion mutants (lanes 1–4, respectively), cut with *Taq*I which cuts the molecules into 8 fragments of which one, containing the Ad2MLP region, extends from position 23 in pBR322 to position 4739 in SV40. The RNA was analyzed by quantitative S_1 nuclease mapping with the *Hind*III–*Xho*I probe as in Fig. 2B. (B) *In vitro* transcription with a WCE. The WCE was prepared as described (Manley *et al.*, 1980). RNA was synthesized in a threefold standard reaction (Manley *et al.*, 1980) in the presence of 15 μg/ml of the same *Taq*I-digested templates as in (A). Lanes 1–4 show the S_1 nuclease mapping analysis [as in (A)] of unlabeled RNA synthesized from pSVPBIA97, 62, 34, and 21, respectively. Lanes 5–8 show the electrophoretic analysis (5% acrylamide–8.3 M urea) of labeled run-off RNA synthesized under the same conditions but in the presence of [α-32P]CTP. A constant amount (6 μg/ml) of a fragment containing the adenovirus type 5 (Ad5) E4 promoter region was added as an internal transcription control. [The Ad5 *Sma*I restriction fragment (98.4 to 100 map units; see Hérissé *et al.*, 1981) was cloned into pBR322; after excision with *Sma*I and *Sph*I, the resulting 0.7 kb DNA fragment was purified and used as template.] The specific transcripts from the Ad2ML and Ad5E4 promoters are indicated by arrowheads (520 and 250 nucleotides in length, respectively). The apparent differences in the position of the MLP + 1 bands in lanes 1–3 of (A) and (B) are due to an electrophoretic distorsion on the edge of the gel. DNA size markers shown in lanes M are 32P-end-labeled pBR322-*Msp*I restriction fragments.

1–3) did not affect specific initiation (MLP+1) from a linear template with the S100 extract, as measured by S_1 nuclease mapping, whereas deletion of the TATA box abolished it (pSVPBIA21, lane 4). In contrast, when the same experiments were carried out with a WCE (Manley *et al.*, 1980), the effect of the upstream sequences was clearly seen using the S_1 nuclease or the run-off assays (Fig. 4B). Deletions of sequences upstream from −62 and −34 resulted, respectively, in a 3- and 20-fold decrease (lanes 1–3 and Table II) of specific transcription, relative to pSVPBIA97 which was as efficiently transcribed as the wild-type pSVPBIA500 (not shown). Similar results were obtained using the run-off assay (Fig. 4B, lanes 5–7). In this experiment transcription of an Ad5E4 linear template was used as an internal control. No specific transcription was detected when the TATA box was deleted (lanes 4 and 8).

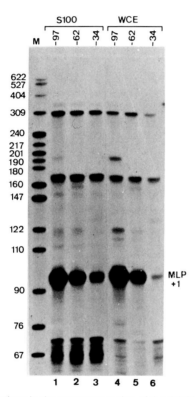

Fig. 5. Effect of deletions in the upstream region of the Ad2ML promoter on specific *in vitro* transcription of circular templates with an S100 or a WCE. The indicated pSVPBIA recombinants were transcribed as circular templates in the presence of S100 (lanes 1 to 3) or WCE (lanes 4 to 6) as described in the legend to Fig. 4. About 70% of the DNA molecules were superhelical. As an internal transcription control, 3 μg/ml (lanes 1–3) and 5 μg/ml (lanes 4–6) of a recombinant plasmid containing the adenovirus type 5 (Ad5) E3 promoter region [the Ad5 *Eco*RI C restriction fragment (Hérissé *et al.*, 1980), inserted into the *Eco*RI site of pBR322] was added and cotranscribed in each reaction. The synthesized RNA was processed and analyzed by S_1 nuclease mapping with the *Hind*III–*Xho*I probe as described in Fig. 2B. The probe used to map the specific E3 transcripts was a single-stranded Sau3A restriction fragment (302 nucleotides) spanning the E3 cap sites and 5′-end-labeled with [32P]. MLP + 1 and E3 refer to the S_1 nuclease-resistant bands which correspond to RNA initiated at the Ad2ML and the Ad5E3 cap sites, respectively. M is as in Fig. 4B.

It has been suggested (Grosschedl and Birstiel, 1982) that the free ends of DNA can serve as entry sites for RNA polymerase B and thereby mask the effect of promoter sequences with similar function. Therefore circular DNAs (mainly superhelical, see legend to Fig. 5 and Section IV) were used with either the S100 or the WCE and specific transcription was measured by S_1 nuclease mapping (Fig. 5). An Ad5E3 template was added to provide an internal control (legend to Fig. 5). With the WCE, deletions of sequences upstream from −34 appeared to have a more pronounced effect with circular than with linear templates (compare Fig. 5, lanes 4–6 with Fig. 4B, lanes 1–3). Using circular templates no specific transcripts were observed with the −21 mutant (not shown). It is noteworthy that the *in vivo* effects of the −62 and −34 deletions (Figs. 3 and 5 and Table II) are faithfully reproduced *in vitro* with the WCE and circular templates. To a lesser degree, an effect of the upstream sequences was also seen with the S100 extract and circular templates (compare lanes 1–3 with 4–6 in Fig. 5), but it is striking that this effect was totally absent when linear templates were used (compare lanes 1–3 in Figs. 5 and 4A).

IV. Discussion

As previously shown for other RNA polymerase B promoters (see Section I) our results demonstrate that sequences located upstream from the TATA box are important for efficient *in vivo* promotion of RNA synthesis from the Ad2ML promoter. Sequences upstream from −97 were not required, whereas sequences located between −97 and −34 played a major role. Our results (Fig. 3) suggest either that two sets of sequences are involved and that the effect of the −62 to −34 region is more important than that of the −97 to −62 region, or that only one sequence, centered on position −62, is implicated. This second possibility is supported by a sequence homology between the Ad2MLP sequence around −62 and the upstream sequence of the rabbit β-globin gene, which is homologous to the upstream consensus sequence previously pointed out (Benoist *et al.*, 1980; Efstratiadis *et al.*, 1980) and was recently shown to be important for efficient transcription *in vivo*.

$$-76$$
$$\text{Rabbit } \beta\text{-globin} \quad 5' - \text{CTGGTGTTGGCCAAT} - 3'$$
$$\text{Ad2MLP} \quad 5' - \text{TAGGTGTAGGCCACG} - 3'$$
$$-62$$

Mutations of both the two Gs (at positions −77 and −76; see Grosveld *et al.*, 1982b) or of either one of the two Cs [at position −75 and −74, (P. Dierks, A. Van Ooyen, C. Weissman, personal communication)] of the rabbit β-globin gene resulted in about a tenfold reduction of *in vivo* RNA synthesis.

As expected (see Section I) additional deletion of the TATA box induced a further decrease in specific *in vivo* transcription. However, even when the TATA box was completely deleted, the residual transcription (0.6% of the wild type) appeared to be still mainly initiated from the Ad2ML cap site. This is in contrast to the *in vitro* situation (Figs. 4 and 5 and Corden *et al.,* 1980) where deletion of the TATA box completely abolished specific transcription. It appears therefore that some sequences located downstream from the TATA box could also be involved in the process which, *in vivo,* directs the transcription machinery to initiate at the cap site.

It is unlikely that insertion of the SV40 72 bp repeat at more than 4 kb from the adenovirus sequence differentially modulates the activity of the different elements of the Ad2ML promoter which appears to be stimulated as a whole. Indeed, the effect of the various deletions was roughly the same, whether it was measured indirectly after microinjection in CV1 cell nuclei of recombinants lacking the 72 bp repeat or directly, at the RNA level, after transfection of HeLa cells with recombinants containing the 72 bp repeat inserted at 4 kb from the Ad2MLP. However, it is clear from the results shown in Fig. 2B that insertion of the 72 bp repeat in a position too close to Ad2MLP elements can mask their effect. These observations, and those which suggest that the effect of the 72 bp repeat is the strongest on initiation from proximal sequences (see results), are in agreement with the hypothesis that the 72 bp repeat could act as an entry site for RNA polymerase B (Moreau *et al.,* 1981). Obviously an element with a similar effect is not present in the first 500 bp upstream from the Ad2ML cap site. Whether it is present further upstream and could play a role in stimulating initiation of transcription from the Ad2MLP during viral infection remains to be established.

The *in vivo* effect of the upstream sequences (-97 to -34) of the Ad2MLP can be faithfully reproduced *in vitro* with circular templates and a transcription system where the source of RNA polymerase B and initiation factor(s) is a WCE (Figs. 3A and 5). However, a circular template is not absolutely required, since an effect of the upstream sequences was also seen with linear templates (Fig. 4B). A similar observation was previously reported for *in vitro* transcription of a sea urchin *H2A* histone gene (Grosschedl and Birnstiel, 1982). In agreement with our previous results (Corden *et al.,* 1980), no effect of the upstream sequences could be demonstrated with linear templates when the WCE was replaced by an S100 extract. Assuming that the free ends of linear templates could functionally replace the upstream sequences (Grosschedl and Birnstiel, 1982), this difference between the WCE and the S100 extract suggests the presence, in the WCE, of protein(s) that bind to DNA ends and are absent in the S100 extract. However, this interpretation does not explain why, on circular templates (Fig. 5), the WCE is more efficient than the S100 extract at mimicking the *in vivo* results. This difference cannot be attributed to the calf thymus RNA polymerase B which is added to the S100 system, since the same results were obtained when transcription was performed by the RNA polymerase B contained in the S100 extract, in the absence of exogenous polymerase (results not shown). Further studies will show whether the WCE contains some factor(s) present in limiting amount in the S100 extract which are required to reveal the effect of the upstream sequences. It is unlikely that the role of such factor(s) would be to participate in the assembly of a chromatin structure necessary to reveal the effect of the upstream sequences. In fact, we analyzed the fate of the superhelical DNA template after various times of incubation and found that it was transformed within 5 minutes into covalently closed relaxed circles (results not shown), whereas if nucleosomes would have been formed, at least some superhelicity should have been conserved (Germond *et al.*, 1975).

Acknowledgments

We are particularly grateful to P. Moreau for many helpful discussions and gifts of materials. We thank W. Schaffner for his help with cell transfection and T. Leff for a critical reading of the manuscript. We gratefully acknowledge the technical assistance of K. Dott, C. Hauss, B. Boulay, E. Badzinski, C. Kutschis, and C. Werlé. This investigation was supported by grants from the CNRS (ATP 006520/50), from the INSERM (CRT 80.1029), from the Association pour le Développement de la Recherche sur le Cancer, and from the Fondation Simone et Cino del Duca. R. Hen is a fellow of the Ligue Nationale Française contre le Cancer and J. Corden of the Université Louis Pasteur—Strasbourg.

References

Akusjärvi, G., and Pettersson, U. (1979). *J. Mol. Biol.* **134**, 143–158.
Banerji, J., Rusconi, S., and Schaffner, W. (1981). *Cell* **27**, 299–308.
Benoist, C., and Chambon, P. (1980). *Proc. Natl. Acad. Sci. U.S.A.* **77**, 3865–3869.
Benoist, C., O'Hare, K., Breathnach, R., and Chambon, P. (1980). *Nucleic Acids Res.* **8**, 127–142.
Breathnach, R., and Chambon, P. (1981). *Annu. Rev. Biochem.* **50**, 349–383.
Corden, J., Wasylyk, B., Buchwalder, A., Sassone-Corsi, P., Kédinger, C., and Chambon, P. (1980). Science **209**, 1406–1414.
De Villiers, J., and Schaffner, W. (1981). *Nucleic Acids Res.* **9**, 6251–6264.
Dierks, P., Van Ooyen, A., Mantei, N., and Weissmann, C. (1981). *Proc. Natl. Acad. Sci. U.S.A.* **78**, 1411–1415.
Efstratiadis, A., Posakony, J. W., Maniatis, T., Lawn, R. M., O'Connell, C., Spritz, R. A., DeRiel, J. K., Forget, B. G., Weissman, S. M., Slightom, J. L., Blechl, A. E., Smithies, O., Baralle, F. E., Shoulders, C. C., and Proudfoot, N. J. (1980). *Cell* **21**, 653–668.
Germond, J. E., Hirt, B., Oudet, P., Gross-Bellard, M., and Chambon, P. (1975). *Proc. Natl. Acad. Sci. U.S.A.* **72**, 1843–1847.
Grosschedl, R., and Birnstiel, M. L. (1980). *Proc. Natl. Acad. Sci. U.S.A.* **77**, 7102–7106.
Grosschedl, R., and Birnstiel, M. L. (1982). *Proc. Natl. Acad. Sci. U.S.A.* **79**, 297–301.
Grosveld, G. C., Shewmaker, C. K., Jat, P., and Flavell, R. A. (1981). *Cell* **25**, 215–226.

Grosveld, G. C., de Boer, E., Shewmaker, C. K., and Flavell, R. A. (1982a). *Nature (London)* **295**, 120–126.

Grosveld, G. C., Rosenthal, A., and Flavell, R. A. (1982b). *Nucleic Acids Res.* **10**, 4951–4971.

Hérissé, J., Courtois, G., and Galibert, F. (1980). *Nucleic Acids Res.* **8**, 2173–2192.

Hérissé, J., Rigolet, M., Dupont de Dinechin, S., and Galibert, F. (1981). *Nucleic Acids Res.* **9**, 4023–4042.

Hu, S.-L., and Manley, J. L. (1981). *Proc. Natl. Acad. Sci. U.S.A.* **78**, 820–824.

Lee, D. C., Roeder, R. G., and Wold, W. S. M. (1982). *Proc. Natl. Acad. Sci. U.S.A.* **79**, 41–45.

McKnight, S. L., Gavis, E. R., Kingsbury, R., and Axel, R. (1981). *Cell* **25**, 385–398.

Manley, J. L., Fire, A., Cano, A., Sharp, P. A., and Gefter, M. L. (1980). *Proc. Natl. Acad. Sci. U.S.A.* **77**, 3855–3859.

Mathis, D. J., and Chambon, P. (1981). *Nature (London)* **290**, 310–315.

Maxam, A., and Gilbert, W. (1980). *In* "Methods in Enzymology. Part I. Nucleic Acids" (L. Grossman, ed.), Vol. 65, pp. 499–580. Academic Press, New York.

Mellon, P., Parker, V., Gluzman, Y., and Maniatis, T. (1981). *Cell* **27**, 279–288.

Moreau, P., Hen, R., Wasylyk, B., Everett, R., Gaub, M. P., and Chambon, P. (1981). *Nucleic Acids Res.* **9**, 6047–6068.

Myers, R. M., Rio, D. C., Robbins, A. K., and Tjian, R. (1981). *Cell* **25**, 373–384.

Sassone-Corsi, P., Corden, J., Kédinger, C., and Chambon, P. (1981). *Nucleic Acids Res.* **9**, 3941–3958.

Struhl, K. (1981). *Proc. Natl. Acad. Sci. U.S.A.* **78**, 4461–4465.

Tsai, S. Y., Tsai, M.-J., and O'Malley, B. W. (1981). *Proc. Natl. Acad. Sci. U.S.A.* **78**, 879–883.

Tsuda, M., and Suzuki, Y. (1981). *Cell* **27**, 175–182.

Wasylyk, B., Kédinger, C., Corden, J., Brison, O., and Chambon, P. (1980). *Nature (London)* **285**, 367–373.

Weil, P. A., Segall, J., Harris, B., Ng, S.-Y., and Roeder, R. G. (1979). *J. Biol. Chem.* **254**, 6163–6173.

Tumor Transforming Genes

GEOFFREY M. COOPER AND MARY-ANN LANE

Dana–Farber Cancer Institute
and Department of Pathology
Harvard Medical School
Boston, Massachusetts

I. Identification and Specificity of Neoplasm Transforming Genes

Transfection of cellular DNAs has demonstrated that a variety of neoplasms contain genes that induce oncogenic transformation of NIH 3T3 mouse cells with high efficiencies. Since DNAs of homologous normal cells lack efficient transforming activity, these findings indicate that the development of some neoplasms involves dominant genetic alterations resulting in the activation of cellular transforming genes that are then detectable in transfection assays.

The neoplasms that contain such activated transforming genes include lymphoid neoplasms of chicken, mouse, and human origin (Cooper and Neiman, 1980; Lane *et al.*, 1982a); rodent and human bladder, colon, lung, and mammary carcinomas (Krontiris and Cooper, 1981; Shih *et al.*, 1981; Lane *et al.*, 1981; Perucho *et al.*, 1981; Murray *et al.*, 1981); rodent and human neuroblastomas (Shih *et al.*, 1981; Perucho *et al.*, 1981); a human promyelocytic leukemia (Murray *et al.*, 1981); and human sarcomas (Pulciani *et al.*, 1982; Marshall *et al.*, 1982). These neoplasms include spontaneously occurring, chemically induced, and virally induced tumors. They also include primary chicken, mouse, and human tumors, as well as tumor-derived cell lines. It thus appears that dominant transforming genes can be activated in a variety of different types of neoplasms induced by different agents. In addition, activation of transforming genes occurs in primary neoplasms and is not restricted to cultured cell lines.

Comparisons of the transforming genes of different types of tumors have indicated that the same transforming gene is activated in most neoplasms of the same differentiated cell type, whereas different transforming genes are activated in most neoplasms of different origins. For example, the transforming activities of DNAs of a human mammary carcinoma cell line, five virus-induced mouse mammary carcinomas, and a chemically induced mouse mammary carcinoma displayed identical patterns of susceptibility to cleavage with seven different restriction endonucleases (Lane *et al.*, 1981). Since the probability of this pattern occurring by chance was less than 10^{-10}, these results indicated that these seven different mammary carcinomas, including spontaneous, virally induced, and chemically induced tumors, contained the same or closely related transforming genes (Lane *et al.*, 1981). This conclusion has been further substantiated by identification of an antigen that is specifically expressed in NIH cells transformed by human or mouse mammary carcinoma DNAs, as well as in primary mouse mammary carcinomas (Becker *et al.*, 1982). Different specific transforming genes have been identified in chemically transformed mouse fibroblasts (Shilo and Weinberg, 1981), human colon and lung carcinomas (Perucho *et al.*, 1981), human and mouse lymphocyte neoplasms (Lane *et al.*, 1982a), and human sarcomas (Marshall *et al.*, 1982).

Analysis of the transforming genes of human and mouse lymphocyte neoplasms has further indicated that different transforming genes are activated in neoplasms representing different stages of normal B and T lymphocyte differentiation (Lane *et al.*, 1982a). For example, a common transforming gene was detected in four human and two mouse pre-B lymphocyte neoplasms (Lane *et al.*, 1982a,b). A different transforming gene was detected in two human and three mouse B cell lymphomas, and a third distinct transforming gene was detected in two human myelomas and two mouse plasmacytomas (Lane *et al.*, 1982a). Two additional distinct transforming genes were activated in human and mouse T lymphocyte neoplasms representing intermediate and mature stages of T cell differentiation (Lane *et al.*, 1982a). These results indicate that specific transforming genes are activated in neoplasms representing different stages of differentiation within common cell lineages.

Taken together, these results indicate a high degree of specificity for the transforming genes activated in neoplasms. One interpretation of this specificity is that only one or a few of the total number of potential transforming genes are susceptible targets for activation in certain differentiated cells. In addition, this specificity suggests that transformation may result from alterations of genes that normally function in control of proliferation of specific differentiated cell types.

II. Transforming Genes of Human Bladder, Colon, and Lung Carcinomas

One class of cellular genes with potential oncogenic activity are the cellular homologs of retrovirus transforming genes. The acute transforming retroviruses contain specific genes responsible for oncogenicity. At least 15 distinct transforming genes have been identified in different virus isolates, all of which are closely related to homologous genes in normal cells (Bishop, 1981). It was therefore of interest to determine whether any of the transforming genes detected by transfection of tumor DNAs were cellular homologs of the transforming genes of retroviruses.

Molecular clones of retrovirus transforming genes were used as probes in blot-hybridization analysis of DNAs of NIH cells transformed by a variety of different tumor DNAs. The results of these experiments have indicated that the transforming genes of human lymphoid neoplasms and mammary carcinomas are not related to the retrovirus transforming genes *src, myc, fes, erb, mos, myb, sis*, or *ras*. However the transforming genes of human bladder, colon and lung carcinomas are cellular homologs of the *ras* retrovirus transforming gene family.

Analysis of NIH cells transformed by DNAs of the human bladder carcinoma cell lines EJ, J82, and T24 indicated that the transforming gene detected by transfection of their DNAs was a cellular homolog of the ras^H gene of Harvey sarcoma virus (Der *et al.*, 1982; Parada *et al.*, 1982; Santos *et al.*, 1982). Recent characterization of these three bladder carcinoma cell lines by HLA typing, however, has indicated that they are cross-contaminated (C. M. O'Toole, personal communication), so that activation of the ras^H transforming gene has been detected in only one independent bladder carcinoma.

The transforming gene detected by transfection of DNA of the LX-1 human lung carcinoma cell line was identified as a cellular homolog of a different member of the *ras* gene family, the ras^K gene of Kirsten sarcoma virus (Der *et al.*, 1982). More recent studies have extended these results to show that the same cellular ras^K gene is also activated in a second human lung carcinoma cell line Calu-1 and in two human colon carcinoma cell lines SW480 and SK-CO-1 (Der and Cooper, 1983). These results confirm earlier findings of Perucho *et al.* (1981) which indicated that the same transforming genes were activated in independent lung and colon carcinomas and identify this common lung/colon carcinoma transforming gene as a cellular ras^K homolog.

Blot-hybridization analysis of DNAs of both human cells and transformed NIH cells has indicated that the same ras^H- and ras^K-containing restriction fragments, which constitute the activated transforming genes of bladder, lung, and colon carcinomas, are present in normal human DNAs (Goldfarb *et al.*, 1982; Shih and Weinberg, 1982; Der *et al.*, 1982; Der and Cooper, 1983). These results indicate that the transforming genes of these neoplasms are derived from genes of normal cells. In addition, activation of the transforming activity of *ras* genes in these human carcinomas does not appear to result from either gene amplification or detectable DNA rearrangements. Instead, activation of these transforming genes appears likely to be a consequence of point mutations or small rearrangements that were not detected by restriction endonuclease analysis.

The ras^H and ras^K genes are members of a family of related genes in vertebrate cells (Ellis *et al.*, 1981). The retrovirus ras^H and ras^K genes encode related proteins of 21,000 daltons that are expressed at high levels in Harvey and Kirsten sarcoma virus-transformed cells (Langbeheim *et al.*, 1980). Similar 21,000 dalton proteins are expressed in a variety of normal vertebrate cells, but at significantly lower levels than in virus-transformed cells (Langbeheim *et al.*, 1980). Molecular clones of normal rat and human ras^H genes do not induce transformation upon transfection, but transforming activity of these normal cell genes can be activated by ligation to viral transcriptional regulatory sequences (DeFeo *et al.*, 1981; Chang *et al.*, 1982). These results indicate that abnormal expression of these cellular ras^H genes is sufficient for induction of oncogenic transformation.

It thus would appear possible that activation of *ras* genes in human carcinomas could be a consequence of mutations in regulatory sequences resulting in abnormal gene expression. Alternatively, however, activation of *ras* genes in carcinomas could involve mutations affecting the structure and activity of their gene products. Due to the availability of monoclonal antibodies against *ras*-encoded proteins (Furth *et al.*, 1982), it has been possible to investigate the expression of these proteins (designated p21s) in human cells and in NIH cells transformed by human carcinoma DNAs.

Immunoprecipitation with anti-p21 monoclonal antibody indicated that p21 proteins were expressed in NIH cells transformed by bladder carcinoma DNA at two- to fourfold higher levels than in NIH 3T3 cells (Der *et al.*, 1982). The level of p21 expression in EJ bladder carcinoma cells was similar to that in NIH cells transformed by EJ DNA (Der *et al.*, 1982). These results indicated that *ras* gene products were expressed in both the human bladder carcinoma cell line and in NIH cells transformed by the activated ras^H gene of this carcinoma. The levels of p21 expression in EJ bladder carcinoma cells were also elevated (three- to eightfold) compared to the levels of p21 expression in primary cultures of normal human bladder epithelial cells (Der and Cooper, 1983). In addition, a similar elevation of p21 expression was observed in a primary culture of a fresh human bladder carcinoma specimen (Der and Cooper, 1983).

To further investigate the possible correlations between gene expression and transforming activity of *ras* genes in neoplasms, these parameters were analyzed in seventeen different human carcinoma cell lines (Der and Cooper, 1983). These cell lines included (1) the EJ bladder carcinoma containing an activated ras^H gene, (2) two colon and two lung carcinomas containing activated ras^K genes, (3) mammary carcinoma, pancreatic carcinoma, and Wilm's tumor cell lines that contained activated transforming genes that were not homologous to either ras^H or ras^K, and (4) nine carcinoma cell lines of bladder, lung, colon, prostate, cervical, and adrenal cortical orgin which did not contain activated transforming genes detectable by transfection of NIH 3T3 cells.

The levels of p21 expression were similar in all of the carcinoma cell lines investigated. In particular, p21 expression in the ras^H-positive EJ bladder carcinoma cell line did not differ significantly from p21 expression in three other bladder carcinoma cell lines whose DNAs lacked transforming activity. Therefoe, the elevated expression of ras gene products in EJ bladder carcinoma cells, as compared to normal bladder epithelial cells, may not be specifically correlated with activation of the transforming activity of ras^H.

The p21 proteins expressed in EJ bladder carcinoma cells were indistinguishable in electrophoretic mobility in one-dimensional SDS–polyacrylamide gels from the p21 proteins expressed in normal human embryo fibroblasts and normal human bladder epithelial cells. Electrophoretically similar p21 proteins were also expressed in all of the other carcinoma cell lines studied, with the exception of the four lung and colon carcinoma cell lines that contained activated ras^K genes.

The two lung and two colon ras^K-positive cell lines all expressed p21 proteins that were distinct in electrophoretic mobility from those detected in other cells. The p21 proteins of these cell lines included abnormal species of p21 with lower electrophoretic mobility than the p21 proteins of other cells. The abnormal p21 proteins of the LX-1 lung and the SW480 and SK-CO-1 colon carcinoma cell lines were similar to each other and migrated with an electrophoretic mobility corresponding to an apparent molecular weight increase of 1500 to 2000 compared to normal p21 proteins. A different abnormal p21 species was expressed in the Calu-1 lung carcinoma cell line. This cell line expressed a p21 migrating with slightly lower electrophoretic mobility than normal cell p21 but with higher electrophoretic mobility than the abnormal p21 species detected in the three other ras^K-positive carcinomas.

To determine whether the abnormal p21 proteins expressed in these lung and colon carcinoma cell lines were encoded by their activated ras^K genes, the p21 proteins expressed in transformed NIH cells were characterized. The p21 proteins expressed in NIH 3T3 cells and in NIH cells transformed by Wilm's tumor, bladder carcinoma, mammary carcinoma, or pancreatic carcinoma DNAs were indistinguishable in electrophoretic mobility. However, NIH cells transformed by LX-1, SW480, and SK-CO-1 DNAs expressed the same abnormal species of p21 as were detected in these human lung and colon carcinomas. In addition, NIH cells transformed by Calu-1 DNA expressed the distinct abnormal p21 species of the Calu-1 lung carinoma cell line. The abnormal p21 proteins expressed in these four lung and colon carcinoma cell lines therefore appeared to be encoded by the cellular ras^K genes whose transforming activity was activated in the carcinomas.

These results indicate that ras^K genes activated in four different carcinomas encode structurally abnormal gene products. Since the two distinct abnormal p21 species observed were both encoded by the same ras^K gene, it appears that activation of ras^K genes in these neoplasms involved mutations that altered the structure of the p21 encoded by these genes. In addition, it would appear that different molecular alterations can lead to activation of ras^K in different individual neoplasms.

Studies of viral ras-encoded p21 proteins have indicated that these proteins are located on the inner surface of the cytoplasmic membrane (Willingham et al., 1980). The Harvey and Kirsten sarcoma virus-encoded p21 proteins are phosphorylated in vivo, bind guanine nucleotides, and display GTP-dependent autokinase activity in vitro (Scolnick et al., 1979; Shih et al., 1980). In contrast, the p21 proteins expressed by either normal cells or encoded by the cellular ras^H and ras^K genes activated in human carcinomas are not phosphorylated (Der and Cooper, 1983). The nature of the molecular alterations occurring in these carcinomas and their effects on the biochemical activities of p21 proteins remain to be determined.

III. Transforming Genes of Chicken B Cell Lymphomas

B Cell lymphomas are induced in chickens by infection with avian lymphoid leukosis virus (LLV), a retrovirus that induces neoplasms with long latent periods and does not contain a specific viral transforming gene. In contrast, acute transforming retroviruses contain specific transforming genes, transform cells in vitro, and induce neoplasms with short latent periods in vivo. Oncogenesis by LLVs thus appears to resemble chemically induced or naturally occurring oncogenesis more closely than oncogenesis by sarcoma and acute leukemia viruses.

Transfection assays of DNAs of LLV-induced B cell lymphomas indicated that these neoplasms contained transforming genes that induced transformation of NIH 3T3 mouse cells with high efficiencies (Cooper and Neiman, 1980). In contrast, DNAs of LLV-infected nonneoplastic cells lacked transforming activity. LLV-induced lymphomagenesis thus appeared to involve dominant genetic alterations leading to activation of cellular transforming genes.

To determine whether the transforming genes detected by transfection of these lymphoma DNAs were linked to viral DNA sequences, transformed NIH cells were analyzed for the presence of LLV DNA by blot hybridization. No viral DNA sequences were detected in NIH cells transformed by LLV-induced lymphoma DNAs using probes either representative of the entire LLV genome or specific for the LLV long terminal redundancy (Cooper and Neiman, 1980). Therefore, the transforming genes of B cell lymphomas detected by transfection were not linked to viral DNA, indicating that lymphomagenesis by LLVs involved indirect activation of cellular transforming genes at some stage of the disease process.

Hayward *et al.* (1981) have reported that approximately 80% of LLV-induced B cell lymphomas contain viral DNA sequences integrated in the vicinity of *c-myc*, the cellular homolog of the transforming gene of the acute leukemia virus MC29. Integration of viral sequences apparently results in increased transcription of *c-myc,* implicating *c-myc* activation as a direct consequence of virus infection in lymphomagenesis (Hayward *et al.*, 1981).

The LLV-induced lymphomas that were used as DNA donors in transfection assays also contain viral DNA sequences integrated near *c-myc* (Cooper and Neiman, 1981). However, further analysis of NIH cells transformed by these lymphomas DNAs indicates that transformation was not mediated by transfer of these activated *c-myc* sequences (Cooper and Neiman, 1981). B Cell lymphomas induced by LLV thus appear to contain at least two different candidate transforming genes: (1) a *c-myc* gene activated by integration of viral DNA sequences and (2) a distinct cellular gene, not linked to viral DNA, which efficiently induces transformation of NIH 3T3 cells.

The long latent period and pathogenesis of lymphomas induced by LLV suggests a process that includes several preneoplastic and neoplastic stages and might, therefore, be expected to involve more than a single transformation event. Multiple preneoplastic follicles are observed in the bursas of most birds within approximately 40 days after LLV infection (Neiman *et al.*, 1980). The majority of these preneoplastic follicles regress, but a small fraction appear to develop into neoplastic nodules that are the presumed precursors of metastatic lymphomas (Neiman *et al.*, 1980). Proliferation of preneoplastic follicles thus appears to be an early event in the disease process that is sometimes followed by progression to neoplasia. Viral activation of *c-myc* may thus be involved in a stage of lymphomagenesis that precedes or complements activation of transforming genes detected by transfection. For example, activation of *c-myc* might be an early event in lymphomagenesis resulting in proliferation of preneoplastic follicles. Progression to neoplasia might then involve mutations or gene rearrangements within cells of this preneoplastic proliferative population resulting in activation of the transforming gene detected by transfection. Neoplastic nodules and metastatic lymphomas contain both activated *c-myc* genes and activated transforming genes detectable in the transfection assay (Cooper and Neiman, 1980, 1981). However, the activity of either of these genes in preneoplastic follicles is not known. Further work will thus be required to elucidate the roles of these two transforming genes in the disease process.

The cellular transforming gene activated in a lymphoma cell line (RP-9) has recently been isolated by molecular cloning (Goubin *et al.*, 1983), DNA of NIH cells transformed by RP-9 DNA was subjected to partial digestion with *Mbo* I and cloned in λ Charon 30 to generate a library of approximately 200,000 phage.

This library was screened by sib selection (Cavalli-Sforza and Lederberg, 1956) using transfection of NIH 3T3 cells to identify recombinant phage populations containing a biologically active transforming gene. A single phage was isolated (designated λChBlym-1) which contains a cellular DNA insert of 4.5 kb and induces transformation with an efficiency of approximately 2000 transformants/μg cell DNA.

Analysis of the transforming activity of λChBlym-1 by cleavage with restriction endonucleases indicated that its transforming gene was localized to a region of less than 1.8 kb. This region contains sequences that are homologous to a family of genes present in normal chicken DNA. Comparative analysis of the organization of these sequences in DNAs of normal cells and lymphomas indicates that, as in the case of *ras* genes activated in human carcinomas, activation of the transforming activity of the λChBlym-1 gene in lymphomas is not a consequence of DNA rearrangements detectable by blot-hybridization analysis. The transforming gene of λChBlym-1 also appears to be homologous to a family of sequences present in normal human DNA, indicating that this gene family is highly conserved in evolution. This transforming sequence is transcribed in chicken lymphoma cells as a small polyadenylated RNA.

Hybridization analysis did not reveal any homology between the transforming gene of λChBlym-1 and the transforming genes of highly oncogenic retroviruses. Therefore, the nucleotide sequence of the λChBlym-1 transforming gene was determined. The positions of polyadenylation and promoter sequences within the transforming region were consistent with the mapping of transforming sequences and with the transcript detected in lymphoma cells by hybridization.

The translation product predicted by this nucleotide sequence is a protein of 65 amino acids with a calculated molecular weight of approximately 7800. The amino acid sequence of this predicted transforming protein displays partial homology (30%) with the amino-terminal regions of transferrin family proteins. Expression of cell surface receptors for transferrin is closely correlated with proliferation of both normal and neoplastic cells, suggesting a possible involvement of these receptors in control of cell proliferation. It is therefore attractive to speculate that, if the homology between the transforming protein and transferrin reflects a functional relationship, this protein may contribute to the neoplastic phenotype via interaction with such a cell regulatory system.

References

Becker, D., Lane, M.-A., and Cooper, G. M. (1982). *Proc. Natl. Acad. Sci. U.S.A.* **79**, 3315–3319.

Bishop, J. M. (1981). *Cell* **23**, 5–6.

Cavalli-Sforza, L. L., and Lederberg, J. (1956). *Genetics* **41**, 367–386.

Chang, E. H., Furth, M. E., Scolnick, E. M., and Lowy, D. R. (1982). *Nature (London)* **297,** 479–483.

Cooper, G. M., and Neiman, P. E. (1980). *Nature (London)* **287,** 656–659.

Cooper, G. M., and Neiman, P. E. (1981). *Nature (London)* **292,** 857–858.

Der, C. J., and Cooper, G. M. (1983). *Cell* **32,** 201–208.

Der, C. J., Krontiris, T. G., and Cooper, G. M. (1982). *Proc. Natl. Acad. Sci. U.S.A.* **79,** 3637–3640.

DeFeo, D., Gonda, M. A., Young, H. A., Chang, E. H., Lowy, D. R., Scolnick, E. M., and Ellis, R. W. (1981). *Proc. Natl. Acad. Sci. U.S.A.* **78,** 3328–3332.

Ellis, R. W., DeFeo, D., Shih, T. Y., Gonda, M. A, Young, H. A., Tsuchida, N., Lowy, D. R., and Scolnick, E. M. (1981). *Nature (London)* **292,** 506–511.

Furth, M. E., Davis, L. J., Fleurdelys, B., and Scolnick, E. M. (1982). *J. Virol.* **43,** 294–304.

Goldfarb, M., Shimizu, K., Perucho, M., and Wigler, M. (1982). *Nature (London)* **296,** 404–409.

Goubin, G., Goldman, D., Luce, J., Neiman, P. E., and Cooper, G. M. (1983). *Nature* **302,** 114–119.

Hayward, W. S., Neel, B. G., and Astrin, S. M. (1981). *Nature (London)* **290,** 475–480.

Krontiris, T. G., and Cooper, G. M. (1981). *Proc. Natl. Acad. Sci. U.S.A.* **78,** 1181–1184.

Lane, M.-A., Sainten, A., and Cooper, G. M. (1981). *Proc. Natl. Acad. Sci. U.S.A.* **78,** 5185–5189.

Lane, M.-A., Sainten, A., and Cooper, G. M. (1982a). *Cell* **28,** 873–880.

Lane, M.-A., Neary, D., and Cooper, G. M. (1982b). *Nature (London)* **300,** 659–661.

Langbeheim, H., Shih, T. Y., and Scolnick, E. M. (1980). *Virology* **106,** 292–300.

Marshall, C. J., Hall, A., and Weiss, R. A. (1982). *Nature (London)* **299,** 171–173.

Murray, M. J., Shilo, B.-Z., Shih, C., Cowing, D., Hsu, H. W., and Weinberg, R. A. (1981). *Cell* **25,** 355–361.

Neiman, P. E., Payne, L. N., Jordan, L., and Weiss, R. A. (1980). *Cold Spring Harbor Conf. Cell Proliferation* **7,** 519–528.

Parada, L. F., Tabin, C. J., Shih, C., and Weinberg, R. A. (1982). *Nature (London)* **297,** 474–478.

Perucho, M., Goldfarb, M., Shimizu, K., Lama, C., Fogh, J., and Wigler, M. (1981). *Cell* **27,** 467–476.

Pulciani, S., Santos, E., Lauver, A. V., Long, L. K., Robbins, K. C., and Barbacid, M. (1982). *Proc. Natl. Acad. Sci. U.S.A.* **79,** 2845–2849.

Santos, E., Tronick, S. R., Aaronson, S. A., Pulciani, S., and Barbacid, M. (1982). *Nature (London)* **298,** 343–347.

Scolnick, E. M., Papageorge, A. G., and Shih, T. Y. (1979). *Proc. Natl. Acad. Sci. U.S.A.* **76,** 5355–5359.

Shih, C., and Weinberg, R. A. (1982). *Cell* **29,** 161–169.

Shih, T. Y., Papageorge, A. G., Stokes, P. E., Weeks, M. O., and Scolnick, E. M. (1980). *Nature (London)* **287,** 686–691.

Shih, C., Padhy, L. C., Murray, M., and Weinberg, R. A. (1981). *Nature (London)* **290,** 261–264.

Shilo, B., and Weinberg, R. A. (1981). *Nature (London)* **289,** 607–609.

Willingham, M. L., Pastan, I., Shih, T. Y., and Scolnick, E. M. (1980). *Cell* **19,** 1005–1014.

PART II

Chromosome Pattern in Animal and Human Tumors

Introduction

JANET D. ROWLEY

Section of Hematology/Oncology
The University of Chicago
Chicago, Illinois

The study of the chromosome pattern in the affected cells of a number of human tumors has been one of the most exciting areas in cancer research over the last 20 years. Major advances in our understanding of the specificity of some of the abnormalities have occurred in the last 10 years with the application of new chromosome banding techniques. These techniques allow the identification of each human chromosome and of parts of chromosomes as well. Thus the hypothesis put forward by Boveri at the turn of the century, namely, that an abnormal chromosome pattern was intimately associated with the malignant phenotype of the tumor cell, can now be tested with substantial hope of obtaining a valid answer (Boveri, 1914).

The study of the chromosome pattern in human leukemias can be divided into two periods: each one covering 10 years. The first lasted from 1960 to 1970 and the second from 1970 to 1980. During the first period, the chromosome abnormalities seen in leukemic cells were identified without banding, and therefore they include the changes in morphology that were detectable in unbanded preparations as well as changes in the modal chromosome number. The most significant observation was the identification of the Philadelphia (Ph[1]) chromosome in leukemic cells from patients with chronic myelogenous leukemia. In 1960, when this abnormality was discovered by Nowell and Hungerford (1960), it appeared to represent a deletion of about half of the long arm of one G group chromosome; whether pair No. 21 or No. 22 was affected was not determined. This observation led to a search for similar abnormalities closely associated with other types of malignant hematologic diseases. The results were quite disappointing in that although the abnormalities seemed to be consistent in any particular patient, the patterns varied greatly from one patient to another. Moreover about one-half of the patients with acute leukemia of both the myeloid and lymphoid types ap-

CHROMOSOMES AND CANCER
57

peared to have a normal karyotype in their leukemic cells (Rowley and Testa, 1982; Mitelman and Levan, 1981; Sandberg, 1980). Thus the accepted notion was that the Ph[1] was a unique example of a consistent karyotypic abnormality, and the general rule was one of marked variability in karyotype. This, in turn, lead most investigators to assume that chromosome changes were a secondary phenomenon not fundamentally involved with the process of malignant transformation.

The evidence obtained during the second period showed that these assumptions were probably not correct. With the use of banding techniques, other specific abnormalities were found to be associated with certain leukemias and lymphomas as well as various types of cancer (Rowley and Testa, 1982). Moreover, banding techniques revealed that the gains and losses of chromosomes were distinctly nonrandom. However, most of the studies during this period used chromosomes that were relatively contracted, and the banding pattern often was fuzzy and poorly defined. For this reason subtle abnormalities such as a deletion or a duplication of one-third of a chromosome band, involving about 3×10^6 nucleotide pairs would not be detectable.

We are now embarking on a third period of analysis that will be characterized by substantial improvements in the quality of the chromosome preparations that are available for analysis. Just recently, these techniques have been adapted for use with bone marrow cells. Yunis *et al.* (1981) have reported that with the use of elongated (prophase) chromosomes from patients with acute nonlymphocytic leukemia (ANLL), every one of 24 patients had an abnormal karyotype. Thus the future emphasis will be to identify the abnormalities we have all overlooked in the past. This is a major challenge for the future.

An even more exciting prospect, however, is the likelihood that within the next few years we will have identified the genes that are located at the breakpoints of the consistent translocations and deletions. Moreover, we will have a substantially clearer understanding of the alterations in the normal functions of these genes that occur with these structural rearrangements.

To assist the noncytogeneticist in understanding the notations used in this section, a brief review of chromosome nomenclature appears appropriate. In virtually all of the presentations in this section, the chromosome aberrations are present in the majority of cells obtained from a particular neoplastic disease, either leukemia or solid tumor. All of the evidence currently available indicates that these abnormalities are clonal in origin. Except for the patients discussed by Dr. Francke, all of the aberrations are limited to the tumor cells and they are, thus, somatic mutations in an otherwise chromosomally normal individual. In the patients discussed by Dr. Francke, some of those with various embryonic tumors have a constitutional chromosome deletion.

The karyotype of patients or tumors is described using the system proposed by the ISCN (1978). The total chromosome number is listed first, followed by the

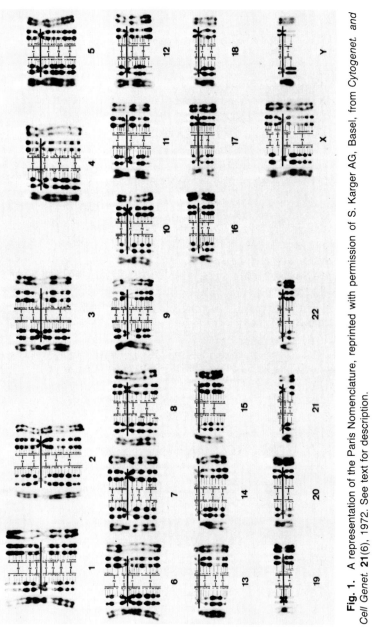

Fig. 1. A representation of the Paris Nomenclature, reprinted with permission of S. Karger AG, Basel, from *Cytogenet. and Cell Genet.* **21**(6), 1972. See text for description.

sex chromosomes and then gains or losses of whole chromosomes followed by structural rearrangements. Gain or loss of a whole chromosome is indicated by a + or −, respectively, before the affected chromosome; gain or loss of part of a chromosome is indicated by a + or − after the affected chromosome. Thus 47,XY,+8 indicates a male whose cells have an extra chromosome 8, which is the most common change in various myeloproliferative diseases. The short and long arm of the chromosome are represented by p and q, respectively. A translocation is indicated by t with the chromosomes involved enclosed within the first set of parentheses and the chromosome band affected by the break enclosed within the second set of parentheses. Thus, t(9;22)(q34;q11) signifies a translocation involving chromosomes 9 and 22, with a break in 9 in the long arm band 34 and in 22 in the long arm band 11. This translocation is the one most commonly identified in chronic myeloid leukemia. A chromosome deletion is abbreviated as del with the chromosome in the first set of brackets and the breakpoint indicated next. Figure 1 is a representation of the Paris Nomenclature. For each chromosome, examples of G and R banding are shown. Reading from left to right an actual photograph of a G-banded chromosome, a schematic drawing and then the Paris system, a schematic drawing of R banding, and finally an actual photograph of an R-banded chromosome. The dark bands obtained with G banding generally appear pale on R banding, and vice versa. The bands are numbered from the centromere to the ends of the short and long arms. Major portions are identified by the larger-sized number between the chromosomes, and individual bands are identified by the smaller number adjacent to each schematic drawing. Thus, the prominent G band in the middle of the long arm of No. 1 is lq31; "1" for the chromosome number, "q" for the long arm, "3" for the region, and "1" for the specific band within that region.

References

Boveri, T. (1914). "Zur Frage der Entstehung Maligner Tumoren." Fischer, Jena.
An International System for Human Cytogenetic Nomenclature (1978). *Cytogenet. Cell Genet.* **21**, 309–404.
Mitelman, F., and Levan, G. (1981). *Hereditas* **95**, 79–139, 1981.
Nowell, P. C., and Hungerford, D. A. (1960). *Science* **132**, 1497.
Paris Conference, 1971. (1972). *Birth Defects: Orig. Artic. Ser.* **8**(7).
Rowley, J. D., and Testa, J. R. (1982). *Adv. Cancer Res.* **36**, 103–148.
Sandberg, A. A. (1980). The "The Chromosome in Human Cancer and Leukemia." Elsevier/North-Holland, New York.
Yunis, J. J., Bloomfield, C. D., and Ensrud, B. S. (1981). *N. Engl. J. Med.* **305**, 135–139, 1981.

Chromosome Patterns in Human Cancer and Leukemia

FELIX MITELMAN

Department of Clinical Genetics
University of Lund
Lund, Sweden

I. Introduction

In 1890, David von Hansemann first drew attention to the frequent occurrence of mitotic irregularities in malignant tissues. He associated them with the origin and development of malignancy and suggested that such nuclear abnormalities could be used as a criterion for diagnosing the malignant state. Such notions formed the basis of the mutation theory of cancer, presented in 1914 by Theodor Boveri in his famous book "Zur Frage der Entstehung Maligner Tumoren," in which chromosomal aberrations were suggested as the cause of the change from normal to malignant growth. This long remained a theoretical idea that could not be put to the test mainly because of the technical difficulties in chromosome preparation that encumbered mammalian cytogenetics throughout the first half of the present century. This was the period during which plant cytogenetics made spectacular progress, largely due to the application of rapid squash and smear methods, which from 1920 has simplified chromosome studies in plants, and also insects, and at the same time disclosed chromosome structures more clearly and often more reliably than was possible with the previously used microtome technique. It was not discovered, however, until around 1950 that a malignant mammalian material, ascites cells from experimental tumors, responded very favorably to the same rapid methods, and this led to the sudden realization that mammalian chromosomes could be just as suitable for detailed analysis as any of the most advantageous plant materials.

At that time, cells in tissue culture were made available as a source of chromosomes. This was possible thanks to the application of vital pretreatment with colchicine and hypotonic salt solution. Now mammalian cytogenetics entered into a period of vivid expansion. During the 1950s and 1960s detailed karyotypes were worked out in a rapidly increasing number of mammalian species, including man, and clear-cut correlations were established between specific chromosome deviations, numerical as well as structural, and a number of constitutional malformation syndromes. Also, the study of chromosomes in animal ascites tumors during the early 1950s, supplemented soon with results from human malignant exudates, laid a firm foundation for modern cancer cytogenetics. The early chromosome studies on malignant cells in mammals, including man, have been summarized by Atkin (1976), Levan et al. (1977), Hsu (1979), and Sandberg (1980).

During this period the rules for chromosome behavior in old, far progressed malignant cell populations were elucidated in detail, and it was clarified that the chromosomal variability was regulated by certain laws: the stem line concept first defined by Winge (1930), the competition between stem lines, and the labile chromosomal equilibria of malignant cell populations responsive to environmental changes. All this led to the important realization that there is a basic similarity cytogenetically between the evolution of tumor stem lines and the natural evolution of organisms. The same event of genetic variability, followed by selection and survival of the fittest, takes place at both levels of evolution (Levan, 1967).

The discovery of these basic mechanisms of tumor cell proliferation was of the utmost importance for a deeper understanding of the chromosome aberrations that prevailed in cancer. The results clearly demonstrated that the chromosome changes observed were an integral part of tumor evolution. However, the ascitic tumors studied were all far progressed metastatic tumor cell populations, in which the chromosomal picture can be assumed to have changed a great deal since the primary oncogenic process. Therefore, few, if any, conclusions could be drawn as to the role of chromosome changes in early tumor stages and/or in the etiology of neoplasia.

In 1960, however, cancer cytogenetics had its first spectacular success: Nowell and Hungerford reported the first consistent chromosome abnormality in a

human cancer; they observed an unusually small G group chromosome in leukemic cells from patients with chronic myeloid leukemia. This chromosome, which
appeared to have lost about one-half of its long arm, was named the Philadelphia
or Ph[1] chromosome in honor of its city of discovery. The question of whether the
deleted portion of the long arm was missing from the cell or whether it was
translocated to another chromosome could not be answered at that time because it
was impossible to identify each human chromosome precisely with the techniques then available.

The discovery of the Ph[1] chromosome in chronic myeloid leukemia seemed to
be the conclusive verification of Boveri's idea: a malignant disorder strictly
correlated to a specific chromosomal change. The finding greatly stimulated
interest in the cytogenetic aspects of cancer, but for several reasons this consistent abnormality long remained an exception among human neoplasms. The
confusing variety of karyotypic changes observed in other cancers during the
1960s strongly suggested that chromosomal abnormalities were epiphenomena in
tumor progression rather than causative factors essential for the initiation of the
malignant state. The enthusiasm for tumor cytogenetics, to a large extent aroused
by the discovery of the Ph[1] chromosome, gradually faded. The significance of
the Ph[1] chromosome was actually counteracted by its uniqueness: why should
there be such a simple association between a chromosomal trait and one malignant disease, when more and more data from other neoplasms accumulated
showed either no chromosome aberrations at all or a confusing mess of apparently meaningless abnormalities?

The first indication of nonrandom karyotypic changes in human tumors was
detected in 1966 independently by Levan and van Steenis. The authors analyzed
the chromosome changes in about 40 published cases, mainly ascitic forms of
gastric, mammary, uterine, and ovarian carcinomas, and found beyond question
that certain chromosome types tended to increase in number and others to decrease. Soon afterward evidence for nonrandom patterns was demonstrated also
in specific types of solid tumors and leukemia. Among the human tumors,
nonrandomness was especially striking in the meningiomas (Zang and Singer,
1967; Mark, 1970). Also during the 1960s a comprehensive study of more than
200 primary sarcomas induced by the Rous sarcoma virus (RSV) in four species
of experimental animals very definitely led to the same conclusion (review in
Mitelman, 1974). Especially in the RSV-induced rat tumors it was seen clearly
that the addition of three specific chromosomes was essential for the evolution of
the malignant stem lines, and it was possible to demonstrate that the chromosomal additions formed a fixed pattern of sequential chromosome evolution (Mitelman, 1971, 1972). From these studies in animal tumors and man it could be
concluded that the chromosome variation observed consisted of two different
kinds: nonrandom variation, specifically affecting the same chromosome types,

and random or background variation, affecting all chromosomes. One of the causes of the slow progress of cancer cytogenetics during this period was that the significant nonrandom variation was always blurred by the background variation.

The introduction of chromosome banding techniques by Caspersson and co-workers in 1970 revolutionized tumor cytogenetics: each human chromosome could now be precisely identified on the basis of its unique banding pattern. Perhaps no area of chromosome research has gained more from the banding technique than cancer cytogenetics. All descriptions of chromosome deviations immediately became more precise and the conclusions accordingly became more stringent. Consequently, a number of cancer-associated chromosomal aberrations, including various specific marker chromosomes, have been disclosed. The major aim of this chapter is to review the nature, occurrence, and significance of such nonrandom and specific chromosome aberrations and to discuss the theoretical implications of these changes for our understanding of what happens at the initiation of a malignant cell.

II. Survey of Chromosome Aberrations

Since the introduction of chromosome banding techniques, we have tried systematically to collect and periodically to summarize data on banded tumor chromosomes in man (Levan and Mitelman, 1975, 1977; Mitelman and Levan, 1976a, 1978, 1981; Mitelman, 1980, 1981a, 1982). The material has been collected from three main sources: published cases ascertained by the aid of three separate computer-based literature scans, unpublished cases from our laboratory, and unpublished cases kindly communicated by numerous colleagues all over the world in answer to our appeals for such data (Mitelman and Levan, 1976b, 1979). The number of tumors contained in this registry has increased exponentially from 114 in the first survey of 1975 to 1871 in the latest published survey of 1981; an additional 973 cases have been included since, and thus the total number of cases contained in the registry is at present 2844 cases.

The total material, subdivided into 15 classes of neoplastic disease according to the diagnosis reported by the original investigator, is shown in Table I. In principle, only cases studied in direct preparations or after short-term *in vitro* culture have been included. However, in a few instances, as in Burkitt's lymphoma and some solid tumors, cell lines were also included. It should be noted, however, that cases with chronic myeloid leukemia and the Ph[1] chromosome as the sole abnormality are not included among the 2844 cases listed in Table I. Owing to technical problems, the application of chromosome banding techniques on solid tumors has just begun; in direct process of tumor biopsies the success rate for obtaining suitable metaphase spreads is very low, and therefore the bulk of cytogenetic data has been gathered from leukemias and various hematological

TABLE I

Subdivision of 2844 Cases of Human Neoplasms with Chromosome Aberrations Identified by Banding Technique

Tumor group	Designation	Tumor type	Number of cases
Myeloproliferative disorders	CML	Chronic myeloid leukemia	
		t(9:22) and other aberrations	549
		aberrant translocations	136
	ANLL	Acute nonlymphocytic leukemia	711
	PV	Polycythemia vera	102
	MD	Myelodysplastic diseases	382
Lymphoproliferative disorders	BL	Burkitt's lymphoma	119
	ML	Malignant lymphoma	174
	ALL	Acute lymphocytic leukemia	234
	CLL	Chronic lymphocytic leukemia	69
	MG	Monoclonal gammopathies	54
Solid tumors	BMT	Benign mesenchymal tumors	65
	BET	Benign epithelial tumors	28
	CA	Carcinomas	171
	SA	Sarcomas	7
	MM	Malignant melanomas	16
	NT	Neurogenic tumors	27

disorders. In the total material, the myeloproliferative disorders comprise 66.1% of all cases, and one leukemia type (acute nonlymphocytic leukemia) contributes with about 25% of all cases; the lymphoproliferative disorders constitute 22.9%, and all solid tumors only 11.0% of the cases ascertained. This undoubtedly is a serious obstacle in evaluating the results, especially in drawing general conclusions. Also, a certain bias cannot be excluded since many cases might be selected from larger series of patients analyzed in a particular center. However, for certain purposes the material is large enough to permit some generalizations. In the following, the main findings in the different tumor types will be briefly summarized. It is not possible in this chapter to include references to all cases; detailed references for 1871 cases can be found in Mitelman and Levan (1981); references for the remaining cases included in the registry may be obtained directly from the author. The data, including information on histopathological diagnosis, sex, age, previous neoplasms or other significant disorders, hereditary disorders, exposure to potential mutagenic and/or carcinogenic agents, chromosome preparation technique, clinical findings, and survival, are at present being computerized. Hopefully, the total organized material, which could be retrieved to compile a catalog, will be available for interested workers in the field during 1983.

A. Myeloproliferative Disorders

1. *Chronic Myeloid Leukemia (CML)*

Bone marrow cells from approximately 90% of patients who have clinically typical CML contain the Ph[1] chromosome, identified by Rowley (1973a) as a translocation of a long arm segment of chromosome 22 to the long arm of chromosome 9. Even though some uncertainty still exists whether the breakpoint in chromosome 22 involved in the formation of the Ph[1] is in band 22q11 or q12, or whether its location varies among cases, the general opinion holds that the breakpoint is in band q11 in all cases. The typical abnormality is an apparently balanced translocation with no loss or gain of genetic material. Some recent observations indicate that that t(9;22) is a reciprocal translocation.

In a minority of CML cases the origin of the Ph[1] is associated with aberrant or variant translocations. These appear to be of two kinds: a simple translocation in which the deleted segment of No. 22 has been translocated onto another chromosome than No. 9, or complex translocations involving three or four different chromosomes. Unusual and complex Ph[1] translocations occurred in 8% of the unselected CML cases recorded at the First International Workshop on Chromosomes in Leukemia (1978a). In the present material, 136 cases were ascertained; 51 simple translocations and 85 complex translocations are listed in Table II. As seen from the table, the Y chromosome is the only one that has not been reported so far to be involved in any unusual Ph[1] translocation. In three cases, the deleted segment was not found translocated to any other chromosome of the complement: in one case the deletion of chromosome 22 was the sole abnormality observed. Even though the number of patients with unusual simple or complex Ph[1] translocations available for analysis is still relatively small, the data collected indicate that the clinical features of these cases do not differ significantly from the CML cases with the standard type of Ph[1] translocation (Sandberg, 1980). Two conclusions can be drawn from these observations: (1) Since CML associated with the aberrant Ph[1] translocations is indistinguishable from the disease with the typical Ph[1] translocation, the crucial event in CML must be the deletion of the long arm of chromosome 22. (2) Since still more than 90% of the Ph[1] translocations involve t(9;22) with apparently identical breakpoints in the two chromosomes in all cases, this obviously is not consistent with any hypothesis of random occurrence of chromosome aberrations followed by selection of cells with the Ph[1] chromosome. The self-evident conclusion is that some mechanism exists that strongly favors the formation of t(9;22). Furthermore, statistical analyses of the deviating types of the Ph[1]-associated translocations, described in detail in Mitelman and Levan (1981), showed that the chromosomes substituting for No. 9 in the unusual simple Ph[1] translocations, and those participating in addition to Nos. 9 and 22 in the complex translocations, exhibited interesting differences in their mechanics of origin. Whereas the former ones showed no

TABLE II

Aberrant Translocation Patterns in 136 Cases of Ph¹-Positive Chronic Myeloid Leukemia (CML)

Translocation	No. of cases	Translocation	No. of cases	Translocation	No. of cases
t(X;22)	1	t(X;9;22)	1	t(X;9;17;22)	1
t(2;22)	2	t(1;9;22)	9	t(1;4;20;22)	1
t(3;22)	1	t(2;9;22)	8	t(3;4;9;22)	1
t(4;22)	2	t(2;22;22)	1	t(3;9;17;22)	1
t(5;22)	1	t(3;9;22)	10	t(4;9;17;22)	1
t(6;22)	2	t(4;9;22)	5	t(6;9;11;22)	1
t(7;22)	2	t(5;9;22)	3	t(7;9;11;22)	1
t(9;22)	1	t(6;9;22)	4	t(9;13;15;22)	1
t(10;22)	4	t(7;9;22)	5	t(9;13;17;22)	1
t(11;22)	2	t(8;9;22)	1	t(9;16;17;22)	1
t(12;22)	5	t(9;10;22)	2	t(9;10;15;19;22)	1
t(13;22)	3	t(9;11;22)	3	del(22)	3
t(14;22)	4	t(9;13;22)	3		
t(15;22)	2	t(9;14;22)	6		
t(16;22)	3	t(9;15;22)	2		
t(17;22)	9	t(9;17;22)	2		
t(18;22)	1	t(9;20;22)	1		
t(19;22)	4	t(10;14;22)	2		
t(21;22)	1	t(11;14;22)	1		
t(22;22)	1	t(17;17;22)	1		
		t(21;22;22)	1		

correlation between their chromosome length and the incidence with which they were formed, the latter showed very strong such correlation. This difference was greatly emphasized by the strikingly different distributions of the translocation sites over the chromosome bodies of the two kinds: in the simple unusual translocations, the absolute majority of translocation sites were at or near the ends of the chromosomes; in the complex translocations, these sites were almost exclusively located interstitially. These observations, in our opinion, give strong support to the idea that the ordinary Ph¹ translocation does not originate as the result of selection among a great number of random chromosomal changes. Also, the unusual translocations apparently do not originate as haphazard errors in the ordinary mechanism: in that case, one would have expected the breakpoints to scatter randomly over available chromosome length.

At the time of blastic crisis, about 75–80% of all patients develop additional chromosome aberrations, superimposed on the karyotype with only the Ph¹ translocation. These secondary aberrations are strictly nonrandom: at least one of three particular changes, +8, iso(17q), and +Ph¹, occur in about 80% of the cases. In this context it may be worth mentioning that only 5 of the 549 cases surveyed had an extra Ph[1] and iso(17q) in the absence of trisomy 8. This is highly unexpected on basis of the frequencies of the other combinations of the three types of aberrations. The reason for this deviation, noted previously (Mitelman *et al.*, 1976), is obscure but it can hardly be fortuitous.

Clinical cytogenetic correlations in CML have been attempted by several investigators (review in Rowley, 1980; Sandberg, 1980). It is well established that patients with Ph[1]-positive CML have a much better prognosis than those with Ph[1]-negative CML, but the prognostic significance of additional karyotypic changes among Ph[1]-positive cases is still controversial (Prigogina *et al.*, 1978; Sonta and Sandberg, 1978; Bernstein *et al.*, 1980; Fleischman *et al.*, 1981; Oláh and Rák, 1981; Alimena *et al.*, 1982). Apparently, more information is needed on this aspect as well as on the possible association between particular karyotypic changes, clinical findings, and other parameters of the disease. Thus, recently obtained results have demonstrated an association between basophilia and presence of iso(17q) (Prigogina *et al.*, 1978; Alimena *et al.*, 1982), appearance of atypical chromosomal changes in patients who received intensive chemotherapy (Alimena *et al.*, 1979), as well as differences in survival between patients with certain specific chromosomal changes and some morphologic characteristics of the blastic cells (Fleischman *et al.*, 1981; Alimena *et al.*, 1982).

2. *Acute Nonlymphocytic Leukemia (ANLL)*

This group includes all types of ANLL, i.e., M1 to M6 according to the FAB classification (Bennett *et al.*, 1976). It has generally been accepted that approximately 50% of untreated patients with ANLL *de novo* have a completely normal karyotype in their bone marrow cells, while 50% exhibit detectable clonal abnormalities (First International Workshop on Chromosomes in Leukemia, 1978b). The incidence of an aneuploid pattern is certainly underestimated: First, bone marrow samples from many of the patients were studied only in direct preparations; current evidence suggests that some of the patients considered to be normal on the basis of a directly processed sample may have a definite abnormal clone in short-term cultures (Berger *et al.*, 1980; Carbonell *et al.*, 1981; Knuutila *et al.*, 1981). Second, most of the patients were analyzed with techniques that do not yield an adequate number of cells with elongated prometaphase chromosomes, and, therefore, subtle rearrangements, such as those recently reported by Yunis *et al.* (1981), would have been overlooked. In the material collected there are 711 cases with chromosome aberrations. The chromosomes most commonly involved in aberrations, either alone or in combination, are Nos. 5, 7, 8, 17, and 21. When the type of chromosome changes is taken into account, the nonrandomness of the abnormalities becomes even more obvious, since there is a striking tendency for aberrations of the same chromosomes to be of similar kinds. Thus, chromosomes 5 and 7 are preferentially affected as deletions of the long arm and as monosomy; in contrast, loss of genetic material from chromosome 8 is rare (accounts only for about 5% of the cases), whereas this chromosome becomes trisomic or engaged in translocations in the majority of cases. Apparently, it is possible to subdivide ANLL into cytogenetically distinct entities, not only according to the chromosome affected, but also to the particular type of aberration, e.g., -5, $5q-$, -7, $7q-$, $+8$. As more patients are studied in greater detail, it may very well turn out that many of these groups can be further subdivided into specific entities according to the exact sizes and locations of the deletions.

In this context it is of great interest that certain consistent structural rearrangements in fact have been related to specific types of ANLL. t(8;21), first reported by Rowley (1973b), is associated with the M2 morphology according to the FAB classification, i.e., myeloblastic with some maturation. t(15;17), first reported by Rowley et al. (1977), appears to be specific for acute promyelocytic leukemia (APL), i.e., M3 according to the FAB classification. t(9;11), recently reported by Berger et al. (1982) and Hagemeijer et al. (1982), has been associated with the poorly differentiated type of M5 (acute monocytic leukemia) (Second International Workshop on Chromosomes in Leukemia, 1980a,b,c; Fourth International Workshop on Chromosomes in Leukemia, 1983).

Clinical cytogenetic correlations in ANLL with special regard to possible associations between specific chromosome abnormalities and prognosis have been the subject of several recent collaborative studies which have provided extremely interesting and important results (First International Workshop on Chromosomes in Leukemia, 1978b; Second International Workshop on Chromosomes in Leukemia, 1980a,b,c; Fourth International Workshop on Chromosomes in Leukemia, 1983). Hopefully, improved prognostic prediction will be obtained in the future by combining cytogenetic findings with other parameters of the leukemic cells, e.g., in vitro growth pattern of clonogenic cells (Gustavsson et al., 1983).

A possible influence of external factors on the karyotypic pattern of leukemic cells was first suggested in a retrospective study of 56 patients with ANLL (Mitelman et al., 1978). Clonal chromosomal aberrations were significantly more common in patients exposed to chemical solvents, insecticides, and petroleum products than in patients with no history of occupational exposure to such agents. More recent evaluations of 162 patients studied by Mitelman et al. 1981) and 74 by Golomb et al. (1982) confirmed the initial observations and also showed that certain specific karyotypic aberrations, such as $-5/5q-$ and $-7/7q-$, were more frequent in the patients for whom a previous occupational exposure to potential mutagenic/carcinogenic agents was evident. Similar conclusions were reached by the pooled data from 15 laboratories reviewed at the Fourth International Workshop on Chromosomes in Leukemia (1983). An interesting observation, found at the Workshop, was that the difference between nonexposed and exposed patients only is evident in patients 30 years and older. In fact, the difference was most notable in the age group 30–69 years. This association with age may be regarded as additional indirect indication that the karyotypic changes are of etiologic significance; with a latency period of about 10 years, one would not expect any relationship with chromosome changes in patients below the age of 30. Other aspects on chromosome changes in relation to age and occupational exposure have been discussed recently by Rowley *et al.* (1982) and Brandt *et al.* (1983).

The late development of acute leukemia, almost always of the nonlymphocytic types, after previous cytotoxic and/or radiation therapy for a primary malignancy, usually malignant lymphoma or multiple myeloma, has been reported with increasing frequency during the past decade (references in Rowley *et al.*, 1981). The great majority of these patients have an abnormal karyotype, and one or both of two consistent chromosome changes have been noted: −5/5q− and −7 (Whang-Peng *et al.*, 1979; Pedersen-Bjergaard *et al.*, 1981; Rowley *et al.*, 1981). It should be recalled that this pattern of abnormality is very similar to that in patients with ANLL *de novo* who have had documented exposure to environmental mutagens and/or carcinogens. In this context it may be relevant to recall that intensive chemotherapy during the chronic phase of chronic myeloid leukemia has been found to produce clones with preferential engagement of chromosome 1 (Alimena *et al.*, 1979).

Geographic heterogeneity of the incidence of specific chromosome changes was first noted by Mitelman and Levan (1978). For this reason we started in our survey to include data on the geographic proveniencies of all cases recorded in order to be able to test whether any significant differences existed between cases from different geographic regions. We also hoped that in case such differences were once established they would exhibit correlations with etiologic factors. Table III shows the frequencies of the major chromosome aberrations in 644 informative cases of ANLL from different regions. Some striking differences may be seen: (1) the incidence of −5/5q− is about 20% in the United States, whereas this aberration is extremely rare in Japan and Africa; (2) −7/7q− is again very rare in Japan, while the incidence in Europe and the United States is about 20%; (3) trisomy 8 has been reported in about 40% of the cases from Australia, but in only about 20% of the cases from Europe, Japan, and Africa; (4) t(8;21) has been found in more than 30% of the cases from Japan, the incidence being about 10% in the rest of the world. The high incidence of t(8;21) in Japan seems now to be well established (Sakurai *et al.*, 1982).

A most striking unusual geographic distribution of the t(15;17), characteristic of acute promyelocytic leukemia, first reported by Teerenhovi *et al.* (1978) and also noted at the Second International Workshop on Chromosomes in Leukemia (1980c), has been confirmed in the present material. As can be seen from Table IV, the incidence of the t(15;17) in this subtype of ANLL has been found to vary from 0 to 100% in different regions.

TABLE III

Percentage Incidence in Different Geographic Regions of Specific Chromosome
Aberrations in 644 Patients with Acute Nonlymphocytic Leukemia (ANLL)

Region	Chromosome aberration				No. of cases
	−5/5q−	−7/7q−	+8	t(8;21)	
Africa	3.6	10.7	17.9	14.3	28
Australia	9.8	9.8	39.0	7.3	41
Europe	12.6	20.8	20.0	8.7	380
Japan	0	3.6	17.9	32.1	56
United States	23.0	25.2	12.9	7.9	139
Total	13.3	19.1	19.4	10.7	644

3. Polycythemia Vera (PV)

The great majority of cases with PV have normal karyotypes. The variation in
different series may to some degree reflect how early in the course of the disease
most patients were investigated, and also whether they had been treated with
mutagenic agents; chromosome aberrations have been noticed in treated patients
much more often than in untreated patients, and cytogenetic abnormalities are
almost invariably present if patients with PV progress to ANLL (Nowell, 1982).

TABLE IV

Incidence of t(15;17) in Acute Promyelocytic Leukemia (APL)

Austral-Asia	
Australia	6/9
New Zealand	5/6
Japan	18/19
South Africa	5/9
Europe	
Belgium	22/26
France	18/24
Holland	4/5
Spain	2/4
Italy	4/16
England	3/12
Scandinavia	3/33
West Germany	0/7
United States	
Chicago, Illinois	25/25
Minneapolis, Minnesota	9/14
Buffalo, New York	1/21

The chromosomes most often involved in aberrations are Nos. 1, 8, 9, and 20. The characteristic aberrations are translocation and/or trisomy for a portion of the long arm of chromosome 1, trisomy 8, trisomy 9, and deletion of the long arm of chromosome 20. The most characteristic feature of this disease is the 20q− marker (Reeves et al., 1972), which has been identified in about 30% of the cases with aberrations; the deleted segment has only exceptionally been found to be translocated onto another chromosome, i.e., No. 5 in one case and No. 11 in another case. In the total material at least one of the four changes mentioned above has been reported in about 75% of the cases.

4. Myelodysplastic Diseases (MD)

This group comprises a variety of hematopoietic disorders that carry an increased risk for the ultimate development of leukemia. The group includes both marrow stem cell dyscrasias characterized by cytopenia (e.g., refractory anemias, granulocytopenia, thrombocytopenia, and pancytopenia), as well as disorders characterized by overproduction of one or more of the marrow elements (e.g., myelofibrosis, myeloproliferative syndrome, and thrombocytosis). Nomenclature and classification of these diseases is confusing because the hematologic findings are variable and overlapping, and the transition to clinical leukemia may be gradual and inconstant. An excellent review, summarizing the major cytogenetic findings in these disorders, emphasizing particularly the more recent results with banding techniques, and possible clinical implications of these observations, has been published (Nowell, 1982).

Chromosome abnormalities are found in approximately 50% of patients at diagnosis. In the largest series reported to date (Second International Workshop on Chromosomes in Leukemia, 1980d), 51% of patients had a cytogenetically abnormal clone in the bone marrow. The chromosomes most often affected are Nos. 5, 7, and 8; the most characteristic aberrations are monosomy 5, 5q−, monosomy 7, 7q−, and trisomy 8. In general, thus, the aberrations in these disorders closely resemble those characteristic of ANLL.

One specific syndrome deserves special mention: the "5q− syndrome" [more specifically an interstitial deletion of the region 5q12–31 as first described by Van Den Berghe et al. (1974)] associated with refractory macrocytic anemia with a uniform pattern of hematologic abnormalities (Sokal et al., 1975; Mahmood et al., 1979). Progression to ANLL is usually associated with cytogenetic changes in addition to the 5q− marker.

No other specific chromosome aberration has been found among the myeloproliferative disorders. The suggested association between primary thrombocythemia and a deletion of the long arm of chromosome 21 has not been substantiated as additional individuals have been investigated (Third International Workshop on Chromosomes in Leukemia, 1981c).

B. Lymphoproliferative Disorders

1. *Burkitt's Lymphoma (BL)*

The cytogenetic findings in BL were recently reviewed in some detail (Mitelman, 1981b), the results may be briefly summarized as follows:

1. The characteristic aberration in BL—endemic and nonendemic—is t(8;14)(q24;q32), i.e., a translocation of the distal segment of chromosome 8 to the terminal segment of the long arm of chromosome 14, producing a characteristic 14q+ marker chromosome (Manolov and Manolova, 1972; Zech *et al.*, 1976). By means of analysis of prophase and prometaphase chromosomes, by which an improved resolution of the G band pattern was achieved, Manolova *et al.* (1979) provided evidence suggesting that the 8;14 translocation is reciprocal, the end segments of chromosomes 8 and 14 being interchanged. This highly interesting observation remains to be confirmed.

2. The t(8;14) is not associated with the Epstein-Barr virus (EBV) genome. This conclusion is supported by the following facts: the translocation has been found in EBV genome-negative BL cell lines and in EBV-negative acute lymphocytic leukemia; the translocation has not been found in infectious mononucleosis lymphocytes, neither in lymphoblastoid cell lines derived from lymphocytes of patients with mononucleosis nor in EBV-transformed peripheral lymphocytes from BL patients.

3. The t(8;14) is not specific for BL; the translocation has been found in other lymphoproliferative disorders, including malignant lymphomas, acute lymphocytic leukemia, and chronic lymphocytic leukemia. However, the t(8;14) has so far only been found in B cell lymphoproliferative disorders, and not in any T or null cell type of leukemia/lymphoma.

4. Two variant translocations, t(2;8) and t(8;22), have been described in endemic as well as nonendemic BL. In all the cases so far reported the breakpoint in chromosome 8 has been located to the same band, q24, as in the 8;14 translocation. Thus, these results strongly indicate that the important karyotypic event associated with the disease may be the deletion of chromosome 8 rather than the site of translocation of the deleted segment.

Studies of the variant BL translocations have provided exciting new information and ideas about the phenotypic effects of chromosomal aberrations in tumor cells. Chromosomes 2 and 22, i.e., the two chromosomes involved in variant translocations, have recently been shown to carry genes for immunoglobulin (Ig), κ and λ light chains (Erikson *et al.*, 1981; Malcolm *et al.*, 1982; McBride *et al.*, 1982), respectively. Moreover, with the use of chromosome hybridization *in situ*, Malcolm *et al.* (1982) mapped the κ light chain genes to band 2p12-13 (the same band that is involved in the 2;8 translocation). Recently, Lenoir *et al.* (1982) reported that when a light chain is expressed in BL cells its type is strictly related, in cases of variant translocation, to the chromosomes involved: all BL cases with t(2;8) that expressed Ig light chains secrete κ light chains and all with an 8;22 translocation secrete λ light chains.

2. Malignant Lymphomas (ML)

The karyotypes of a total of 174 non-Hodgkin, non-Burkitt lymphomas have been ascertained. No attempt has been made to subdivide the cases according to histopathologic type, mainly because detailed histopathologic description is available only for very few of them; also, no uniform system of classification of lymphomas has been accepted, and thus cases are described using at least three different systems of nomenclature. This leads to great difficulty in comparing and classifying the cases with cytogenetic findings published in the literature. Also, the cytogenetic data obtained with banding are usually based on a relatively small number of cells studied and are often incomplete or consist of very complex changes containing multiple unidentified markers. These problems have recently been discussed by Sandberg (1981).

All chromosome types may be affected in ML. However, one chromosome (No. 14) is affected decidedly more often than the others, and one specific type of aberration, a 14q+ marker chromosome, is the single most common abnormality in lymphomas of all varieties; a 14q+ marker has been found in 56% of the cases with aberrations. The exact mode of origin of the 14q+ has been established in approximately one-third of the cases. It seems that most chromosome types may be engaged as donors of the segment translocated to chromosome 14. However, it is obvious that certain chromosome types act as donors decidedly more often than others, in particular chromosomes 1, 8, 11, and 18. Certain correlations have been reported between the histopathologic type of lymphoma, on the one hand, and the presence of 14q+ marker and also the type of translocation producing the 14q+, on the other (Fukuhara et al., 1979; Reeves and Pickup, 1980). Thus, the extremely interesting possibility exists that lymphomas may ultimately be characterized in terms of the nature of the 14q+ translocation. In general, the potential of karyotype analysis in lymphoma lies in this possibility that such data may considerably clarify the complicated status of classification of these diseases. The use of fine needle aspiration biopsy offers an excellent opportunity to obtain such information (Kristoffersson et al., 1981).

A possible prognostic significance of the chromosome aberrations in ML has recently been reported. Kaneko et al. (1982) found that patients with markers of unknown origin had a poorer prognosis than patients without such markers, and, in a study by Kristoffersson et al. (1983), patients with gains or structural changes of chromosome 7, especially in combination with numerical changes of chromosome 20, had a particularly poor prognosis; these tumors were morphologically classified as high-grade as well as low-grade malignant lymphomas according to the Kiel classification; however, all the low-grade lymphomas were of the centroblastic/centrocytic diffuse type. Furthermore, all three patients with the specific translocation t(14;18)(q32;q21) had a remarkably favorable prognosis; all three were histologically low-grade malignant lymphomas of centroblastic/centrocytic follicular type. Thus, the findings suggest that in non-Hodgkin lymphomas, as in malignant hematologic disorders, the chromosome banding pattern may be an important independent prognostic factor. Further prospective studies are needed on this important aspect.

3. *Acute Lymphocytic Leukemia (ALL)*

The chromosomal pattern in ALL was recently dealt with extensively by the Third International Workshop on Chromosomes in Leukemia (1981a,b). The major aims of the Workshop were (1) to determine the detailed karyotypic patterns in the malignant cells of patients with ALL, studied by modern chromosome banding techniques, and (2) to correlate the karyotype of patients with ALL with a number of clinical parameters, including sex, age, white blood cell count, hemoglobin value, platelet count, percent blast cells, morphology of the blast cells according to the criteria of the FAB classification, lymphocyte surface markers, lymphadenopathy, splenomegaly, central nervous system involvement, type of treatment, complete remission rate, and survival.

The total Workshop material, provided by 17 laboratories around the world, amounted to 330 patients with ALL. The results have been reported in detail (Third International Workshop on Chromosomes in Leukemia, 1981a,b), and therefore only some of the major findings will be summarized:

1. The Workshop confirmed the association between ALL and certain chromosomal aberrations and revealed the presence of a number of nonrandom changes that were previously unrecorded. Of the 216 cases of ALL with chromosome abnormalities, 46% had one of the following specific structural abnormalities: t(9;22) 17.9%, t(4;11) 8.2%, t(8;14) 7.3%, 14q+ 6.9%, and 6q− 6.0%.

2. The Workshop rigorously demonstrated for the first time that the karyotype is an important prognostic factor in ALL. Furthermore, the data suggest that the karyotype is an independent risk factor, since it correlated with survival, even when other well-known risk factors were considered, such as age, white blood cell count, and FAB type. The data also suggest that children and adults with the same specific chromosome abnormalities will respond identically to treatment. Thus, among patients with t(9;22), t(4;11), and t(8;14), the survival curves of children and adults were similar. A follow-up study of the patients alive at the time of the Workshop is at present in progress.

4. Chronic Lymphocytic Leukemia (CLL)

Information regarding chromosome changes in CLL is meager; only 69 cases with aberrations have been ascertained. This is primarily due to the fact that approximately 90% of the CLL cases are of B cell type, and until recently it has not been possible to induce divisions in such cells. These methodological difficulties explain why almost all cases reported in the past have exhibited normal diploid karyotype—the result of stimulation of nonleukemic normal T cells by conventional mitogens such as phytohemagglutinin.

Recently division of the malignant B cells have been induced in lymphocytes of patients with CLL by polyclonal B cell mitogens, such as lipopolysaccharide B from *E. coli* or the Epstein-Barr virus (EBV) (Gahrton *et al.*, 1980; Morita *et al.*, 1981; Schröder *et al.*, 1981). The number of cases is still too small to permit any definite conclusions, but it appears that chromosomal aberrations are present in at least half of the patients with chronic B-cell type CLL. The most common aberration is an extra chromosome 12, which may appear alone or together with other numerical or structural aberrations. Other characteristic and possibly nonrandom aberrations have been noted less frequently: a 14q+ marker chromosome, including t(8;14), an extra chromosome 3, iso(17q), and 6q−.

C. Solid Tumors

Because of technical problems in the preparation of solid tumor chromosomes, very little information is available on this heterogeneous group of neoplasms, comprising both benign and malignant mesenchymal, neurogenic, and epithelial tumors, the latter being quantitatively the largest tumor group in man. Furthermore, among the solid tumors studied, the great majority have been metastatic tumors, mostly effusions; the extremely complex karyotypic rearrangements found in most of these cases makes it necessary to examine a much larger number of tumors before the chromosomal findings can be at all interpreted in terms of nonrandomness and association to site of origin or histopathologic type. It is, therefore, promising and of extreme interest that an increasing number of associations between certain tumor types and more or less specific chromosome changes actually have been found during recent years.

1. Meningioma

This is the most extensively studied solid tumor in man. The cytogenetics of this benign tumor was recently reviewed in detail by Zang (1982). At least 89 tumors have been studied with banding; 24 of these had completely normal karyotype. Sixty-three of the 65 cases with aberrations (96.9%) have the specific aberration originally demonstrated by Mark *et al.* (1972) and Zankl and Zang (1972), i.e., monosomy 22 or, exceptionally, a deletion of the long arm of this chromosome; 18 of the 65 tumors had lost one chromosome 8.

TABLE V

Incidence of Monosomy 8 and Monosomy 22 in Meningiomas

Region	Type of aberration		No. of cases
	−8	−22	
Germany	0	33 (97.1%)	34
Sweden	17 (65.4%)	25 (96.2%)	26

A striking geographic heterogeneity of the karyotypic pattern may be noted between the two series of patients studied in Germany and Sweden. The pertinent data are summarized in Table V, showing that monosomy 22 has the same high incidence in the two regions; monosomy 8, however, has been found in 65% of the Swedish cases but in none of the 34 German.

2. Pleomorphic Adenoma

Among a total of 30 benign mixed salivary gland tumors studied by Mark *et al.* (1982), 18 had normal karyotype. Nine of the 12 cases with aberrations showed an engagement of the segment 8q12-q22; 6 of the adenomas had, in fact, a specific translocation, i.e., t(3;8)(p21;q12).

3. Neuroblastoma

Deletions or rearrangements of the terminal portion of the short arm of chromosome 1 have been reported in the majority of neuroblastoma tumors and cell lines (Brodeur *et al.*, 1981; Gilbert *et al.*, 1982). The breakpoint identified most frequently was 1p32, and the particular segment missing in all deletions and included in all rearrangements was distal to 1p31, always 1p34 to 1pter.

4. Cervical Carcinoma

Structural aberrations, usually of the long arm, of chromosome 1 were reported in each of 26 cervical carcinomas (Atkin and Baker, 1979). A survey of 343 breakpoints that led to abnormalities of chromosome 1 in 218 neoplasms, including cervical carcinomas, showed that 49.9% were located in or immediately adjacent to the centromeric heterochromatin (Brito-Babapulle and Atkin, 1981).

5. Lung Cancer

Chromosome studies of 16 cell lines, 3 short-term cultures and one direct bone marrow preparation, representing 18 different patients with small cell lung cancer, showed a common deletion of the short arm of chromosome 3 in all samples; the common deletion was in the region p14-23 (Whang-Peng *et al.*, 1982).

6. Ovarian Cancer

A specific karyotypic change, t(6;14)(q21;q24), i.e., a reciprocal translocation between chromosomes 6 and 14, has been found in ovarian papillary serous cystadenocarcinomas by Wake et al. (1980). The two marker chromosomes resulting from this translocation, 6q− and 14q+, coexisted in the cells of 8 of 12 cases studied; either of the two markers was present in all remaining four cases.

7. Embryonic Tumors

Two tumors, retinoblastoma and the aniridia–Wilms' tumor syndrome, are each associated with a specific chromosomal abnormality: interstitial deletion of band q14 in the long arm of chromosome 13 (Yunis and Ramsay, 1978; Motegi, 1981) and deletion of band p13 in the short arm of chromosome 11 (Riccardi et al., 1980), respectively. However, these chromosome changes, when observed, are constitutional changes, i.e., the aberration is observed in all somatic cells and is not confined to the tumor cells. Results of karyotype analyses of the malignant cells are so far conflicting (Gardner et al., 1982; Balaban et al., 1982).

III. General Conclusions

On the basis of the analysis of 2844 human neoplasms, reported in well above 600 published papers and by a great many personal communications, the following main conclusions may be proposed:

1. The chromosome aberrations are strictly nonrandom within each group of tumors, and consistent specific aberrations have been discovered in an increasing number of tumor types; the most characteristic specific aberrations are summarized in Table VI. These findings provide convincing evidence for the fundamental role of chromosome changes in the initiation of the malignant process.

2. A survey of the distribution of specific aberrations shows that only one of the specific marker chromosomes, the 14q+ marker produced by the t(8;14), is limited to just one cell type, the B cell lymphocyte. Although all the other types of markers are usually much more frequent in one or a couple of disorders, it is very striking that they may also be found in several other tumor types. The entire situation has been summarized in Mitelman and Levan (1981). An overall pattern is gradually beginning to materialize, in which diseases affecting related cell types are more similar in the chromosomal variation than those affecting unrelated cell types, but there appears to be little or no target cell specificity of the specific aberrations.

3. Some chromosomes are preferentially engaged in aberrations decidedly more often than others. This tendency for aberrations to cluster to certain chromosome types was pointed out in our earlier surveys (Mitelman and Levan,

TABLE VI

Specific Chromosome Aberrations in Human Neoplasia

Tumor type	Chromosome aberration	References
Myeloproliferative disorders		
Chronic myeloid leukemia	t(9;22)	Nowell and Hungerford (1960), Rowley (1973a)
Acute myeloid leukemia	t(8;21)	Rowley (1973b)
Acute promyelocytic leukemia	t(15;17)	Rowley et al. (1977)
Acute monocytic leukemia	t(9;11)	Berger et al. (1982), Hagemeijer et al. (1982)
Refractory anemia	del(5)(q12q31)	Van Den Berghe et al. (1974)
Polycythemia vera	del(20)(q11)	Reeves et al. (1972)
Lymphoproliferative disorders		
Burkitt's lymphoma	t(8;14)	Manolov and Manolova (1972), Zech et al. (1976)
Acute lymphocytic leukemia	t(9;22) t(4;11) t(8;14)	Third International Workshop on Chromosomes in Leukemia (1981a)
Chronic lymphocytic leukemia	+12	Gahrton et al. (1980), Morita et al. (1981)
Solid tumors		
Meningioma	−22	Mark et al. (1972), Zankl and Zang (1972)
Pleomorphic adenoma	t(3;8)	Mark et al. (1982)
Neuroblastoma	del(1)(p32)	Brodeur et al. (1981), Gilbert et al. (1982)
Cervical carcinoma	?1q	Atkin and Baker (1979)
Lung cancer	del(3)(p14-23)	Whang-Peng et al. (1982)
Ovarian cancer	t(6;14)	Wake et al. (1980)
Retinoblastoma	del(13)(q14)	Yunis and Ramsay (1978)
Wilms' tumor—aniridia	del(11)(p13)	Riccardi et al. (1980)

1981), and the picture is unchanged when constructed on the basis of the 2844 cases now analyzed. It is striking that all tumor types cluster to 15 of the 24 chromosome types, and that eight chromosome types are involved each with at least three disorders. Each of the chromosomes 1, 8, and 14 is involved with seven disorders, while the chromosomes 2, 4, 10, 15, 16, 18, 19, X and Y show no selective involvement. It may be mentioned that the clustering tendency, first observed in 1975 in our material of 114 neoplasms, is even more pronounced now with the 25-fold number of cases. This could hardly be fortuitous, and our interpretation is that the chromosomes most often affected carry genetic material which is important in the regulation of cell proliferation and/or differentiation and which needs to be manipulated in the process of malignant transformation.

4. Many cases both of experimental and human malignancy are known in which specific chromosome segments tend to be involved in duplication or deletion. Often the same type of change affects many cases of the same malignant disease, even though the exact size of the added or deleted segment may vary. Thus, we observed (Levan *et al.*, 1974) that a common segment of rat chromosome 2 was duplicated in several cases of sarcoma induced by polycyclic hydrocarbons, and Rowley (1977) demonstrated in a series of 34 patients with myeloproliferative disorders that, among a variety of chromosomal aberrations in their malignant karyotypes, all shared trisomy for a certain segment of chromosome 1. A similar picture emanated when the deletions of chromosomes 5, 6, and 7, recorded in our previous survey of 1871 cases (Mitelman and Levan, 1981), were examined in detail. It was striking that although the breakpoints obviously showed little specificity, common deleted segments were found in all three chromosomes. In fact, among the 125 cases scrutinized, only two fell outside of these common deleted segments. Again, it may be speculated that genes of importance for transformation of a normal cell to a malignant cell are concentrated to such regions.

5. Results from experimental studies suggest that at least in certain instances the inducing factor may be suspected to induce specific chromosome patterns (references in Mitelman, 1981a). It is extremely difficult to find avenues of approach toward this question as far as human neoplasias are concerned. Tumors associated with known environmental carcinogens are uncommon, and so far none has been subjected to chromosome analysis. However, two observations suggest that such correlations may in fact exist in man. First, the demonstration that differences in the chromosome picture of the malignant cells may be found between patients who have been exposed to potential mutagenic/carcinogenic agents and those without any known such exposure. At least, this no doubt indicates that the karyotypic pattern of malignant cells may be influenced by external factors. Second, the striking geographic heterogeneity of the patterns of chromosome variation. This would be compatible with the idea that different oncogenic agents may have an uneven geographic distribution. Admittedly, the material is too small and also deficient in various respects to allow definite conclusions, but still it is a very promising area of study, which may give important results as more data are accumulated.

6. The systematic survey of the chromosome aberrations in malignant cells has made us propose the idea that chromosome aberrations associated with malignancy could be of essentially two distinct kinds with different modes of origin (Mitelman and Levan, 1978, 1981). According to this idea, one kind of aberration, the primary or active, arises from direct interaction between the inducing agent and the genetic material of the target cell. The primary aberrations are therefore located in specific chromosome areas, the Ph[1] translocation being the typical instance of this kind. The other kind of aberration, the secondary or passive, arises by chance disturbances of mitosis. However, only those

secondary changes that happen to enhance the effect of a primary change will have selective value and, thus, will accumulate in the tumor cell population. Therefore, also the passive changes exhibit distinct nonrandom patterns that reflect the primary changes. In our opinion, the assumption of two essentially different kinds of chromosome aberrations fits nicely to the actual situation observed in neoplastic conditions of animals and man and also to recently proposed models of carcinogenesis by genetic transpositions and gene amplification (Cairns, 1981; Klein, 1981; Mitelman and Levan, 1981; Pall, 1981; Rowley, 1982).

Acknowledgments

Original work presented in this chapter was supported by grants from the Swedish Cancer Society and the John and Augusta Persson Foundation for Medical Research.

References

Alimena, G., Brandt, L., Dallapiccola, B., Mitelman, F., and Nilsson, P. G. (1979). *Cancer Genet. Cytogenet.* **1,** 79–85.

Alimena, G., Dallapiccola, B., Gastaldi, R., Mandelli, F., Brandt, L., Mitelman, F., and Nilsson P. G. (1982). *Scand. J. Haematol.* **28,** 103–117.

Atkin, N. B. (1976). *Exp. Biol. Med.* **6,** 1–171.

Atkin, N. B., and Baker, M. C. (1979). *Cancer (Philadelphia)* **44,** 604–613.

Balaban, G., Gilbert, F., Nichols, W., Meadows, A. T., and Shields, J. (1982). *Cancer Genet. Cytogenet.* **6,** 213–221.

Bennett, J. M., Catovsky, D., Daniel, M.-T., Flandrin, G., Galton, D. A. G., Gralnick, H. R., and Sultan, C. (1976). *Br. J. Haematol.* **33,** 451–458.

Berger, R., Bernheim, A., and Flandrin, G. (1980). *C. R. Acad. Sci. Paris* **290,** 1557–1559.

Berger, R., Bernheim, A., Sigaux, F., Daniel, M.-T., Valensi, F., and Flandrin, G. (1982). *Leuk. Res.* **6,** 17–26.

Bernstein, R., Morcom, G., Pinto, M. R., Mendelow, B., Dukes, I., Penfold, G., and Bezwoda, W. (1980). *Cancer Genet. Cytogenet.* **2,** 23–37.

Boveri, T. (1914). "Zur Frage der Entstehung Maligner Tumoren." Fischer, Jena.

Brandt, L., Mitelman, F., and Nilsson, P. G. (1983). *Scand. J. Haematol.* **30,** 227–231.

Brito-Babapulle, V., and Atkin, N. B. (1981). *Cancer Genet. Cytogenet.* **4,** 215–225.

Brodeur, G. M., Green, A. A., Hayes, F. A., Williams, K. J., Williams, D. L., and Tsiatis, A. A. (1981). *Cancer Res.* **41,** 4678–4686.

Cairns, J. (1981). *Nature (London)* **289,** 353–357.

Carbonell, F., Grilli, G., and Fliedner, T. M. (1981). *Leuk. Res.* **5,** 395–398.

Caspersson, T., Zech, L., and Johansson, C. (1970). *Exp. Cell Res.* **60,** 315–319.

Erikson, J., Martinis, J., and Croce, C. M. (1981). *Nature (London)* **294,** 173–175.

First International Workshop on Chromosomes in Leukemia (1978a). *Br. J. Haematol.* **39,** 305–309.

First International Workshop on Chromsomes in Leukemia (1978b). *Br. J. Haematol.* **39,** 311–316.

Fleischman, E. W., Prigogina, E. L., Volkova, M. A., Frenkel, M. A., Zakhartchenko, N. A., Konstantinova, L. N., Puchkova, G. P., and Balakirev, S. A. (1981). *Hum. Genet.* **58,** 285–293.

Fourth International Workshop on Chromosomes in Leukemia, 1982 (1983). *Cancer Genet. Cytogenet.* (in press).

Fukuhara, S., Rowley, J. D., Variakojis, D., and Golomb, H. M. (1979). *Cancer Res.* **39**, 3119–3128.

Gahrton, G., Robert, K. H., Friberg, K., Zech, L., and Bird, A. G. (1980). *Blood* **56**, 640–647.

Gardner, H. A., Gallie, B. L., Knight, L. A., and Phillips, R. A. (1982). *Cancer Genet. Cytogenet.* **6**, 201–211.

Gilbert, F., Balaban, G., Moorhead, P., Bianchi, D., and Schlesinger, H. (1982). *Cancer Genet. Cytogenet.* **7**, 33–42.

Golomb, H. M., Alimena, G., Rowley, J. D., Vardiman, J. W., Testa, J. R., and Sovik, C. (1982). *Blood* **60**, 404–411.

Gustavsson, A., Mitelman, F., Olofsson, T., and Olsson, I. (1983). *Scand. J. Haematol.* (in press)

Hagemeijer, A., Hählen, K., Sizoo, W., and Abels, J. (1982). *Cancer Genet. Cytogenet.* **5**, 95–105.

Hsu, T. C. (1979). "Human and Mammalian Cytogenetics." Springer-Verlag, Berlin and New York.

Kaneko, Y., Abe, R., Sampi, K., and Sakurai, M. (1982). *Cancer Genet. Cytogenet.* **5**, 107–121.

Klein, G. (1981). *Nature (London)* **294**, 313–318.

Knuutila, S., Vuopio, P., Elonen, E., Siimes, M., Kovanen, R., Borgström, G. H., and de la Chapelle, A. (1981). *Blood* **58**, 369–375.

Kristoffersson, U., Olsson, H., Mark-Vendel, E., and Mitelman, F. (1981). *Cancer Genet. Cytogenet.* **4**, 53–60.

Kristoffersson, U., Mitelman, F., Olsson, H., Gullberg, B., and Åkerman, M. (1983). *Cancer Genet. Cytogenet.* (in press)

Lenoir, G. M., Preud'homme, J. L., Bernheim, A., and Berger, R. (1982). *Nature (London)* **298**, 474–476.

Levan, A. (1966). *Hereditas* **55**, 28–38.

Levan, A. (1967). *Hereditas* **57**, 343–355.

Levan, G., and Mitelman, F. (1975). *Hereditas* **79**, 156–160.

Levan, G., and Mitelman, F. (1977). *In* "Chromosomes Today" (A. de la Chapelle and M. Sorsa, eds.), pp. 363–371. Elsevier/North-Holland Biomedical Press, Amsterdam.

Levan, G., Ahlström, U., and Mitelman, F. (1974). *Hereditas* **77**, 263–280.

Levan, A., Levan, G., and Mitelman, F. (1977). *Hereditas* **86**, 15–30.

McBride, O. W., Swan, D., Leder, P., Hieter, P., and Hollis, G. (1982). *Cytogenet. Cell Genet.* **32**, 297–298.

Mahmood, T., Robinson, W. A., Hamstra, R. D., and Wallner, S. F. (1979). *Am. J. Med.* **66**, 946–950.

Malcolm, S., Barton, P., Bentley, D. L., Ferguson-Smith, M. A., Murphy, C. S., and Rabbitts, T. H. (1982). *Cytogenet. Cell Genet.* **32**, 296.

Manolov, G., and Manolova, Y. (1972). *Nature (London)* **237**, 33–34.

Manolova, Y., Manolov, G., Kieler, J., Levan, A., and Klein, G. (1979). *Hereditas* **90**, 5–10.

Mark, J. (1970). *Eur. J. Cancer* **6**, 489–498.

Mark, J., Levan, G., and Mitelman, F. (1972). *Hereditas* **71**, 163–168.

Mark, J., Dahlenfors, R., Ekedahl, C., and Stenman, G. (1982). *Hereditas* **96**, 141–148.

Mitelman, F. (1971). *Hereditas* **69**, 155–186.

Mitelman, F. (1972). *Acta Pathol. Microbiol. Scand., Sect. A* **80A**, 313–328.

Mitelman, F. (1974). *In* "Chromosomes and Cancer" (J. German, ed.), pp. 675–693. Wiley, New York.

Mitelman, F. (1980). *Clin. Haematol.* **9**, 195–219.

Mitelman, F. (1981a). *In* "Genes, Chromosomes and Neoplasia" (F. E. Arrighi, P. N. Rau, and E. Stubblefield, eds.), pp. 335–350. Raven, New York.

Mitelman, F. (1981b). *Adv. Cancer Res.* **34**, 141–170.

Mitelman, F. (1982). *IARC Scientific Publ. No. 39, IARC, Lyon,* 481–496.

Mitelman, F., and Levan, G. (1976a). *Hereditas* **82**, 167–174.

Mitelman, F., and Levan, G. (1976b). *Lancet* **ii**, 264.

Mitelman, F., and Levan, G. (1978). *Hereditas* **89**, 207–232.

Mitelman, F., and Levan, G. (1979). *Cancer Genet. Cytogenet.* **1**, 29–32.

Mitelman, F., and Levan, G. (1981). *Hereditas* **95**, 79–139.

Mitelman, F., Levan, G., Nilsson, P. G., and Brandt, L. (1976). *Int. J. Cancer* **18**, 24–30.

Mitelman, F., Brandt, L., and Nilsson, P. G. (1978). *Blood* **52**, 1229–1237.

Mitelman, F., Nilsson, P. G., Brandt, L., Alimena, G., Gastaldi, R., and Dallapiccola, B. (1981). *Cancer Genet. Cytogenet.* **4**, 197–214.

Morita, M., Minowada, J., and Sandberg, A. A. (1981). *Cancer Genet. Cytogenet.* **3**, 293–306.

Motegi, T. (1981). *Hum. Genet.* **58**, 168–173.

Nowell, P. C. (1982). *Cancer Genet. Cytogenet.* **5**, 265–278.

Nowell, P. C., and Hungerford, D. A. (1960). *Science* **132**, 1497.

Oláh, E., and Rák, K. (1981). *Int. J. Cancer* **27**, 287–295.

Pall, M. L. (1981). *Proc. Natl. Acad. Sci. U.S.A.* **78**, 2465–2468.

Pedersen-Bjergaard, J., Philip, P., Thing Mortensen, B., Ersbøll, J., Jensen, G., Panduro, J., and Thomsen, M. (1981). *Blood* **57**, 712–723.

Prigogina, E. L., Fleischman, E. W., Volkova, M. A., and Frenkel, M. A. (1978). *Hum. Genet.* **41**, 143–156.

Reeves, B. R., and Pickup, V. L. (1980). *Hum. Genet.* **53**, 349–355.

Reeves, B. R., Lobb, D. S., and Lawler, S. D. (1972). *Humangenetik* **14**, 159–161,

Riccardi, V. M., Hittner, H. M., Francke, U., Yunis, J. J., Ledbetter, D., and Borges, W. (1980). *Cancer Genet. Cytogenet.* **2**, 131–137.

Rowley, J. D. (1973a). *Nature (London)* **243**, 290–293.

Rowley, J. D. (1973b). *Ann. Genet.* **16**, 109–112.

Rowley, J. D. (1977). *Proc. Natl. Acad. Sci. U.S.A.* **74**, 5729–5733.

Rowley, J. D. (1980). *Clin. Haematol.* **9**, 55–86.

Rowley, J. D. (1982). *Science* **216**, 749–751.

Rowley, J. D., Golomb, H. M., and Dougherty, C. (1977). *Lancet* **i**, 549–550.

Rowley, J. D., Golomb, H. M., and Vardiman, J. W. (1981). *Blood* **58**, 759–767.

Rowley, J. D., Alimena, G., Garson, O. M., Hagemeijer, A., Mitelman, F., and Prigogina, E. L. (1982). *Blood* **59**, 1013–1022.

Sakurai, M., Sasaki, M., Kamada, N., Okada, M., Oshimura, M., Ishihara, T., and Shiraishi, Y. (1982). *Cancer Genet. Cytogenet.* **7**, 59–65.

Sandberg, A. A. (1980). "The Chromosomes in Human Cancer and Leukemia." Elsevier/North-Holland, New York.

Sandberg, A. A. (1981). *Hum. Pathol.* **12**, 531–540.

Schröder, J., Vuopio, P., and Autio, K. (1981). *Cancer Genet. Cytogenet.* **4**, 11–21.

Second International Workshop on Chromosomes in Leukemia, 1979 (1980a). *Cancer Genet. Cytogenet.* **2**, 97–98

Second International Workshop on Chromosomes in Leukemia, 1979 (1980b). *Cancer Genet. Cytogenet.* **2**, 99–102.

Second International Workshop on Chromosomes in Leukemia, 1979 (1980c). *Cancer Genet. Cytogenet.* **2**, 103–107.

Second International Workshop on Chromosomes in Leukemia, 1979 (1980d). *Cancer Genet. Cytogenet.* **2**, 108–113.

Sokal, G., Michaux, J. L., Van Den Berghe, H., Cordier, A., Rodhain, J., Ferrant, A., Moriau, M., de Bruyère, M., and Sonnet, J. (1975). *Blood* **46**, 519–533.

Sonta, S., and Sandberg, A. A. (1978). *Cancer (Philadelphia)* **41,** 153–163.

Teerenhovi, L., Borgström, G. H., Mitelman, F., Brandt, L., Vuopio, P., Timonen, T., Almqvist, A., and de la Chapelle, A. (1978). *Lancet* **ii,** 797.

Third International Workshop on Chromosomes in Leukemia, 1980 (1981a). *Cancer Genet. Cytogenet.* **4,** 101–110.

Third International Workshop on Chromosomes in Leukemia, 1980 (1981b). *Cancer Genet. Cytogenet.* **4,** 111–137.

Third International Workshop on Chromosomes in Leukemia, 1980 (1981c). *Cancer Genet. Cytogenet.* **4,** 138–142.

Van Den Berghe, H., Cassiman, J. J., David, G., Fryns, J. P., Michaux, J. L., and Sokal, G. (1974). *Nature (London)* **251,** 437.

van Steenis, H. (1966). *Nature (London)* **209,** 819–821.

von Hansemann, D. (1890). *Virchows Arch. A Pathol. Anat.* **119,** 299–326.

Wake, N., Hreshchyshyn, M. M., Piver, S. M., Matsui, S., and Sandberg, A. A. (1980). *Cancer Res.* **40,** 4512–4518.

Whang-Peng, J., Knutsen, T., O'Donnell, J. F., and Brereton, H. D. (1979). *Cancer (Philadelphia)* **44,** 1592–1600.

Whang-Peng, J., Bunn, P. A., Jr., Kao-Shan, C. S., Lee, E. C., Carney, D. N., Gazdar, A., and Minna, J. D. (1982). *Cancer Genet. Cytogenet.* **6,** 119–134.

Winge. Ö. (1930). *Z. Zellforsch. Mikrosk. Anat.* **10,** 683–735.

Yunis, J. J., and Ramsay, N. (1978). *Am. J. Dis. Child.* **132,** 161–163.

Yunis, J. J., Bloomfield, C. D., and Ensrud, K. (1981). *N. Engl. J. Med.* **305,** 135–139.

Zang, K. D. (1982). *Cancer Genet. Cytogenet.* **6,** 249–274.

Zang, K. D., and Singer, H. (1967). *Nature (London)* **216,** 84–85.

Zankl, H., and Zang, K. D. (1972). *Humangenetik* **14,** 167–169.

Zech, L., Haglund, U., Nilsson, K., and Klein, G. (1976). *Int. J. Cancer* **17,** 47–56.

Similar Translocation Pattern in B Cell Derived Tumors of Human, Mouse, and Rat Origin

JACK SPIRA

Department of Tumor Biology
Karolinska Institute
Stockholm, Sweden

I. Introduction

The specific chromosome changes that are found in certain human hematopoetic tumors, especially the Philadelphia chromosome in chronic myeloid leukemia, contributes to the diagnosis and prognosis of the disease (Mitelman and Levan, 1981; Rowley, 1980). Although chromosome aberrations are present in this and many other tumors, their role in tumor development still remains uncertain. The question of whether the aberrations are cause or consequence is still open, even in chronic myeloid leukemia.

Recent cytogenetic studies in mouse and rat lymphomas and plasmacytomas, and in human Burkitt's lymphomas have provided new results that emphasize the role of chromosome alterations in tumorigenesis. They also give impulses toward a more functional explanation of how the genetic transposition can act in the cell. This chapter briefly summarizes part of these findings, concentrating upon nonrandom chromosome rearrangements in the mouse T cell lymphoma and the mouse plasmacytoma. The similarity between their aberration pattern and the pattern in rat lymphoma and plasmacytoma and human Burkitt's lymphoma is highly remarkable.

II. Chromosome 15 Trisomy in Murine Lymphomas

Trisomy of chromosome 15 is the most common and often the only cytogenetic change in murine T cell leukemias. It was first described in the spontaneous leukemias of AKR mice (Dofoku et al., 1975) and subsequently in 7,12-dimethylbenz(a)anthracene (DMBA); benzo(a)pyrene(BP); X-ray–Moloney and radiation–leukemia virus-induced leukemias in various mouse strains (Wiener et al., 1978a; Chan et al., 1979; Chang et al., 1977; Spira et al., 1981a; Wiener et al., 1978b). Evidently the 15 trisomy arises regardless of whether the inducing agent is a viral or chemical carcinogen or is a spontaneous tumor. Although often present, the percentage of trisomic cells in individual tumors and the number of trisomic versus normal diploid tumors in different experiments varies (Kodama et al., 1978, 1981). The age of the animal during the carcinogenic exposure, exposure type (e.g., injecting intraperitoneally, stomach feeding), as well as strain susceptibility seem to be the three major factors determining the proportion of trisomic versus diploid leukemias (Chan et al., 1981). In leukemias with hyperdiploid cells the trisomy 15 is a regular feature in all studies.

Chromosome 15 trisomy is not limited to T cell leukemias. It has also been found in radiation induced B cell tumors in Balb/FR (N2) mice or spontaneous (BALB×feral)F_1 mice (Fialkow et al., 1980). Similar results were found in spontaneous B cell tumors of aged BALB/c mice (Wiener et al., 1981). The B cell tumor, in contrast to the T cell tumors, usually carry multiple other chromosome changes, including trisomies and unidentified marker chromosomes. The significance of trisomy 15 in the B cell tumors is therefore uncertain.

The regular occurrence of trisomy 15 suggested that duplication of a specific gene locus was essential for leukemogenesis. Could its location on the chromosome be mapped? If so it would substantiate this view. In order to try to map the genes leukemias were induced with DMBA in CBAT6T6 mice (Wiener et al., 1978c). These mice are homozygous for a translocation in which part of chromosome 15 is translocated to chromosome 14, thereby creating the T(14;15) chromosome. A small centric portion possibly with a tiny piece of chromosome 14 makes up the remaining part of the 15 chromosome. Five of six leukemias were trisomic for the translocation chromosome T(14;15), i.e., the distal part of chromosome 15 was duplicated. This shows that the genes of importance for leukemia development are located below the translocation breakpoint (see Fig. 1) and excludes trisomy 15 as being due to some abnormal behavior of this chromosome that would make it undergo nondisjunction more often than other chromosomes.

The location of the leukemia-associated locus was further pinpointed by the cryptic trisomy 15 in T cell leukemias of SJL mice. (Spira *et al.*, 1980). The duplicated segment was located below band 15C. A schematic representation of the breakpoint is shown in Fig. 1.

In another experiment T cell leukemias were induced in Robertsonian translocation mice in which chromosome 15 was fused at the centromere with autosomes 1, 5, and 6, respectively (Spira *et al.*, 1979). DMBA- and Moloney virus-induced tumors were trisomic for the entire translocation chromosome. These results were confirmed in the inbred AKR(6;15) strain (Herbst *et al.*, 1981). Trisomy 15 is also present in leukemias in Robertsonian mice where chromosome 15 is "free" and other autosomes are fused. An example of such a leukemia is shown in Fig. 2.

Two conclusions were drawn from these results. Trisomy of chromosome 1, 5, or 6 does not restrict cell viability or proliferation, and trisomy of chromosome 15 is of such importance that it forces other attached autosomes to become

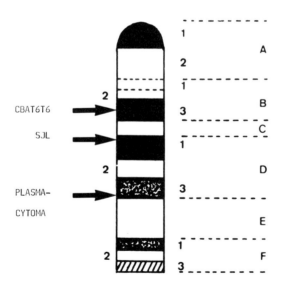

Fig. 1. Schematic figure of mouse chromosome 15. Top arrow shows the breakpoint in CBAT6T6 mice, middle arrow in T cell leukemias of SJL mice, and the lowest arrow in murine plasmacytomas.

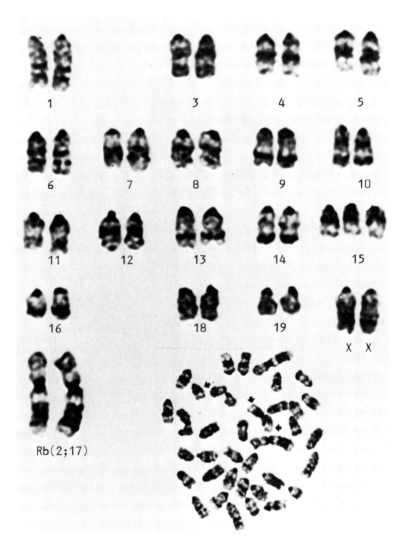

Fig. 2. Karyotype of a T cell leukemia induced in a noninbred mouse homozygous for the Rb (2;17) chromosome. Note the presence of trisomy 15.

trisomic as well. That it is not due to the translocated state is clear from Fig. 2 (see above). This chromosome duplication behavior in the leukemias indicates that trisomy 15 is an important event in leukemogenesis.

In further experiments Wiener and co-workers (Wiener *et al.*, 1979, 1980a; F. Wiener and J. Spira, unpublished results) assessed whether there was any genetic factor involved in the T cell leukemia-associated chromosome 15 duplication.

This was achieved by crossing mice carrying different translocations involving chromosome 15 with inbred mice in such a manner that it was cytogenetically possible to distinguish the parental origin of the chromosome 15. Leukemias were induced by DMBA or N-methylnitrosourea (MNU) stomach feeding. In the leukemias the question was asked, which of the parental chromosome 15 was most often duplicated or was the chromosome 15 duplication in a random fashion? The results showed that only in two crosses, (AKR×AKR6;15)F_1 and (CBA×CBAT6T6)F_1, where there is only a morphological difference and not a genetical difference between the chromosome 15, was duplication random. In all other crosses one parental chromosome 15 was preferentially duplicated. A certain "hierarchy" of duplication preference could be made, as depicted in Fig. 3. Arrows between the strains indicate performed crosses. The strain located at the highest level in a certain cross will have the greatest frequency of duplication. Strains at the same level will duplicate their chromosome 15 at random. This indicates that there exists a genetic variance between the leukemia-associated gene in the various strains. Thus duplication of chromosome 15 of certain strains is more likely to be tumorigenic. It is of interest that the high leukemogenic AKR strain holds the highest position in the hierarchy.

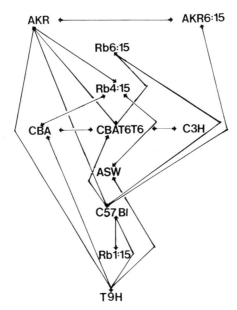

Fig. 3. Hierarchy of duplication in trisomic T cell leukemias of various mouse strains. Rb(6;15),Rb(4;15) are noninbred Robertsonian translocation stocks homozygous for the chromosomes fused at the centromere. The T9H strain has a reciprocal translocation between chromosomes 7 and 15. For explanation see text.

The difference between the strains raises another question: Is there a difference between a normal derived chromosome 15 and a tumor duplicated one? Two different approaches were used to study this question. In the first, three different T cell leukemia-derived cell lines were karyotyped with the early replicative banding (ERB) method (Somssich *et al.*, 1982). The method is based upon growing the cells in presence of bromodeoxyuridine(BrdU) during a defined period of the S phase and staining with either acridine orange or Giemsa (Perry and Wolf, 1974). When comparing the ERB pattern of the leukemia-derived chromosome 15 with that of normal derived homologs a clear difference was observed. In the majority (more than 90%) of tumor metaphase cells, the E band was missing from chromosome 15. Late replicating studies and normal R and G banding showed a normal pattern, indicating that the band not was deleted. It is interesting that 15E is in the region that is associated with T cell leukemia duplication (see Fig. 1). It is still unknown if the ERB change implies functional activation or not.

Another approach to study if there is a genetical difference between normal and leukemic chromosome 15 is by somatic cell hybrids. We performed such a study by fusing a chromosome 15 trisomic highly leukemogenic T cell line of AKR origin with normal fibroblasts or lymphocytes from CBAT6T6 (Spira *et al.*, 1981b). Due to the cytogenetic difference between tumor-derived chromosome 15 (normal morphology) and normal-derived homolog [carried as the T(14;15) translocation chromosome] it was possible to distinguish the origin of chromosome 15 in the hybrids. High and low tumorigenic hybrids were compared with trypsin–Giemsa banding. In the high tumorigenic hybrids there was an impressive increase in the number of tumor-derived chromosome 15 copies from the expected 3 to 5–6 copies, where the number of normal derived T(14;15) chromosomes was decreased from expected 2 to 1 copy. A random high tumorigenic karyotype is shown in Fig. 4. Low tumorigenic hybrids showed an opposite pattern. They contained 2–3 tumor-derived chromosome 15 copies and 2 normal-derived T(14;15) (very close to the expected number in a 1 : 1 hybrid). The few *in vivo* growing segregants of the low tumorigenic hybrids changed their chromosome 15 content toward the high tumorigenic situation; tumor-derived chromosome 15 copies increased in number to 4–5 and normal-derived homologs decreased to 1 copy.

The ERB pattern study and the somatic cell hybrid study implicate a functional difference between the normal- and tumor-derived chromosome 15. Because only the tumor-derived chromosomes were amplified in tumorigenic hybrids, they must be different from normal chromosomes. On the contrary, it appeared that the normal derived homolog to a certain extent suppressed the tumorigenic phenotype.

In conclusion, the results indicate that in murine leukemias, chromosome 15 may contain a leukemia-associated oncogene as postulated by Klein (1981). The

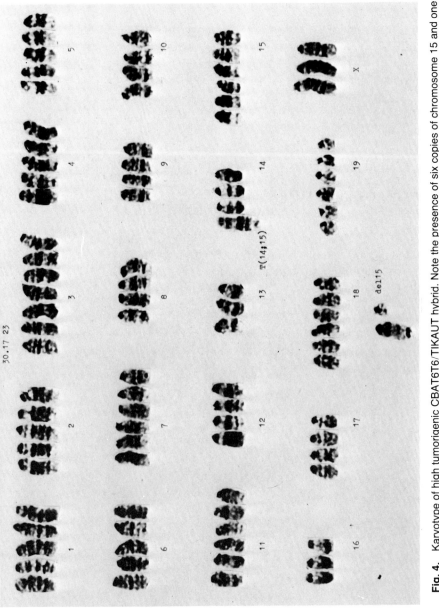

Fig. 4. Karyotype of high tumorigenic CBAT6T6/TIKAUT hybrid. Note the presence of six copies of chromosome 15 and one T(14;15).

oncogene would be activated by mutation, by insertion of a proviral promotor (Hayward *et al.*, 1981) near to the postulated oncogene, or by sister chromatid exchanges [as has been postulated for human retinoblastoma (Kinsella and Radman, 1978)]. The change would affect one chromosome first, and after duplication by nondisjunction the cell would be transformed. The latter step would be an easy way of overcoming the trans-acting suppression of the normal homolog.

III. Chromosome Translocation in Murine Plasmacytomas

Mouse plasmacytoma is a B cell-derived tumor, usually induced by intraperitoneal injection of pristane oil into susceptible strains such as BALB/c or NZB. Early karyotypic observations in long transplanted *in vivo* tumors and established cell lines described a deletion of the terminal segment of chromosome 15 (Shepard *et al.*, 1974, 1978; Yoshida *et al.*, 1978). In some cases a translocation to chromosome 12 was seen, and in one case (Shepard *et al.*, 1978), a translocation to chromosome 6. The tumors and cell lines exhibited many other changes as well. Recently the finding was confirmed and further clarified (Ohno *et al.*, 1979; Wiener *et al.*, 1980b). Primary and early passage immunoglobulin A (IgA) κ and λ light chain-producing plasmacytomas were karyotyped. All plasmacytomas contained one of two translocations. The more common one, seen in both κ and λ chain producers, was the transposition of the distal segment of chromosome 15 to chromosome 12 [T(12;15) with breakpoints (12F2,15D3)]. In a minority of cases, only κ producers, a reciprocal 6;15 translocation was seen. It had the same chromosome 15 breakpoint as that in the T(12;15) translocation, 15D3, and on chromosome 6 at band C. In near diploid tumors, only one of the two homologs is involved in the translocation. In tetraploid tumors, two of the four homologs are affected. The translocation therefore probably arose before polyploidization. The translocated chromosome segment in plasmacytomas is within the region that regularly becomes trisomic in the T and B cell leukemias (see Fig. 1). Since this region is closely associated with lymphoid tumorigenesis it is possible that it contains a gene that not only controls lymphocyte growth but also plasmacyte growth or differentiation. It may also, as postulated previously, contain a retrovirus-related oncogene.

The immunoglobulin (Ig) heavy chain locus is located on chromosome 12 of the mouse, and the kappa light chain gene is on chromosome 6 (Hengartner *et al.*, 1978; Swan *et al.*, 1979). The heavy chain genes are located on the chromosome close to the plasmacytoma related breakpoint (Meo *et al.*, 1980). Based on this observation it is possible that a gene located on chromosome 15 may come under the influence of a highly active Ig related promotor on chromosome 6 or 12. It is of interest to determine whether the translocation affects the allelically excluded chromosome 12 or the expressed homolog. This can be achieved by studying plasmacytomas in mice with the appropriate cytogenetic and Ig allotype markers.

As a conclusion to the nonrandom chromosome aberrations in mouse lymphomas and plasmacytomas, rearrangements of chromosome 15 is the common feature. In T and B cell lymphomas it is trisomic. This not only implies a 50% increase in gene dosage but, as shown in the early replicative banding and the somatic cell hybrid study, also a qualitative change of the chromosome 15-associated leukemia promoting gene. Duplication of the altered chromosome is necessary for full expression of the leukemic phenotype. In the plasmacytoma this is achieved by transposing the same (?) gene to the neighborhood of the highly active Ig related promotor on either chromosome 6 or 12. Further experiments are needed to verify this hypothesis.

IV. Trisomy in Rat Tumors

The most common aberration found in carcinogen-induced rat leukemias, sarcomas, and carcinomas is trisomy of chromosome 2 (Kurita et al., 1968; Ahlström, 1974; Sugiyama, 1978; Mitelman and Levan, 1972). As in the case of the mouse a varying proportion of the tumors has a normal diploid pattern, depending on carcinogens, dosages, etc. Mouse virus-induced sarcomas show a different pattern with trisomy 7 as the dominating change (Mitelman, 1971). The tumors of the rat thus show an agent-specific aberration pattern, whereas the mouse pattern is more of a tissue-specific aberration (Spira et al., 1980).

V. Translocation in Rat Plasmacytomas

So far the most consistent chromosome aberration in rat is the recently described T(6;7) translocation in rat plasmacytomas (Wiener et al., 1982). The distal part of the 7q arm is translocated to the end of chromosome 6. The T(6;7) chromosome was consistently present in all seven spontaneous primary or early passage IgE-producing immunoglomas in the inbred LOU/C/Wsl strain. The translocation is similar to that in the mouse in two ways: First, a distal fragment of one chromosome is translocated to a similar position in both cases. Second, the donor fragments are associated with tumorigenesis in other tumors in both hosts: Mouse chromosome 15 with leukemias, rat chromosome 7 with virus-induced sarcomas. Where is the Ig gene of the rat located? In hybridoma studies, expression of the rat heavy chain immunoglobulin was associated with the presence of rat chromosome 14 (Schröder et al., 1980).

If one compares the banding pattern of mouse and rat chromosomes some regions are very homologous. This is especially true for mouse chromosome 12 and rat chromosome 6, and mouse chromosome 15 and rat chromosome arm 7q. Based on the close homology between these chromosomes and the close homology between the plasmacytoma translocations, we predict that the heavy chain gene is located on chromosome 6 in the rat. Combined cytogenetic and molecular hybridization studies, using appropriate hybrids and DNA probes are required to map the rat Ig genes definitively. Such experiments are presently being performed in our laboratory.

VI. Trisomy in Human Tumors

The human chromosome number 8 is, next to number 1, the chromosome most often rearranged in human tumors (Mitelman and Levan, 1981). It is associated with no less than seven different neoplasms. The aberrations include translocations in Burkitt's lymphoma, acute myelocytic leukemia, acute lymphatic leukemia and trisomy in acute myelocytic leukemia, chronic myelocytic leukemia, polyeythemia vera, myeloproliferative syndromes, siderblastic anemia, and preleukemic syndromes. In many tumors, trisomy 8 is present as a common "additional" chromosome change, for instance, in Philadelphia positive chronic myelocytic leukemia.

VII. Translocations in Human Burkitt's Lymphomas

The most consistent chromosome abnormality involving chromosome 8 is seen in human Burkitt's lymphomas (BL), a B cell derived tumor. Irrespective of whether the tumor cells carry the Epstein–Barr virus, 90% of the tumors and derived cell lines carry a specific translocation, in which the distal chromosome 8 below band 8q24 is translocated to the terminal band q32 on chromosome 14. (Manolov and Manolova, 1972; Zech et al., 1976; Manolova et al., 1979). The translocation is probably reciprocal (Manolova et al., 1979). Human heavy chain genes have been mapped to chromosome 14 (Croce et al., 1979) and in situ hybridization has localized the cluster to band 14q32 (McBride et al., 1981). This is the same band as the breakpoint in the tumors.

In 10% of BL there are variant translocations. The donor segment is the same as in the 8;14 translocation that is 8q24 to 8qter. The recipients are chromosomes 2 or 22 at the breakpoints 2p12 and 22q11, respectively (Van den Berghe et al., 1979; Miyoshi et al., 1979; Berger et al., 1979). Moreover chromosome 2 carries the κ gene locus (McBride et al., 1982) and chromosome 22 the λ gene locus (McBride et al., 1982; Eriksson et al., 1981). In situ experiments mapped the κ chains to band 2p11–2p13. (Malcolm *et al.*, 1981). This is the same chromosome band as the tumor-associated breakpoint in the 2;8 variant translocation.

In the variant translocations seven of eight 2;8 translocation carrying BL all made κ light chains, whereas three of five 8;22 carrying BL made λ light chains (Lenoir *et al.*, 1982). The remaining tumors in each group (one and two, respectively) were functionally inactive. The regular correlation between the immunoglobulin light chain type expressed and the translocation pattern indicate that the functional Ig locus is important in the translocation process.

These results suggest that a similar oncogene that was postulated to be present on mouse chromosome 15 and rat chromosome 7 may be carried by human chromosome 8. Similar mechanisms seem to be responsible for the activation of the B cell into Ig-producing tumors in the three species.

Many parts of this scenario remain to be proved. By combining modern techniques of molecular cloning genetics, cytogenetics, and transfection the verification of the hypothesis is possible.

VIII. Summary

The chromosome aberration pattern of certain human, rat, and mouse hematopoetic tumors are very similar. B Cell-derived tumors, such as human Burkitt's lymphoma and mouse and rat plasmacytomas, present the most consistent pattern. In human Burkitt's lymphoma a distal segment of chromosome 8 is translocated to chromosome 14, or in a minority of cases to chromosome 2 or 22. In rat plasmacytomas the terminal part of chromosome 7 is joined with chromosome 6, and in mouse plasmacytomas a distal part of chromosome 15 is transposed to chromosome 6 or 12. The donor chromosome, human 8, rat 7, and mouse 15 are often amplified and are rearranged in other ways in many other tumors of their respective host. The resemblance is further emphasized by the location of immunoglobulin heavy or light chain genes on the recipient chromosomes in the human and mouse translocations.

The similarity between the species and the preciseness of the translocations indicate that the transposition of genetic material occurs by a specific mechanism and that they play a significant role in the development of certain tumors.

Acknowledgments

The studies at the laboratory of Tumor Biology in this field have been supported by Grant 2R01 CA 14054-10 awarded by the National Cancer Institute and by Grant 83:151 from the Swedish Cancer Society.

References

Ahlström, U. (1974). *Hereditas* **78**, 235–244.

Berger, R., Bernheim, A., Weh, H. J., Flandrin, G., Daniel, M. T., Brouet, J. C., and Colbert, A. (1979). *Hum. Genet.* **53**, 111–112.

Chan, F. P. H., Ball, J. K., and Sergovich, V. (1979). *J. Natl. Cancer Inst.* **62**, 605–610.

Chan, F. P. H., Ens, B., and Frei, J. V. (1981). *Cancer Genet. Cytogenet.* **4**, 337–344.

Chang, T. D., Biedler, J. L., Stockert, E., and Old, L. J. (1977). *Proc. Natl. Am. Assoc. Cancer Res.* **18**, 225.

Croce, C. M., Strander, M. A., Martinis, J., Cicurel, L., D'Ancona, G. G., Dolby, T. W., and Koprowski, H. (1979). *Proc. Natl. Acad. Sci. U.S.A.* **76**, 3416–3419.

Dofoku, R., Biedler, J. L., Spenbler, B. A., and Old, L. J. (1975). *Proc. Natl. Acad. Sci. U.S.A.* **72**, 1515–1517.

Eriksson, J., Martinis, J., and Croce, C. M. (1981). *Nature (London)* **294**, 173–175.

Fialkow, P. J., Reddy, A. L., and Bryant, J. I. (1980). *Int. J. Cancer,* **26**, 603–608.

Hayward, W. S., Neel, B. G., and Astrin, S. M. (1981). *Nature (London)* **290**, 475–479.

Hengartner, H., Meo, T., and Muller, E. (1978). *Proc. Natl. Acad. Sci. U.S.A.* **75**, 4494–4498.

Herbst, E. W., Gropp, A., and Tietgen, C. (1981). *Int. J. Cancer* **28**, 805–810.

Kinsella, A. R., and Radman, M. (1978). *Proc. Natl. Acad. Sci. U.S.A.* **75**, 6149–6153.

Klein, G. (1981). *Nature (London)* **294**, 313–318.

Kodama, Y., Yoshida, M. C., and Sasaki, M. (1978). *Proc. Jpn. Acad., Ser. B* **54B**, 222–227.

Kodama, Y., Takagi, N., Yoshida, M. C., and Sasaki, M. (1981). *Cancer Genet. Cytogenet.* **3**, 237–242.

Kurita, Y., Sugiyama, T., and Nishizuka, Y. (1968). *Cancer Res.* **28**, 1738–1752.

Lenoir, G. M., Preud'homme, J. L., Bernheim, A., and Berger, R. (1982). *Nature (London)* **298**, 474–476.

McBride, O. W., Swan, D., Leder, P., Hieter, P., and Hollis, G. (1981). *In* "Human Gene Mapping, VI" Karper, Basel.

McBride, O. W., Heiter, P. A., Hollis, G. F., Swan, D., Otray, M. C., and Leder, P. (1982). *J. Exp. Med.* **155**, 1480–1490.

Malcom, S., Barton, P., Bentley, D. L., Ferguson-Smith, M. A., Murphy, C. S., and Rabbits, T. H. (1981). *In* "Human Gene Mapping, VI" Karger, Basel.

Manolov, G., and Manolova, Y. (1972). *Nature (London)* **237**, 33–34.

Manolova, T., Manolov, G., Kieler, J., Levan, A., and Klein, G. (1979). *Hereditas* **90**, 1–20.

Meo, T., Johnson, J., Beechey, C. V., Andrews, S. J., Peters, J., and Searle, G. (1980). *Proc. Natl. Acad. Sci. U.S.A.* **77**, 550–553.

Mitelman, F. (1971). *Hereditas* **69**, 155–186.

Mitelman, F., and Levan, G. (1972). *Hereditas,* **71**, 325–334.

Mitelman, F., and Levan, G. (1981). *Hereditas* **95**, 79–139.

Miyoshi, I., Hiraki, S., Kimura, L., Miyamoto, K., and Sato, J. (1979). *Experientia* **35**, 742–743.

Ohno, S., Babonits, M., Wiener, F., Spira, J., Klein, G., and Potter, M. (1979). *Cell* **18**, 1001–1007.

Perry, P., and Wolf, S. (1974). *Nature (London)* **251**, 156–158.

Rowley, J. D. (1980). *Cancer Genet. Cytogenet.* **2**, 175–198.

Schröder, J., Autio, K., Junis, J. M., and Milstein, C. (1980). *Immunogenetics (N.Y.)* **10**, 125–131.

Shepard, J. S., Wurster-Hill, D. S., Pettengill, O. S., and Sorensen, G. D. (1974). *Cytogenet. Cell Genet.* **13**, 279–309.

Shepard, J. S., Pettengill, O. S., Wurster-Hill, D. S., and Sörensen, G. D. (1978). *J. Natl. Cancer Inst.* **61**, 255–258.

Somssich, I. E., Spira, J., Hameister, H., and Klein, G. (1982). *Chromosoma* (in press).

Spira, J., Wiener, F., Ohno, S., and Klein, G. (1979). *Proc. Natl. Acad. Sci. U.S.A.* **76,** 6619–6621.

Spira, J., Babonits, M., Wiener, F., Ohno, S., Wirschubski, Z., Haran-Ghera, N., and Klein, G. (1980). *Cancer Res.* **40,** 2609–2616.

Spira, J. Åsjö, B., Cochran, A., Shen, F. W., Wiener, F., and Klein, G. (1981a). *Leuk. Res.* **5,** 113–121.

Spira, J., Wiener, F., Babonits, M., Gamble, J., Miller, J., and Klein, G. (1981b). *Int. J. Cancer* **28,** 785–798.

Sugiyama, T., Uenaka, H., Ueda, N., Fukuhara, S., and Meda, S. (1978). *J. Natl. Cancer Inst.* **60,** 153–160.

Swan, D., D'Eustachio, P., Leinwand, L., Seidman, J., Keithley, D., and Ruddle, F. H. (1979). *Proc. Natl. Acad. Sci. U.S.A.* **76,** 2735–2739.

Van den Berghe, H., Parloir, A., Gosseye, S., Englebienne, V., Cornu, G., and Sokal, G. (1979). *Cancer Genet. Cytogenet.* **1,** 9–14.

Wiener, F., Spira, J., Ohno, S., Haran-Ghera, N., and Klein, G. (1978a). *Int. J. Cancer* **22,** 447–453.

Wiener, F., Ohno, S., Spira, J., Haran-Ghera, N., and Klein, G. (1978b). *J. Natl. Cancer Inst.* **60,** 227–232.

Wiener, F., Spira, J., Ohno, S., Haran-Ghera, N., and Klein, G. (1978c). *Nature (London)* **275,** 658–660.

Wiener, F., Spira, J., Ohno, S., Haran-Ghera, N., and Klein, G. (1979). *Int. J. Cancer* **23,** 504–507.

Wiener, F., Spira, J., Babonits, M., Haran-Ghera, N., and Klein, G. (1980a). *Int. J. Cancer* **26,** 661–668.

Wiener, F., Babonits, M., Spira, J., Klein, G., and Potter, M. (1980b). *Somatic Cell Genet.* **6,** 731–738.

Wiener, F., Babonits, M., Spira, J., Bregula, U., Klein, G., Merwin, R. M., Asofsky, R., Lynes, M., and Haughton, G. (1981). *Int. J. Cancer* **27,** 51–58.

Wiener, F., Babonits, M., Spira, J., Klein, G., and Bazin, H. (1982). *Int. J. Cancer* **29,** 431–437.

Yoshida, M. C., Moriwaki, K., and Migita, S. (1978). *J. Natl. Cancer Inst.* **60,** 235–238.

Zech, L., Haglund, U., Nilsson, K., and Klein, G. (1976). *Int. J. Cancer* **17,** 47–56.

Specific Chromosome Changes in the Human Heritable Tumors Retinoblastoma and Nephroblastoma

UTA FRANCKE

Department of Human Genetics
Yale University School of Medicine
New Haven, Connecticut

I. Introduction

Specific constitutional structural chromosome changes in carriers of heritable tumors may pinpoint the location of DNA sequences that are involved in genetic predisposition to certain types of cancer. The identification of individuals who have deletions, translocations, or duplications of the respective chromosome regions not only provides genetic counseling for the family involved, but may also suggest general mechanisms of cancer predisposition, and may provide experimental material for the isolation and cloning of the respective sequences.

I will illustrate these points using the two best documented examples of human hereditary tumors associated with specific chromosome abnormalities, retinoblastoma with a gene in chromosome band 13q14, and the aniridia–Wilms' tumor predisposition associated with deletion of chromosome band 11q13.

Evidence that places gene(s) predisposing to the human embryonic tumor retinoblastoma to a precise location on human chromosome 13 (band 13q14.1) includes (a) prezygotic heterozygous chromosome deletions, (b) apparently balanced chromosome translocations, (c) mapping of the autosomal dominant retinoblastoma locus to band 13q14 by close linkage to the esterase D locus in the same band, and (d) deletions involving 13q14 in chromosome preparations from retinoblastoma tumor tissue. Heterozygosity for 13q14 deletion with hemizygous representation of the respective sequences leads to retinoblastoma formation.

Nephroblastoma (Wilms' tumor, WT), an embryonic kidney tumor, is in some cases associated with heterozygous deletion of a distinct region of the short arm of chromosome 11. The deletion confers a roughly 30% risk for Wilms' tumor and a near 100% risk for aniridia, a developmental defect of iris formation. The locus for the enzyme catalase is in the same band 11p13. The gene for the autosomal dominant form of WT has not yet been localized.

II. Retinoblastoma (RB)

A. Frequency and Genetics

This embryonal tumor of immature, incompletely differentiated retinal cell elements occurs in between 1 and 16,000 and 1 and 20,000 children. It is usually diagnosed within the first 2 to 3 years of life. The hereditary form, thought to be present in about 40% of cases, is caused by an autosomal dominant mutation with high penetrance. The majority of the hereditary cases (68%) are bilateral (multifocal) and 32% are unilateral. All sporadic bilateral cases are considered to be new mutants. The nonhereditary form is more common (60%). These cases are unilateral and tend to have a later mean age of diagnosis than the familial and bilateral cases. It is of importance for genetic counseling that 10–12% of sporadic unilateral cases are germ cell mutants with a 45% risk of having affected offspring. The formal genetics of retinoblastoma has been reviewed by Francois *et al.* (1975), Vogel (1979), and Matsunaga (1980).

B. Constitutional Chromosome Abnormalities in RB Patients

Retinoblastoma has been reported in patients with constitutional numerical chromosome abnormalities, in particular, supernumerary X chromosomes and trisomy 21 (Table I). A structural chromosome aberration, namely, a deletion of a D group chromosome in a case of retinoblastoma was first reported in 1963 (Lele *et al.*, 1963). The chromosome involved was identified as a chromosome 13 in additional cases. In 1976, after reviewing the extent of the deletions in the three published cases, and in one we had identified, I concluded that the only deleted region shared in common by the unequivocally identified cases involved the faintly staining band 13q14 (Francke, 1976). Speculating about the nature of the relevant genetic material located in 13q14, I suggested that if the relevant gene had a function in normal retinal development, deletion could cause a shortage of the gene product necessary for a stage of retinal differentiation; incompletely differentiated embryonic cells could be more susceptible to tumor formation. I also suggested that families with autosomal dominant retinoblastoma should be studied for linkage of the *RB* locus to *esterase D,* an enzyme locus mapped to chromosome 13q, in order to determine whether the autosomal dominant gene resides in the same region (Francke, 1976). In the meantime, close to 50 patients with interstitial deletions of 13q have been reported, with unilateral or bilateral retinoblastomas and a clinical syndrome of short stature, minor dysmorphic features and various degrees of mental retardation, but not consistent malformations (Francke and Kung, 1976; Howard, 1982). The breakpoints and sizes of the deletions are variable, but they all involve a part of 13q14. The larger deletions are associated with more severe retardation, while a very small one just involving a subband of q14 may be associated with normal development (Yunis and Ramsay, 1978). The development of retinoblastoma seems to

TABLE I

Constitutional Chromosome Abnormalities in Retinoblastoma

Chromosome abnormality	No. of patients
46,13q−	45
47,+13	1
47,+21	7
47,XXY	4
47,XXX	1
48,XXX,+21	1
48,XXY,+21	1
49,XXXXY	1

be a uniform consequence of deletion of the proximal part of band 13q14. No convincing evidence has been reported of patients who have a deletion of that specific region and lack retinoblastoma.

The deletion of the relevant genes in 13q14 may arise by different mechanisms (Table II). In most cases the deletion 13q is *de novo* and present in all cells, suggesting a prezygotic event during germ cell maturation. A few patients have been identified who had chromosomally normal cells in addition to cells with the deletion. In one such mosaic patient, the RB tumor cells all contained the deleted 13 (M. Harrison and U. Francke, unpublished observations). Motegi (1982) detected deletion 13q14 mosaicism by high resolution chromosome banding techniques in 3 of 15 RB cases studied. However, such data have to be interpreted with caution because apparent "nonhomology" due to asynchrony in chromosome condensation is frequently seen in homologous chromosome pairs studied at early mitotic stages. Additional evidence is required, such as consistent presence of the deletion 13q14 in the same homolog identified by a 13p heteromorphism or decreased versus normal esterase D activity in cloned fibroblast populations that can be correlated with the presence or absence of the del (13) chromosome.

The deletion 13q may also be inherited, as for example, in unbalanced offspring of balanced carriers of inversions or insertions. Four such families have been reported, one with a paracentric inversion within the long arm of 13 and three with insertions of a region involving the critical band of 13q into another autosome, such as chromosomes 3, 12 (Fig. 1), or 20 (Table II). The carriers of these presumably balanced rearrangements did not have retinoblastoma. However, their children who inherited the chromosome 13 with missing interstitial

TABLE II

Different Mechanisms Can Lead to Deletion of Chromosome Band 13q14 in Retinoblastoma Patients

1. Nonhereditary deletions	
del 13q *de novo*, prezygotic	(Francke, 1976)
del 13q mosaic, postzygotic	(Motegi, 1981)
2. Hereditary deletions	
Unbalanced offspring of balanced carriers of	
inv(13)(q12q22)	(Sparkes *et al.*, 1979)
ins(12;13)(p11.21;q12.3q22.1)	(Riccardi *et al.*, 1979)
ins(3;13)(p12;q13.1q14.3)	(Strong *et al.*, 1981)
ins(20;13)(p21;q1307q14.3)	(Rivera *et al.*, 1981)
3. Translocations *de novo*, apparently balanced	
t(X;13)(p22;q12)	(Nichols *et al.*, 1980)
t(X;13)(p22;q12)	(Hida *et al.*, 1980)
t(1;13)(p22;q12)	(Davison *et al.*, 1979)
t(13;18)(q14.1;q12.2)	(Motegi *et al.*, 1982)

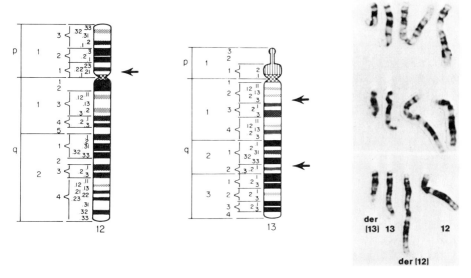

Fig. 1. Balanced insertion of proximal half of long arm of a chromosome 13 (region q 12.3 → q 22.1) into short arm of a chromosome 12 at band p11.21. The inserted piece is not inverted with respect to the centromere. In the three partial karyotypes prepared with trypsin-Giemsa banding the derivative 13 [der(13)] and the normal 13 have been placed upside down to facilitate comparison with the inserted material in the derivative 12 [der(12)]. The breakpoints have been renumbered according to ISCN (1981). The ideograms are from U. Francke, *Cytogenet. Cell Genet.* **31**, 24 (1981). An unbalanced offspring of this insertion carrier had deletion of 13q12.3 → q22.1 and bilateral retinoblastoma (Riccardi *et al.*, 1979).

material, but not the autosome in which the material had been inserted, did develop tumors. In two of the families the breaks have been localized into the distal subband of 13q14 (band q14.3, ISCN 1981). Thus, the missing material *proximal* to these break points and *not* the breakage event itself has to be implicated in tumor predisposition.

In contrast, four patients have been reported with *de novo* apparently balanced reciprocal translocations involving chromosome 13, who also had RB in the absence of a positive family history for the tumor. In two unrelated patients the chromosome rearrangements were very similar with a break in 13q12 and translocation of the distal part of 13q to the short arm of the X chromosome (Cross *et al.*, 1977; Hida *et al.*, 1980). X chromosome replication studies have shown that in a proportion of these patients' cells the translocated X is late replicating and that the late replication pattern is spreading into the translocated part of 13q (Nichols *et al.*, 1980; Ejima *et al.*, 1982a). Mohandas and colleagues (1982) have demonstrated that the *esterase D* locus, also mapped to chromosome band 13q14 was inactivated as a result of inactivation spreading into the 13q region. It

is therefore attractive to speculate that in the two patients with t(X;13) translocations the relevant sequences in 13q14 have become inactivated in a proportion of
retinal cells. This inactivation has led to retinoblastoma predisposition equal to
that conveyed by physical deletion of this part of the chromosome.

Patients with *de novo* balanced translocations and RB may be especially informative with respect to the precise localization of the gene. In one case of RB and
a *de novo* t(1;13) translocation the breakpoint on 13 was interpreted to be in band
q12 (Davison *et al.,* 1979). However, the published karyotypes suggest that
alternative interpretations (e.g., q14) are possible. Recently, Motegi and colleagues (1982) have reported a new mutation of retinoblastoma associated with a
de novo t(13;18) translocation studied with high-resolution banding. The breakpoint on 13 was localized into the most proximal subband 13q14.1. There was no
apparent deletion of chromosomal material. The authors suggested that this
breakpoint might pinpoint precisely the localization of the retinoblastoma gene,
in analogy to the female patients with Duchenne muscular dystrophy who have
de novo X/autosome translocations with breakpoints in Xp21 (Jacobs *et al.,*
1981). According to this hypothesis the break in 13q14.1 would disrupt or render
inactive a sequence of DNA whose function is necessary for proper differentiation of retinal cells.

C. Nature of DNA Sequences at 13q14.1

1. *Mapping of the Autosomal Dominant Retinoblastoma Locus by Family Linkage Studies*

Because of a paucity of genetic markers assigned to chromosome 13, the
initial linkage studies used heteromorphic chromosome variants, such as strongly
fluorescent regions on the short arm in quinacrine stained preparations. The
segregation of chromosomes 13 that were distinguishable by Q-band fluorescence with retinoblastoma has been studied in six families. The recombination
fraction did not differ significantly from 50% (Knight *et al.,* 1980; Morten *et al.,*
1982). These findings are consistent with meiotic chiasma distribution data that
estimated a recombination fraction of 0.27 to 0.37 in males, and possibly 0.5 in
females, between 13p fluorescent markers and the proposed RB locus at 13q14
(Palmer and Hulten, 1982). The conclusion from these studies is that fluorescent
13p heteromorphisms are not suitable for identification of gene carriers in RB
families. The reported studies also failed to provide any evidence with respect to
localization of the autosomal dominant RB gene.

Most recently, however, linkage studies carried out by R. S. Sparkes and
associates in Los Angeles have demonstrated very close linkage of the RB gene
with *esterase D,* a polymorphic enyzme whose locus has previously been
mapped to the same band 13q14 (Sparkes *et al.,* 1980). The lod score is above 3

at a recombination fraction of 0 (Sparkes *et al.,* 1983). These results suggest that the autosomal dominant RB mutation may affect the same DNA sequences that are responsible for RB in the 13q deletion cases.

2. *Function of the Normal Allele at the RB Locus*

a. The RB Gene Acts on the Nontumorous Retina. The proposition that the product of this locus is necessary for normal retinal development has been supported by the histologic and ultrastructural changes found in the nontumorous retina of a 13q deletion/retinoblastoma patient (Hittner *et al.,* 1980). However, one could argue that in this patient with a visible 13q deletion, additional genes on 13q have been deleted that could have been involved in causing the observed histologic changes. Similar studies will have to be done on patients with hereditary retinoblastoma and normal constitutional karyotypes in order to clarify this point.

b. The RB Gene Acts on Extraocular Tissues. There is strong evidence that patients with genetic predisposition to RB, either due to a dominant mutation or a chromosome deletion, have a significantly greater risk for the development of other tumors later in life. Rare malignancies, especially osteosarcoma or soft tissue sarcoma, may occur 10 to 15 years after successful treatment of RB, preferentially in irradiated areas, but often in unirradiated ones as well. There is at least one obligate gene carrier in a retinoblastoma family who developed osteosarcoma without evidence of RB (Francois *et al.,* 1980). The occurrence of pineoblastomas, tumors of the pineal gland that are histologically similar to retinoblastoma, has been reported in 13 cases with multifocal retinoblastoma (Bader *et al.,* 1982). Since the pineal gland is evolutionarily related to photoreceptors in the retina, the argument can be made that pineoblastoma is another manifestation of the retinoblastoma gene in a closely related target tissue. For the other rare tumors, sarcomas of bone and/or soft tissue that occur in 10 to 15% of survivors of heritable retinoblastoma, the argument of multicentric foci of retinoblastoma cannot be made. These are true second primary neoplasms. The risk for osteogenic sarcoma is 500 times greater for RB patients, with or without prior radiation therapy, than for the normal population. It thus appears that the development of these lethal secondary extraocular tumors is directly related to the function of the *RB* locus itself, or possibly to a very closely linked DNA sequence.

The search for a mechanism to explain the second primary tumors led to *in vitro* studies of radiosensitivity of fibroblasts from retinoblastoma patients (Nove *èt al.,* 1980). It has been reported that fibroblasts from patients with hereditary RB and 13q− with RB are more radiosensitive than fibroblasts from patients with sporadic RB or normal controls (Weichselbaum *et al.,* 1979). These findings have led to the postulation of a DNA repair locus, specific for radiation-induced DNA damage, that is closely linked to the RB gene on 13q. In contrast, recent studies by Ejima *et al.* (1982b) on fibroblast strains from 14 patients with various forms of RB have determined that all of these strains were within the normal range of radiosensitivity as determined by clonogenic assay. Cells from a patient with ataxia telangectasia, an autosomal recessive condition with increased X-ray sensitivity were used as "affected" controls. The authors concluded that RB cannot be classified as a radiosensitive genetic disease and that there is no evidence for a DNA repair locus on chromosome 13. At this time there is no generally accepted mechanism that explains the occurrence of late extraocular tumors in individuals with hereditary RB, but the possibility remains that the normal allele at the *RB* locus is expressed in other tissues besides retinal precursor cells.

III. Nephroblastoma (Wilms' Tumor, WT)

A. Frequency and Genetics

Nephroblastoma, an embryonic tumor of the kidney, has an incidence of 1 in 10,000 and is one of the most common tumors in childhood. The great majority of cases are sporadic and the familial nature of the disease was more difficult to establish than for RB, for two reasons: There are fewer survivors who have offspring, and penetrance is incomplete. In 1972, Knudson and Strong suggested a model for Wilms' tumor (WT) analogous to the one developed for RB (Knudson, 1971). They postulated a hereditary form present in 38% of cases, due to an autosomal dominant mutation with 63% penetrance. The majority of individuals with this mutation have unilateral tumors (79%), and 21% have bilateral multifocal nephroblastomas. Five percent of the sporadic cases are bilateral, and these may be new mutants of the autosomal dominant form. As in RB, the nonhereditary form is more common (62%). The median age of diagnosis is 3.8 years. In proven familial cases the age of diagnosis is around 2 years. This apparent difference may in part be due to ascertainment bias, i.e., more careful examination of children born to nephroblastoma families.

As in RB, the dominant WT mutation may predispose to other malignancies as well, as suggested by a recent survey of offspring and siblings of WT patients (Kantor *et al.,* 1982).

B. The Aniridia–Wilms' Tumor Association (AWTA) and Deletion of Chromosome Band 11p13

It has long been known that children with WT have an increased incidence of associated abnormalities, mainly hemihypertrophy, genitourinary abnormalities, and mental retardation. In 1964, Miller and associates identified six cases with aniridia (congenital absence or underdevelopment of the iris) in 440 WT cases whose medical records they reviewed. Aniridia is an extremely rare condition, occurring in approximately 1 in 50,000 individuals. However, there is an autosomal dominant aniridia gene that is also expressed in the form of other ocular malformations (Ferrell *et al.*, 1980). Miller's cases had sporadic aniridia. Therefore, the occurrence of sporadic aniridia must be even rarer, possibly in the range of 1 in 75,000. The finding of sporadic aniridia in 1 of 73 patients with WT represents an incidence 1000 times greater than expected and points to a highly significant association. The aniridia–Wilms' tumor association (AWTA) has since become a known clinical syndrome with more than 50 patients reported until, in 1978, a small interstitial deletion of band 11p13 was found to be the underlying defect (Riccardi *et al.*, 1978). Three male patients were studied who had mental retardation, genitourinary abnormalities, and aniridia, and only one of them had WT. All of them had interstitial deletions of 11p that were nonidentical but partially overlapping. The only band shared by all the deletions was band 11p13 (Fig. 2). One patient (C) whose deletion extended into 11p12 also had lactate dehydrogenase A (LDH A) deficiency consistent with a gene dosage effect of this locus assigned to 11p12 (Francke *et al.*, 1977). The region respon-

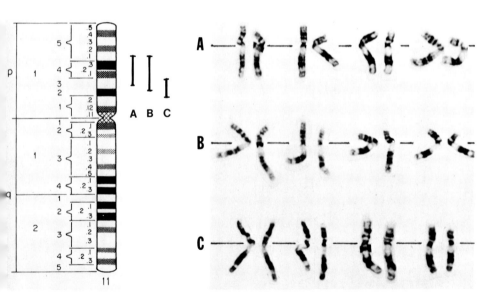

Fig. 2.   Four pairs of chromosome 11 from 3 male patients A, B, and C who had aniridia, genitourinary abnormalities, and mental retardation [AGR triad (Riccardi *et al.*, 1978)]; patient B had Wilms' tumor. The right members of each pair of chromosomes 11 have the deletion. Ideogram from U. Francke, *Cytogenet. Cell Genet.* **31,** 24 (1981), consistent with the 850 band stage of the International System for Human Cytogenetic Nomenclature (1981), shows extents of the three different deletions. Only band 11p13 is shared by all of them.

sible for the phenotype has been confirmed and more precisely defined in subsequent studies (Francke *et al.*, 1979; Yunis and Ramsay, 1980; Riccardi *et al.*, 1980).

In analogy to the findings in RB, many of the patients with AWTA and deletion 11p13 had *de novo* deletions, but several had unbalanced chromosomes inherited from a balanced translocation carrier, such as a t(8;11) translocation (Goedde-Salz and Behnke, 1981), a balanced shift within chromosome 11 (Hittner *et al.*, 1979), or an insertion of a very small part of 11p into a chromosome 2 (Yunis and Ramsay, 1980). One patient had a complex chromosome rearrangement, involving at least three breaks in chromosomes 8 and 11, which had been previously reported as resulting in a net deletion of 8p but was reinterpreted as showing a deletion of 11p (Francke *et al.*, 1979).

At this time 27 cases have been reported with aniridia and del 11p13 (Table III). Twelve of them had WT and two had gonadoblastoma (Anderson *et al.*, 1978; Turleau *et al.*, 1981). Genitourinary abnormalities, such as hypospadias, cryptorchidism, or ambiguous genitalia, were present in most of the 17 males. Mental retardation was reported in 23 of the 24 patients old enough to be assessed. The sex ratio of 17 males to 10 females may be biased by increased likelihood of ascertainment of males who had genitourinary abnormalities, in female patients the genitalia are less conspicuous. In a limited series of patients ascertained through the presence of aniridia, no sex difference was observed (Marshall *et al.*, 1982).

In contrast to RB, where the tumor is a uniform consequence of deletion 13q14, the development of WT is not a necessary consequence of deletion 11p13. This point has been illustrated by a pair of monozygous female twins with aniridia and 11p deletion of whom only one developed WT (Cotlier *et al.*, 1978; Maurer *et al.*, 1979; Riccardi *et al.*, 1980). The numbers observed are still close to the originally derived 33% risk for the development of WT in patients with sporadic aniridia.

TABLE III

Aniridia–Wilms' Tumor Association (AWTA) or Aniridia–Genitourinary Abnormalities–Retardation (AGR) Triad with Deletion 11p13[a]

Aniridia	27	Biochemical markers	
Wilms' tumor	12	↓ Catalase activity	6/6
Gonadoblastoma	2	↓ LDH A activity	4/11
Genitourinary abnormalities	12		
Retardation	23/24		

[a] Twenty-seven cases, 17 male and 10 female, including the 14 cases summarized by Gilgenkrantz *et al.* (1982), and those reported by De Grouchy *et al.* (1980), Jordania *et al.* (1981), Kousseff and Agatucci (1981), Waziri *et al.* (1981), Motegi (1981), and Marshall *et al.* (1982).

It is attractive to speculate that the lower penetrance of the autosomal dominant WT gene, as compared to the autosomal dominant RB gene, might be related to the lower risk for WT in deletion 11p13 cases as compared to the high risk for RB in deletion 13q14 cases. Using Knudson's model of the two separate mutations necessary for tumor formation, one may assume that in WT the second "hit" does not occur as regularly as in RB. This could be due to one of two possibilities: First, the locus is not as mutable, or, second, the number of cells that carry the first mutation and are available for "transformation" to tumor cells by the second mutation is smaller. With the population incidence of WT being slightly greater than the incidence of RB, and the relative proportion of hereditary versus nonhereditary cases estimated as being about the same, there is no evidence to support the notion that the *WT* locus is less susceptible to mutation.

In hereditary RB the number of available retinal cells that are susceptible to the second mutation is apparently greater than average mutation rates. This forms the basis for multiple tumors in gene carriers. In the case of WT, the number of developing renal parenchymal cells that are available for a second mutation is not clear. In the macroscopically normal kidneys of patients with familial or bilateral WT, lesions called "nodular renal blastema" may represent manifestations of the autosomal dominant WT gene (Machin, 1980). Such lesions are also found in normal infants less than 4 months of age, but they do persist in WT patients for years (reviewed in Knudson and Strong, 1972). Nodular renal blastema may represent cells arrested during differentiation that are susceptible to WT formation after a second mutational event.

IV. Enzyme Markers: Esterase D for 13q14 and Catalase for 11p13

In analogy to the localization of *esterase D* to the same chromosome band as RB, the locus for the enzyme catalase has been mapped to band 11p13 (Wieacker *et al.,* 1980; Junien *et al.,* 1980). In all six patients with AWTA and deletion 11p in whose blood cells or fibroblasts catalase activity has been measured, it was found to be 50% of normal. Excluding the possibility of a null allele by family studies, these results indicate a gene dosage effect due to loss of one allele coding for catalase. In contrast, LDH A activity was reduced in only four of eleven patients studied, consistent with the mapping of this locus to the more proximal band 11p12 (Francke *et al.,* 1977).

Therefore, quantitative measurements of esterase D and catalase activities can be used as screening tools in patients with RB or aniridia, respectively, in whom a deletion is suspected. If the enzyme activities are found to be low, chromosome studies will have to be done. On the other hand, if chromosomes were studied first and appeared normal, activity measurements of these enzymes will be useful in determining whether a small submicroscopic deletion of the respective chromosome band may be present. Therefore, the study of the respective enzyme marker is recommended as an integral part of the workup of patients presenting with RB or with aniridia, even in the absence of associated abnormalities or mental retardation. Dosage studies of tumor tissue in patients with normal constitutional enzyme activity levels could provide clues as to the nature of the somatic mutation (*vide infra*).

V. The Mechanism of Carcinogenesis in RB and WT

In considering possible mechanisms of carcinogenesis, one that is made attractive by recent research findings discussed in other chapters, invokes the *increased* expression of a normal gene. This increased expression may be brought about by one of the following mechanisms:

1. A point mutation in the coding region, leading to a gene product with increased activity or increased stability
2. A mutation (base change or deletion) in the 5' untranscribed control region, leading to an increased rate of transcription
3. Transposition of a normal gene under the control of an active promoter such as a viral LTR or immunoglobulin switch region leading to increased transcription
4. Gene amplification (i.e., increased numbers of gene copies) that may be associated with specific chromosome changes, such as homogeneously staining regions (HSRs) or double minutes (DM)

In all these mechanisms a single step mutation or translocation may lead to an altered phenotype that acts in a dominant fashion at the cellular level. That such altered genes can be biologically active has been shown by serial transfection and purification of transforming genes from human tumor cell lines that were subsequently found to be homologous to cellular oncogenes (reviewed by Cooper, 1982).

The observations in the two model systems of embryonic tumors, RB and WT, considered here cannot be explained by any of these mechanisms. A hypothesis, that is more suitable to explain the observed results, postulates *decreased* or *absent* expression of a normal gene: The function of a particular locus has to be completely abolished by two successive mutational steps that involve both homologous loci on both members of the homologous chromosome pairs. Mutational events that have been documented, or can be postulated, include the following:

1. A point mutation, leading to an absent or inactive gene product
2. A submicroscopic deletion, which may be present in a patient with RB and 50% esterase D activity but no detectable chromosome deletion

3. Inactivation (position effect) as demonstrated by the two female patients with t(X;13) translocations described above
4. An apparently balanced chromosome rearrangement, leading to a submicroscopic deletion, to disruption of a relevant DNA sequence, or to inactivation of the gene
5. A cytologically visible deletion, as has been documented in numerous cases with RB and del 13q, and AWTA and del 11p

Any initial event of the kind listed under 1 through 5 above that involves one member of a homologous chromosome pair will confer a *dominant* phenotype of tumor susceptibility, but it has to be followed by a second event, which involves the homologous locus on the other member of the chromosome pair, for the mutation to be expressed. If the first mutation is submicroscopic, the second may be a cytologically visible deletion. Cytogenetic studies on direct preparations from these embryonic tumors have, in fact, demonstrated the presence of a partially deleted chromosome 13 in a number of RB cases (Balaban–Malenbaum *et al.*, 1981). Similar studies on WT cells in individuals who had normal constitutional karyotypes have shown numerous changes in chromosome 11, involving deletions of the short arm, and one stem line has been found in which both chromosomes 11 were abnormal with breaks in both short arms (Slater and de Kraker, 1982).

The most elegant evidence in support of the above hypothesis comes from studies of an RB patient who had normal chromosomes and 50% esterase D activity in nontumor cells. Thus, the first mutational event may have been a submicroscopic deletion of part of band q14 in one chromosome 13. In the tumor itself, however, esterase D activity was zero, and one chromosome 13 was consistently missing. Most likely, loss of the normal chromosome 13 represented the "second hit" (Benedict *et al.*, 1983).

The hypothesis outlined above is entirely consistent with Knudson's "two hit" model for development of these embryonic tumors (Knudson, 1971; Knudson and Strong, 1972). However, I would like to stress that the 13q deletion form of RB is not a separate rare subgroup of the disorder but that there is a spectrum of possible genetic change that ranges from base changes, submicroscopic deletions, and gene disruption or inactivation by translocations or insertions, to cytologically visible deletion. All of these events can be biological substrates for the postulated "hits," either the first or the second. We may conclude that the embryonic heritable tumors, RB and WT, behave as dominant traits in the individual but as recessive traits in the cell.

As for aniridia, which is a consistent consequence of 11p13 deletion, the heterozygous deletion seems to act as basis for the dominant phenotype. The locus for another form of autosomal dominant aniridia has been provisionally assigned to chromosome 2 (Ferrell *et al.*, 1980).

Evidence in favor of the above hypothesis is stronger for RB than for WT. It is not known whether the *WT* locus resides on 11p. Linkage studies in autosomal dominant WT families have not yet been reported. Such studies are complicated by the reduced penetrance of the WT gene and the relatively recent occurrence of WT patients surviving to childbearing age. The map of the chromosome 11 short arm contains a large number of genes for which cloned DNA probes are available that detect restriction fragment length polymorphisms (Human Gene Mapping 6, 1982). These include β-, γ-, and δ-globin genes; the insulin gene; a polymorphic locus of unknown function; and the Harvey-*ras* 1 cellular oncogene (DeMartinville *et al.*, 1983). While none of the available polymorphic marker loci may have a direct relationship to the sequences involved in aniridia and WT predisposition, they should provide a series of useful markers for linkage studies in both WT and aniridia families.

Furthermore, patients with AWTA and small deletions of 11p13, patients with RB and small deletions of 13q14, and members of their families who have balanced rearrangements with breaks in the relevant bands provide very useful material for the identification of DNA sequences that map in the deleted region, via somatic cell hybridization, by chromosome sorting, or by *in situ* hybridization methods. Thus, the molecular and cellular genetic tools exist for a direct attack on the isolation and characterization of the genes responsible for these embryonic tumors.

VI. Delayed Mutation or Premutation

I would like to conclude with observations made in both WT and RB families that present one of the most intriguing problems in the study of human mutation, a problem that can be approached as soon as molecular probes are available.

For both WT (Cordero *et al.*, 1980) and RB (Herrmann, 1976; Bundey and Morten, 1981), families have been reported with multiple affected first or second cousins that are related through a common grandparent or great grandparent. The striking observation is the absence of affected individuals in the second generation that contains numerous gene carriers identified by their affected offspring (Fig. 3). Considering the high penetrance, particularly of the RB gene, these findings require an explanation by a different model. The hypothesis of premutation or delayed mutation (Auerbach, 1956) involves the existence of an unstable gene that individuals in generation II have inherited from one of their parents. This premutation does not lead to the tumor phenotype. In the following generation the premutated gene has been changed by the "telomutation" (Herrmann, 1976) which leads to tumors in offspring who inherit it. Occasionally, the first affected individual is found in the third generation, which leads one to postulate that the unstable premutation can be passed on as such. Once the tumor is expressed, the mutation behaves as a regular autosomal dominant trait in the

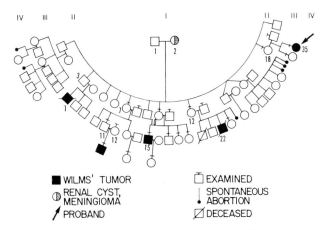

■ WILMS' TUMOR
◕ RENAL CYST, MENINGIOMA
✦ PROBAND
⬚ EXAMINED
SPONTANEOUS ABORTION
⬚ DECEASED

Fig. 3. Pedigree showing the occurrence of Wilms' tumor in five cousins with none of their parents being affected, consistent with the hypothesis of "premutation" or "delayed mutation." (From Cordero et al., Pediatrics **66**, 717, 1980; Copyright American Academy of Pediatrics.)

offspring of the affected individuals. The molecular correlate of the "premutation" remains unknown. Possibilities include transposition, inversion or some form of unstable arrangement at the DNA level. Given the fact that these families are rare, it seems worthwhile to obtain and store cells from gene carriers in the unaffected generation II as well as from their affected and unaffected offspring, in order to generate material for future molecular genetic studies.

Acknowledgments

I thank Drs. R. S. Sparkes, W. F. Benedict, and R. O. Howard for making available their manuscripts in press.

References

Anderson, S. R., Geertinger, P., Larsen, H. W., Mikkelsen, M., Parvings, A., Vestermark, S., and Warburg, M. (1978). *Ophthalmologica* **176**, 171–177.
Auerbach, C. (1956). *Ann. Hum. Genet.* **20**, 266–269.
Bader, J. L., Meadows, A. T., Zimmerman, L. E., Rorke, L. B., Voute, P. A., Champion, L. A., and Miller, R. W. (1982). *Cancer Genet. Cytogenet.* **5**, 203–213.
Balaban-Malenbaum, G., Gilbert, F., Nichols, W. W., Hill, R., Shields, J., and Meadows, A. T. (1981). *Cancer Genet. Cytogenet.* **3**, 243–250.
Benedict, W. F., Murphree, A. L., Banerjee, A., Spina, C., Sparkes, M. C., and Sparkes, R. S. (1983). *Science* **219**, 973–975.

114 UTA FRANCKE

Bundey, S., and Morten, J. E. N. (1981). *Hum. Genet.* **59**, 434–436.
Cooper, G. M. (1982). *Science* **218**, 801–806.
Cordero, J. F., Li, F. P., Holmes, L. B., and Gerald, P. S. (1980). *Pediatrics* **66**, 716–719.
Cotlier, E., Rose, M., and Moel, S. A. (1978). *Am. J. Ophthalmol.* **85**, 129–132.
Cross, H. E., Hansen, R. C., Morrow, G., and Davis, J. R. (1977). *Am. J. Ophthalmol.* **84**, 548–554.
Davison, E. V., Gibbons, B., Aherne, G. E. S., and Roberts, D. F. (1979). *Clin. Genet.* **15**, 505–508.
De Grouchy, J., Turleau, C., Cabanis, M. O., and Richardet, J. M. (1980). *Arch. Fr. Pediatr.* **37**, 531–535.
DeMartinville, B., Giacalone, J., Shih, C., Weinberg, R. A., and Francke, U. (1983). *Science* **219**, 498–501.
Ejima, Y., Sasaki, M. S., Kaneko, A., Tanooka, H., Hara, Y., Hida, T., and Kinoshita, Y. (1982a). *Clin. Genet.* **21**, 357–361.
Ejima, Y., Sasaki, M. S., Utsumi, H., Kaneko, A., and Tanooka, H. (1982b). *Mutat. Res.* **103**, 177–184.
Ferrell, R. E., Chakravarti, A., Hittner, H. M., and Riccardi, V. M. (1980). *Proc. Natl. Acad. Sci. U.S.A.* **77**, 1580–1582.
Francke, U. (1976). *Cytogenet. Cell Genet.* **16**, 131–134.
Francke, U., and Kung, F. (1976). *Med. Pediatr. Oncol.* **2**, 379–385.
Francke, U., George, D. L., Brown, M. G., and Riccardi, V. M. (1977). *Cytogenet. Cell. Genet.* **19**, 197–207.
Francke, U., Holmes, L. B., Atkins, L., and Riccardi, V. M. (1979). *Cytogenet. Cell Genet.* **24**, 185–192.
François, J., Matton, M. T., de Bie, S., Tanaka, Y., and Vandenbulcke, D. (1975). *Ophthalmologica* **170**, 405–425.
François, J., de Sutter, E., Coppieters, R., and de Bie, S. (1980). *Ophthalmologica* **181**, 93–99.
Gilgenkrantz, S., Vigneron, C., Gregoire, M. J., Pernot, C., and Raspiller, A. (1982). *Am. J. Med. Genet.* **13**, 39–49.
Goedde-Salz, E., and Behnke, H. (1981). *Eur. J. Pediatr.* **136**, 93–96.
Herrmann, J. (1976). *Birth Defects, Orig. Artic. Ser.* **XII**, No. 1, 79–90.
Hida, T., Kinoshita, Y., Matsumoto, R., Suzuki, N., and Tanaka, H. (1980). *J. Pediatr. Ophthalmol. Strabismus* **17**, 144–146.
Hittner, H. M., Riccardi, V. M., and Francke, U. (1979). *Ophthalmology (Rochester, Minn.)* **86**, 1173–1183.
Hittner, H. M., Riccardi, V. M., Kretzer, F. L., Levy, C. H., and Moura, R. A. (1980). *Doc. Ophthalmol.* **48**, 345–362.
Howard, R. O. (1982). *Birth Defects, Orig. Artic. Ser.* **18**, No. 6, 703–727.
Human Gene Mapping 6 (1982). *Cytogenet. Cell Genet* **32**, 1–334.
International System for Human Cytogenetic Nomenclature, ISCN (1981). *Cytogenet. Cell Genet.* **31**, 1–32.
Jacobs, P. A., Hunt, P. A., Mayer, M., and Bart, R. D. (1981). *Am. J. Hum. Genet.* **33**, 513–518.
Jordania, R. V., Kulagina, O. E., Buchny, A. E., and Sotnikova, E. N. (1981). *Genetika (Moscow)* **XVII**, 1315–1317.
Junien, C., Turleau, C., de Grouchy, J., Said, R., Rethore, M. O., Tenconi, R., and Dufier, J. L. (1980). *Ann. Genet.* **29**, 165–168.
Kantor, A. F., Li, F. P., Fraumeni, J. F., Jr., Curnen, M. G. M., and Flannery, J. T. (1982). *Med. Pediatr. Oncol.* **10**, 85–89.
Knight, L. A., Gardner, H. A., and Gallie, B. L. (1980). *Am. J. Hum. Genet.* **32**, 194–201.
Knudson, A. G., Jr. (1971). *Proc. Natl. Acad. Sci. U.S.A.* **68**, 820–823.

Knudson, A. G., and Strong, L. C. (1972). *J. Natl. Cancer Inst.* **48**, 313–324
Kousseff, B. G., and Agatucci, A. (1981). *J. Pediat. (St. Louis)* **98**, 676–678.
Lele, K. P., Penrose, L. S., and Stallard, H. B. (1963). *Ann. Hum. Genet.* **27**, 171–174.
Machin, G. A. (1980). *Amer. J. Pediatr. Hemat./Oncol.* **2**, 105–172, 253–301.
Marshall, L. S., Qureshi, A. R., DiGeorge, A. M., Kistenmacher, M. L., and Punnett, H. H. (1982). *Am. J. Hum. Genet.* **34**, 74A.
Matsunaga, E. (1980). *Hum. Genet.* **56**, 53–58.
Maurer, H. S., Pendergrass, T. W., Borges, W., and Honig, G. R. (1979). *Cancer (Philadelphia)* **43**, 295–308.
Miller, R. W., Fraumeni, J. F., and Mannin, M. D. (1964). *N. Engl. J. Med* **270**, 922–927.
Mohandas, T., Sparkes, R. J., and Shapiro, L. J. (1982). *Am. J. Hum. Genet.* **34**, 811–817.
Morten, J. E. N., Harnden, D. G., and Bundey, S. (1982). *J. Med. Genet.* **19**, 120–124.
Motegi, T. (1981). *Hum. Genet.* **38**, 168–173.
Motegi, T. (1982). *Hum. Genet.* **61**, 95–97.
Motegi, T., Komatsu, M., Nakazato, Y., Ohuchi, M., and Minoda, K. (1982). *Hum. Genet.* **60**, 193–195.
Nichols, W. W., Miller, R. C., Sobel, M., Hoffman, E., Sparkes, R. S., Mohandas, T., Veomett, I., and Davis, J. R. (1980). *Am. J. Ophthalmol.* **89**, 621–627.
Nove, J., Weichselbaum, R. R., Nichols, W. W., Albert, D. M., and Little, J. B. (1980). *Int. Ophthalmol. Clin.* **20**, 211–222.
Palmer, R. W., and Hulten, M. A. (1982). *J. Med. Genet.* **19**, 125–129.
Riccardi, V. M., Sujansky, E., Smith, A. C., and Francke, U. (1978). *Pediatrics* **61**, 604–610.
Riccardi, V. M., Hittner, H. M., Francke, U., Pippin, S., Holmquist, G. P., Kretzer, F. L., and Ferrell, R. (1979). *Clin. Genet.* **15**, 332–345.
Riccardi, V. M., Hittner, H. M., Francke, U., Yunis, J. J., Ledbetter, D., and Borges, W. (1980). *Cancer Genet. Cytogenet.* **2**, 131–137.
Rivera, H., Turleau, C., de Grouchy, J., Junien, C., Depoisse, S., and Zucker, J. M. (1981). *Hum. Genet.* **59**, 211–214.
Slater, R. M., and de Kraker, J. (1982). *Cancer Genet. Cytogenet.* **5**, 237–245.
Sparkes, R. S., Muller, H., and Klisak, I. (1979). *Science* **203**, 1027–1029.
Sparkes, R. S., Sparkes, M. C., Wilson, M. G., Towner, J. W., Benedict, W. F., Murphree, A. L., and Yunis, J. J. (1980). *Science* **208**, 1042–1044.
Sparkes, R. S., Murphree, A. L., Lingua, R. W., Field, L. L., Sparkes, M. C., Funderburk, S. J., and Benedict, W. F. (1983). *Science* **219**, 971–973.
Strong, L. C., Riccardi, V. M., Ferrell, R. E., and Sparkes, R. S. (1981). *Science* **213**, 1501–1503.
Turleau, C., de Grouchy, J., Dufier, J. L., Hoang-Phuc, L., Schmelck, P. H., Rappaport, R., Nihoul-Fekete, C., and Diebold, N. (1981). *Hum. Genet.* **57**, 300–306.
Vogel, F. (1979). *Hum. Genet.* **52**, 1–54.
Waziri, M., Patil, S. R., and Hanson, J. W. (1981). *Am. J. Hum. Genet.* **33**, 125A.
Weichselbaum, R. R., Zakov, Z. N., Albert, D. M., Friedman, A. H., Nove, J., and Little, J. B. (1979). *Ophthalmology (Rochester, Minn.)* **86**, 1191–1201.
Wieacker, P., Mueller, C. R., Mayerova, A., Grzeschik, K. H., and Ropers, H. H. (1980). *Ann. Genet.* **23**, 73–77.
Yunis, J. J., and Ramsay, N. (1978). *Am. J. Dis. Child.* **132**, 161–163.
Yunis, J. J., and Ramsay, N. K. C. (1980). *J. Pediatr. (St. Louis)* **96**, 1027–1030.

7

Chromosome Abnormalities and Gene Amplification: Comparison of Antifolate-Resistant and Human Neuroblastoma Cell Systems

JUNE L. BIEDLER,* PETER W. MELERA,†
AND BARBARA A. SPENGLER*

Memorial Sloan-Kettering Cancer Center
New York, New York

*Laboratory of Cellular and Biochemical Genetics.
†Laboratory of RNA Synthesis and Regulation.

CHROMOSOMES AND CANCER
117

I. Introduction

The first indication of gene amplification as a phenomenon occurring in somatic mammalian cells came from cytogenetic studies of experimentally derived sublines of Chinese hamster lung cells (CHL) with high levels of resistance to folic acid antagonists (Biedler and Spengler, 1976a,b). As revealed by the trypsin–Giemsa banding technique, the drug-resistant sublines with the greatest increases in target enzyme dihydrofolate reductase (DHFR) activity had long, nonbanding, uniformly staining chromosome segments that were not present in the antifolate-resistant sublines with lower enzyme levels. Such homogeneously staining regions (HSRs) were also observed to be consistent chromosomal features of several human neuroblastoma cell lines (Biedler and Spengler, 1976a,b). Thus it seemed that the HSRs were functionally involved with excessive production of DHFR in the drug-resistant cells and, for the human tumor lines, a protein(s) specific to malignant neuronal cells (Biedler and Spengler, 1976a). Following these initial reports it was demonstrated by molecular methods that in mouse S180 and L1210 cells overproduction of DHFR was paralleled by an increase in cellular concentration of DHFR-specific mRNA and an increase in the number of DHFR-encoding genes (Alt et al., 1978). Moreover, hybridization of radiolabeled DNA probe complementary to DHFR-specific mRNA to metaphase chromosomes in situ localized the amplified genes to the HSRs of drug-resistant Chinese hamster ovary (CHO) and mouse lymphoblastoid cells (Nunberg et al., 1978; Dolnick et al., 1979). There is now a considerable body of direct or strong circumstantial evidence that, in antifolate-resistant cells that overproduce the target enzyme, HSRs and their cytological counterparts, the small, acentric, chromatic segments known as double-minute chromosomes (DMs) as first reported by Kaufman et al. (1979), contain amplified DHFR genes.

But what is the significance of HSRs in human neuroblastoma cells that do not overproduce DHFR and are under no recognized selection pressure? The presence of this type of aberrant chromosome structure in cell lines established in culture from patients with neuroblastoma was soon confirmed in the laboratory of Balaban-Malenbaum and Gilbert (1977), who also postulated that DMs, present in a proportion of HSR-lacking cells of one of the tumor lines, appeared to be related structures. HSRs or large numbers of DMs are now known to be common features of human neuroblastoma cells lines (Biedler et al., 1979, 1980c; Balaban-Malenbaum and Gilbert, 1980) and to be relatively uncommon in other types of human tumor cells (reviewed by Biedler et al., 1983b). Nevertheless, the nature of the putatively amplified DNA sequences in neuroblastoma cells and whether or not they code for one or more gene products are presently unknown.

Homogeneously staining regions and DMs represent a relatively new class of chromosomal abnormality that is essentially different from well-known structural aberrations, such as deletions, translocations, or inversions, and numerical aberrations, such as monosomy and trisomy. This chapter will describe HSRs, DMs, and additional structural abnormalities that are the consequence of selective amplification of the DHFR gene and will assess and compare these structures with the types of aberrant structures that are particularly prevalent in human neuroblastoma cells. Although the biological significance of gene amplification-associated chromosomal abnormalities in the human tumor cells is not yet known, such an assessment may provide a background for new investigative approaches.

II. Dihydrofolate Reductase (DHFR) Gene Amplification in Antifolate-Resistant Cells

A. Cytological Manifestations of Amplified DHFR Genes

The first cytogenetic abnormality identified as signaling the presence of amplified DHFR genes was the HSR (Biedler and Spengler, 1976a); this observation was soon followed by the recognition that DMs also are distinct and prevalent indicators of DHFR gene amplification (Kaufman et al., 1979). More recent studies have demonstrated an even wider spectrum of amplification-related chromosomal abnormalities (Table I). From karyotype analyses of 17 antifolate-resistant Chinese hamster sublines generated independently by multistep exposure to methotrexate or methasquin, we observed that CHL sublines with increases in DHFR activity greater than 85-fold had HSRs, whereas those sublines with activity increases ranging from 3- to 50-fold had distinctive G banded regions with abnormal band patterns (Biedler et al., 1980b). Since both types of

TABLE I

Types of Abnormal Chromosome Structures Associated with DHFR Gene Amplification in Antifolate-Resistant Cells

Chromosomal abnormality	Reference
HSR (homogeneously staining region)	Biedler and Spengler (1976a)
DMs (double minute chromosomes)	Kaufman et al. (1979)
ABR (abnormally banding region)	Biedler et al. (1980b)
Banded fragments	Bostock and Tyler-Smith (1981)
Homogeneously staining chromosomes	Bostock and Tyler-Smith (1981)
Homogeneously staining rings or ring HSRs	Bostock and Tyler-Smith (1981)

abnormality were preferentially located on the long (q) arm of Chinese hamster chromosome 2 and since the HSRs of methotrexate-resistant CHO cells had indeed been shown to comprise amplified DHFR genes (Nunberg *et al.*, 1978), it was reasonble to conclude that both types of abnormally banding regions were the consequence of DHFR gene amplification. As described further in Section II,B, we now have direct evidence that the abnormally banding regions, here termed ABRs, of the CHL cells with low levels of target enzyme overproduction are, like HSRs, the sites of amplified DHFR genes (Biedler, 1982; Lewis *et al.*, 1982). Figure 1 illustrates the three types of abnormalities mentioned so far: HSRs, ABRs, and DMs (Table I).

As previously discussed and illustrated (Biedler *et al.*, 1980b), there is not always a sharp distinction between HSRs and ABRs. In certain of the antifolate-resistant CHL lines the HSRs are consistently homogeneous in staining quality. The HSRs of other sublines contain fine or indistinct interstitial bands, which are constant in location for any one subline, and are sometimes bordered by one or a few distinctive but nonidentifiable G-positive or G-negative bands. Others have likewise described various degrees of banding of the nonetheless comparatively homogeneously staining abnormal chromosome regions in DHFR-overproducing cells (Bostock *et al.*, 1979; Berenson *et al.*, 1981; Milbrandt *et al.*, 1981). The ABRs of CHL cells with low levels of DHFR overproduction occasionally have, on the other hand, subregions that are HSR-like insofar as they stain with an intermediate intensity and are larger than any of the ''mid-gray'' bands normally present in Chinese hamster chromosomes (Biedler *et al.*, 1980b). In general, long chromosomal segments that are moderately or very homogeneous in appearance, i.e., HSRs, are found in antifolate-resistant cells with large increases in DHFR activity and corresponding increases in DHFR gene copy number, whereas abnormally banding regions with strong but anomalous band patterns, i.e., ABRs, are found in cells with comparatively low levels of enzyme activity and DHFR gene amplification. This was particularly evident in our CHL cell system (Biedler *et al.*, 1980b), as shown for the representative sublines included in Table II.

The detection of ABRs in low enzyme lines (see Table II) was facilitated by the fact that the readily detectable HSRs were located on chromosome 2q in most of the sublines with high DHFR levels. We thus focused our attention on this chromosome arm for the eight sublines with less than 85-fold increases in DHFR and, in G banded cells of adequate quality, were able to discern the specific, abnormally banded regions. It appears likely that ABRs, if present, would not be readily identifiable as such in antifolate-resistant sublines with less than about 50-fold increases in DHFR activity or in cells with a considerable degree of structural chromosome rearrangement, e.g., CHO cells and various heteroploid mouse and human cell lines, or when occurring as a (nonspecific) result of drug exposure.

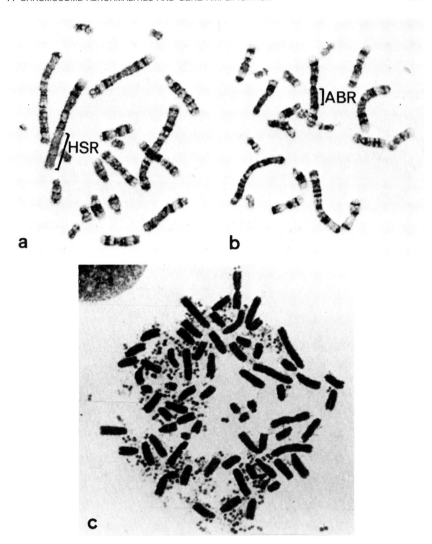

Fig. 1. Amplification-associated cytogenetic abnormalities of antifolate-resistant Chinese hamster and mouse cells stained by trypsin–Giemsa (a) and (b) or conventional (c) techniques. (a) DC-3F/Ab-17 cell with a 281-fold increase in DHFR activity. Bracket delineates the HSR on chromosome 2q. (b) DC-3F8/A55 cell with low level gene amplification (Table II) has an abnormally banding region (ABR) (bracket). The ABR-containing marker chromosome 2 also exhibits a paracentric inversion in the short arm. (c) Antifolate-resistant mouse MAZ/A/MQ60 cell with large numbers of frequently large sized double-minute chromosomes (DMs).

TABLE II

Antifolate-Resistant Chinese Hamster Lung Cell Sublines

Cell line	Relative DHFR activity[a]	Relative DHFR gene copy no.[b]	Abnormal chromosome region[c]		
			Type	Location	Relative length
DC-3F	1	1	None		
DC-3F/MQ10	2.9	6	ABR	2q	0.74
DC-3F/MQ31	3.9	6	ABR	2q	2.2
DC-3F8/A55	4.6	2	ABR	2q	0.62
DC-3F/MQ20	49	40	ABR	2q	2.0
DC-3F/MQ8	144		HSR	2q	0.92
DC-3F/MQ19	151	120	HSR	2q	1.1
DC-3F/A3	170	53	HSR	2q	0.97
A3-P Revertant	18	7	None		
DC-3F/Ab-17	281		HSR	2q	1.0

[a] Data from Biedler *et al.* (1972, 1978, 1980b).
[b] Data from Melera *et al.* (1980) and Lewis *et al.* (1982).
[c] Data from Biedler *et al.* (1980b).

Double-minute chromosomes, rarely observed in DHFR-overproducing Chinese hamster cells, are often the major gene amplification-related abnormality of methotrexate-resistant mouse sublines (e.g., Kaufman *et al.*, 1979; Bostock and Tyler-Smith, 1981; Brown *et al.*, 1981; Martinsson *et al.*, 1982; Biedler *et al.*, 1983a) and human sublines (Masters *et al.*, 1982). However, there are also other chromosome anomalies found in mouse cells, either in addition to or in place of DMs (Biedler *et al.*, 1980a; Bostock and Tyler-Smith, 1981).

The variety of abnormal chromosome structures that may occur in cells with amplified DFHR genes is exemplified by the findings of Bostock and Tyler-Smith (1981) for five different methotrexate-resistant mouse lymphoma lines. In addition to the near-diploid complement of chromosomes characterizing drug-sensitive control cells, resistant cells had one or more of the types of abnormal chromosome structures listed in Table I. Cells of one subline, for example, were characterized by the presence of a variable number (mean, 42.8) of acentric fragments which were banded following trypsin–Giemsa staining. Cells of another subline contained usually seven homogeneously staining subtelocentric chromosomes. Several sublines comprised some proportion (7 to 48%) of cells with homogeneously staining ring chromosomes with no apparent centromere or pericentric heterochromatin. Variable numbers of DMs, with mean numbers per cell ranging from 44 to 63, were also observed in several sublines and were not usually present in cells with one or another of the other types of aberrant chromosome structures. These sublines were selected at extremely high concentrations of methotrexate (0.5 and 1.0 mg/ml) and showed high increases in DHFR activity (886- to 5800-fold) and in number of DHFR genes (825- to 1360-fold) (Tyler-Smith and Alderson, 1981). Thus, high levels of DHFR gene amplification were associated with large numbers of abnormal structures, such as DMs, banded fragments, and homogeneously staining chromosomes, and newly observed, somewhat bizarre forms, such as the fragments and homogeneously staining rings.

A notable feature of methotrexate- and methasquin-resistant cells with high levels of DHFR overproduction is that the resistant phenotype tends to be unstable when cells are grown in absence of drug. In studies of DM-containing antifolate-resistant sublines (e.g., Kaufman et al., 1981; Biedler et al., 1983a), drug resistance, DHFR activity, or amplified gene number declined in magnitude as the acentric DMs progressively declined in number, probably through unequal segregation of DMs and selective advantage of cells with lower numbers of DMs. Our studies indicate that, in absence of drug, HSRs also are unstable structures that break down gradually and are lost from the cell (Biedler et al., 1980b, 1983a). Comparison of reversion patterns of DM- and HSR-containing cells (Biedler et al., 1983a) indicated that although the resistant phenotype in cells where the amplified genes are contained on an HSR rather than on extrachromosomal DMs may have had greater short-term stability and/or a somewhat slower rate of reversion in absence of drug selection pressure, resistance eventually and progressively declined in both types of cells. Thus the distinction between HSRs as indicators of stably amplified genes and DMs as indicators of unstably amplified genes (e.g., Nunberg et al., 1978; Haber and Schimke, 1981) is not a sharp one. On the other hand, ABR-containing cells with low numbers of amplified genes (Lewis et al., 1981; Biedler et al., 1983a), methotrexate-resistant S180 R_1C cells with 50 amplified genes distributed in clusters among 1–3 chromosomes (Kaufman et al., 1981), and revertant cells retaining low level resistance, DHFR activity, and gene amplification (Biedler et al., 1980b; Melera et al., 1980) appear to be phenotypically stable. Thus, whereas integration of large numbers of tandemly duplicated genes and associated DNA sequences results in a somewhat unstable HSR, chromosomal integration of relatively low numbers of amplified genes results in a seemingly stable chromosome structure.

B. Chromosomal Location of Amplified DHFR Genes

As noted in Section II,A, our studies of resistance to antifolate associated with overproduction of target enzyme DHFR have been carried out principally with 17 Chinese hamster lines independently selected with either methasquin or methotrexate. Only those CHL sublines with DHFR activity increases greater than 100-fold had HSRs, usually present on Chinese hamster chromosome 2q (Biedler et al., 1974; Biedler and Spengler, 1976a,b; Biedler et al., 1980b), whereas

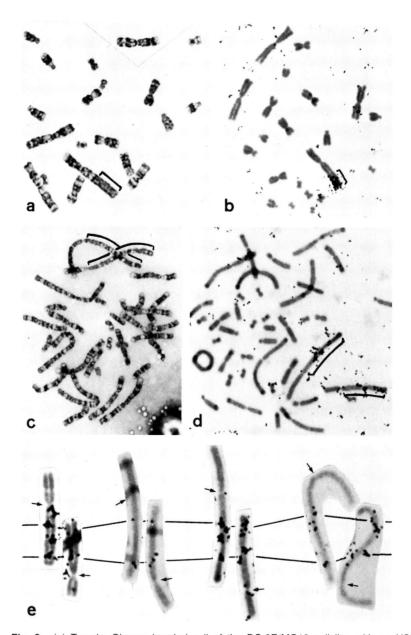

Fig. 2. (a) Trypsin–Giemsa banded cell of the DC-3F/MQ19 cell line with an HSR terminally located on a chromosome 2q (bracket). (b) DC-3F/MQ19 cell hybridized *in situ* with Chinese hamster DHFR-specific pDHFR6 probe. Hybridization was with 67 ng/ml ^{125}I-labeled probe, specific activity of 9×10^8 dpm/μg, for 18 hours at 37°C in 50% formamide, $4\times$ SSC, 10% dextran sulfate; exposure time, 1 month. The HSR (bracket) is heavily and apparently uniformly labeled. (c) Trypsin–Giemsa banded cell of the ABR-containing DC-3F/MQ20 cell line. Brackets indicate the two ABRs. (d) DC-3F/MQ20 cell hybridized with

sublines with less than 85-fold increases in DHFR activity contained ABRs which also were preferentially located on a single chromosome 2q homolog (Biedler *et al.*, 1980b), as exemplified by the data of Table II. These observations and the involvement of chromosome 2q in the methotrexate-resistant CHO line described by Nunberg *et al.* (1978) implicate this chromosome as the carrier of the native DHFR gene(s). Mapping studies likewise implicate chromosome 2 as the native gene site (Roberts *et al.*, 1980; Worton *et al.*, 1981).

In view of this evidence it is interesting to consider the instances where HSRs and ABRs have been found on chromosomes other than No. 2. Among the 15 antifolate-resistant CHL lines with HSRs and/or ABRs (Biedler *et al.*, 1980b), 11 had abnormal regions exclusively on chromosome 2q whereas four sublines had HSRs or ABRs on one or two of four different chromosome arms. Likewise the highly resistant CHO cells described by Milbrandt *et al.* (1981) contained an estimated 700–1000 DHFR genes that were shown by chromosome banding analysis and/or *in situ* hybridization studies to be distributed on three different chromosomes not including chromosome 2 and not corresponding to the HSR and ABR sites of our CHL lines. Although one explanation of these results is that Chinese hamster cells contain a number of DHFR genes located on five different chromosomes at least, a more reasonable explanation is that the amplifying DHFR genes can undergo chromosomal relocation. Therefore, HSR or ABR location may not be an accurate indicator of the permanent location of a gene.

Another line of evidence suggesting that DHFR genes may not amplify *in loco* comes from karyotype analysis of our antifolate-resistant CHL lines. As discernible from the illustrations of the HSRs and ABRs of these sublines (Biedler *et al.*, 1980b) and as described in part in several reports (Biedler *et al.*, 1980c; Biedler, 1982), both HSRs and ABRs are located at many different sites along the 2q arm. Although consistent within any one subline or subpopulation, the abnormal regions characterizing the various cell lines were found in at least 13 different locations as estimated from standard G banded cells. Among a total of 13 bands identified on the 2q arm, from band 1 proximal to the centromere and to terminal band 13, only three (bands 10–12) did not have an HSR or ABR sited either somewhere within a band or at its interface with another band (Biedler, 1982). The nonuniform location of HSRs and ABRs on chromosome 2q again suggests either that there is a family of DHFR genes distributed along the q arm or, more likely, amplification of the DHFR gene did not occur *in loco*.

---

[125]I-labeled Chinese hamster DHFR probe. Clusters of silver grains overlie both ABRs. Exposure time, 2 months. (e) Pairs of ABR-containing marker chromosomes from four different DC-3F/MQ20 cells hybridized with Chinese hamster DHFR probe. Within pairs, chromosomes are positioned so as to align band patterns of the ABRs; arrows indicate centromeres. Silver grains indicate clusters of DHFR genes at at least two distinct sites in each ABR. The relative positions of the clusters are similar both between the two ABR "homologues" in any one cell and between cells.

In continuing investigations in our laboratory, published in brief (Biedler, 1982; Biedler et al., 1983a), we have obtained direct evidence that the HSRs of our antifolate-resistant CHL lines are the sites of the amplified DHFR genes demonstrated by Melera et al. (1980). The recombinant plasmid pDHFR6 containing a 650 bp Chinese hamster DHFR cDNA insert (Lewis et al., 1981) was used as a molecular probe in in situ hybridization studies. As illustrated in Fig. 2a and b, the amplified DHFR genes of DC-3F/MQ19 cells (Table II) are located at least predominantly in the HSR.

More interesting questions, however, have been whether the ABRs of sublines with relatively low levels of DHFR overproduction are indeed sites of DHFR genes, as originally surmised (Biedler et al., 1980b), and how the sometimes greater length of the ABR in cells with low DHFR levels and presumably low numbers of amplified gene copies could be reconciled with the relatively shorter length of the HSR in cells with high DHFR levels and gene copy numbers (Table II). The hybridization kinetic data reported by Lewis et al. (1982) indicate that ABR-containing DC-3F/MQ10, DC-3F/MQ31, and DC-3F8/A55 cells contain two- to sixfold increases in DHFR gene copy numbers relative to control DC-3F cells. When nick-translated pDHFR6 was used as probe in hybridization of DNA to metaphase chromosomes in situ, clusters of grains were found over chromosome regions corresponding to the ABRs of both DC-3F/MQ10 and DC-3F8/A55 cells (Lewis et al., 1981) (DC-3F/MQ31 cells were not tested).

More recently we have focused attention on the DC-3F/MQ20 subline (Table II) which is estimated to have a 40-fold increase in DHFR gene copy number (a revised calculation) and similar increases in DHFR activity and DHFR-specific mRNA (Melera et al., 1980). Cells of this near-tetraploid subline initially possessed one ABR-bearing, structurally rearranged chromosome 2 with a relatively long ABR (Biedler et al., 1980b; Table II) but currently contain two ABR-bearing chromosomes which are nearly identical with respect to the (abnormal) banding pattern of the ABR but differ in other regions of the chromosome (Fig. 2c). Initial in situ hybridization experiments utilizing pDHFR6 as probe gave evidence of discrete clusters of silver grains within the unusually long ABR (Biedler, 1982), and recent experiments indicated that the clustering effect was manifested by both HSRs, as illustrated in Fig. 2d, even after prolonged radio-autographic exposure times (4 to 5 months). When the hybridized ABR-bearing chromosomes are aligned according to band positions gauged from banding patterns and centromere position in G banded cells, considerable correspondence in position of grain clusters along ABRs both within and between cells is discernible (Fig. 2e). These results suggest strongly that ABRs do not simply contain tandemly repeated units of DNA (amplified DHFR genes and associated DNA sequences) as are thought to compose HSRs. These preliminary findings suggest that, assuming that the DHFR gene(s) is located on Chinese hamster chromosome 2q, initial amplification of the gene may occur extrachromosomally (by a copy or excision process) and the amplified sequences are then reintegrated into the chromosome(s), generally at or near the site of the native gene.

C. Extrachromosomal DHFR Gene Amplification Model

All of the independently derived antifolate-resistant Chinese hamster sublines under study in our laboratories have their amplified DHFR genes integrated into chromosomes and usually into only one homologue per diploid chromosome complement. We have observed DMs only rarely, even in phenotypically unstable cells undergoing selection or reversion in absence of drug. Similarly, methotrexate-resistant Chinese hamster sublines developed in other laboratories also have amplified DHFR genes in a chromosomal rather than extrachromosomal location (Nunberg *et al.*, 1978; Milbrandt *et al.*, 1981). These findings contrast with those for antifolate-resistant mouse cells, which most frequently appear to carry amplified DHFR genes on extrachromosomal DMS (e.g., Kaufman *et al.*, 1979; Bostock and Tyler-Smith, 1981), although a substantial number of mouse sublines comprising cells with HSRs (or ABRs) have also been identified (e.g., Dolnick *et al.*, 1979; Bostock and Tyler-Smith, 1981). The basis for this apparent species difference is not known. However, our data suggest that the process of amplification of DHFR and associated DNA sequences may not appreciably differ in HSR-containing CHL versus DM-containing mouse cells, but that Chinese hamster cells have a greater tendency for reinsertion of extrachromosomally amplified sequences. Several observations, as described in the previous section, support this notion:

1. Among our antifolate-resistant CHL sublines, HSRs and ABRs are sometimes located on chromosomes other than chromosome 2q, the putative site of the native DHFR gene(s). A reasonable explanation is that the initially extrachromosomal amplification unit (possibly a DM) reintegrates at a site that is distant from the native DHFR gene and amplification proceeds in the new location. An alternative explanation is chromosomal translocation of HSRs and ABRs during the selection process.

2. HSRs and ABRs are positioned at many different sites along chromosome 2. DHFR genes or gene sets with associated DNA, comprising the unit of amplification, are initially and transiently extrachromosomal, but become rapidly integrated into a 2q chromosome at a site near but not necessarily at the site of the native DHFR gene(s) (Biedler, 1982).

3. In the ABR-containing CHL cells with demonstrably very low DHFR gene copy numbers, the sometimes long regions with strong but abnormal band patterns suggest multiple insertions of DHFR gene and other amplified sequences (Lewis *et al.*, 1982). The observation of DHFR gene clusters on chromosome 2q of DC-3F/MQ20 cells (Fig. 2d and e) support this notion. These data, too, are

consistent with the idea that the amplified genes undergo an extrachromosomal phase and are reinserted into the chromosome.

III. Cytogenetics of Human Neuroblastoma Cells

A. Chromosomal Evidence of DNA Sequence Amplification

In a line of investigation initially unrelated to cell genetic studies of antifolate resistance, we established in cell culture and characterized four tumor lines from three patients with the diagnosis of neuroblastoma (Biedler *et al.*, 1973, 1978). Neuroblastoma is the most common solid tumor of children and arises from cells that form the adrenal medulla and sympathetic nervous system. It is a highly malignant tumor, one in which, however, spontaneous regression may occur in a small proportion of cases, and is essentially refractory to therapeutic control. Prior to 1973 only two continuous lines of human neuroblastoma cells had been established (Goldstein, 1968; Tumilowicz *et al.*, 1970). However, since that time, in addition to the lines SK-N-SH, SK-N-MC, SK-N-BE(1), and SK-N-BE(2) that were established at our institution, over 25 cell lines have been described in the literature (reviewed by Biedler *et al.*, 1983b). Upon reanalysis of our four lines as well as the IMR-32 line of Tumilowicz *et al.* (1970) with banding techniques, we found that SK-N-BE(2) and IMR-32 cells contained HSRs (Biedler and Spengler, 1976a,b). In G banded cells the HSRs characterizing the SK-N-BE(2) line are particularly homogeneous in appearance, thereby resembling strikingly the HSRs of certain of the DHFR-overproducing Chinese hamster sublines (Biedler and Spengler, 1976a,b). All of the near-diploid SK-N-BE(2) cells examined had one or two HSRs as a constant feature. Near-diploid IMR-32 cells had two apparently identical No. 1 chromosomes with an HSR on the short arm as well as a normal chromosome 1. Subsequent reports of new human neuroblastoma cell lines from three other laboratories provided substantiation and additional evidence for the frequent presence of HSRs in cells of this tumor type. Pseudodiploid CHP-134 and CHP-126 cells were found to contain one and two HSRs, respectively, whereas cells of the hypotetraploid NMB line had two to three HSR-bearing chromosomes (Balaban-Malenbaum and Gilbert, 1977). Seeger *et al.* (1977) reported that a large acrocentric marker chromosome, the entire length of which stained homogeneously, was present in 92% of hypotetraploid LA-N-1 cells. Recent studies in our laboratory have demonstrated that LA-N-1 cells now contain 1-3 HSRs (Fig. 3a). Brodeur *et al.* (1977, 1981) has described two near-diploid lines, NGP and NCG, with one HSR per cell.

Balaban-Malenbaum and Gilbert (1977) made the important observation that the CHP-126 line comprised two cell populations, one with an HSR on a chromosome 5 homolog and no DMs, the other with variable numbers of DMs and

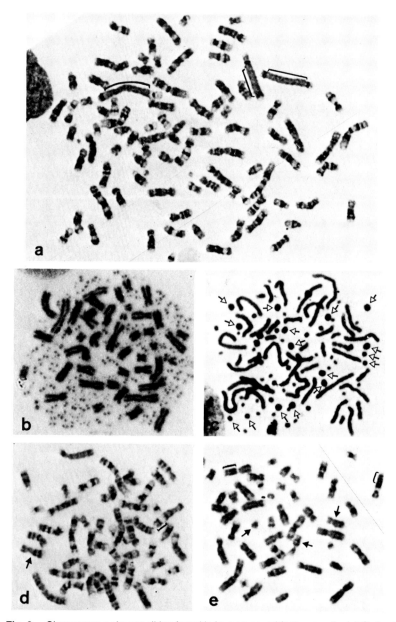

Fig. 3. Chromosome abnormalities found in human neuroblastoma cells. (a) Cells of the LA-N-1 cell line contain multiple, long HSRs on one to three different chromosomes and no DMs. (b) and (c) Cells of the CHP-234 line, stained by conventional techniques, are characterized by large numbers of DMs (b), and/or by the presence of ring chromosomes (arrows) (c). (d) SK-N-SH cells have one chromosome 9 homolog with a distinctive banded segment (bracket) distal to band 9q34 that cannot be identified even in high resolution banding preparations; the arrow indicates a normal chromosome 9. (e) SMS-KANR cells, likewise, have several possible ABRs. Cells of this line do not yield high quality metaphase preparations. Segments located on chromosomes 11q and 13p (brackets) and on three as yet unidentifiable marker chromosomes (arrows) may be ABRs.

normal No. 5 chromosomes. Since HSR- and DM-containing cells shared several structurally abnormal marker chromosomes, it was concluded that the DMs of CHP-126 cells originated from the HSR. Several findings in our laboratory also suggest a relationship between the two types of aberrant chromosome structures, HSRs and DMs. For example, when examined initially, about 70% of SK-N-MC cells had DMs. The frequency of DM-containing cells in this line declined with time in culture (Biedler *et al.*, 1973), and some years later DMs were no longer observed; however, most cells now had short HSRs (Biedler *et al.*, 1980c). Likewise, the SK-N-BE(1) line, the first of two established from the same patient (Biedler *et al.*, 1978), exhibits 10 to 50 DMs per cell, whereas the subsequently isolated SK-N-BE(2) line has HSRs and no DMs; shared marker chromsomes again indicate a common cellular origin of these lines (Biedler *et al.*, 1979). Still another line, designated NAP, initially consisted of cells containing large numbers of DMs (Biedler *et al.*, 1980c). After 3 years of continuous cultivation, most cells were observed to have one or two HSRs and no DMs. These various karyotypic observations suggest that in any one neuroblastoma cell line with both HSR- and DM-containing cells (HSRs and DMs are not usually found together in the same cell), the two types of chromosomal abnormality are alternative cytological manifestations of the same underlying phenomenon. Moreover, the progression from DMs to HSRs or to multiple HSRs suggest that, as in antifolate-resistant cells, HSRs appear to provide selective advantage and/or greater phenotypic stability.

As noted earlier, the HSRs of the neuronal tumor cells tend to stain uniformly, i.e., there is little indication of interstitial banding, and resemble the HSRs of many antifolate-resistant Chinese hamster and mouse cells. The HSRs characterizing the two unrelated systems are similar in other respects as well. Analysis of chromosome replication patterns demonstrated that HSRs of SK-N-BE(2) cells, like those of several resistant CHL sublines, begin replication early and at many sites synchronously and complete replication by the midpoint of the S phase (Biedler and Spengler, 1976a,b). This result is consistent with the idea that the HSRs in SK-N-BE(2) cells, like those of the drug-resistant hamster cells, are regions of transcriptional activity. Another point of similarity between the HSRs of the two different cell systems, to be detailed elsewhere (Biedler *et al.*, submitted), is HSR length. For antifolate-resistant CHL and human neuroblastoma sublines (with the exception of SK-N-MC), HSR length relative to the total length of the autosomal diploid chromosome complement ranges from 3 to 6%.

We have recently and systematically examined 16 neuroblastoma lines, established *in vitro* from 13 patients, for the presence of HSRs and DMs (Table III). Five of these lines comprised HSR-containing cells at one or another time in their culture history, whereas 11 lines had only DM-containing cells or initially contained DMs and, later, HSRs (Biedler *et al.*, 1980c, 1983b). Only two lines, SK-N-SH and SMS-KANR, have never displayed either HSRs or DMs. In contrast

TABLE III

Gene Amplification-Associated Chromosome Abnormalities in Human Neuroblastoma Cell Lines[a]

Cell line	Prior therapy[b]	Chromosomal abnormality		
		HSRs	DMs	Possible ABRs
SK-N-SH	RT, CT	−	−	+
SK-N-MC	RT, CT	+	+	−
SK-N-BE(1)	None	−	+	−
SK-N-BE(2)	RT, CT	+	−	−
IMR-32	None	+	−	+
NAP		+	+	+
LA-N-1	CT	+	−	+
LA-N-2	None	−	+	−
CHP-212	None	−	+	−
CHP-234	None	−	+	+
SMS-KAN	None	−	+	−
SMS-KANR	CT	−	−	+
SMS-MSN	None	−	+	+
SMS-SAN	None	−	+	+
SMS-KCN	None	−	+	−
SMS-KCNR	CT	−	+	−

[a] Adapted from Biedler et al. (1979, 1980c, 1983b).
[b] RT, radiotherapy; CT, chemotherapy.

to the phenotypic instability of antifolate-resistant cells in absence of drug (Section II,A), HSRs and DMs of neuroblastoma cells are consistent and stable features, even though the human cells are under no known selective pressure.

A notable feature of DM-containing human neuroblastoma lines is that DMs, although variable in number, are found in all or most cells, are present often in high numbers (Fig. 3b and Table IV), and are sometimes unusually large in size (Biedler et al., 1980c, 1983b). In general, the human lines had mean numbers of DMs in a range similar to that found for methotrexate-resistant mouse tumor cells with high levels of DHFR activity and, where determined, with large increases in DHFR gene copy numbers (e.g., Kaufman et al., 1979; Bostock and Tyler-Smith, 1981). Two of the lines, SMS-KAN and SMS-MSN, however, were found to have on average more than 100 DMs per cell, comparable to antifolate-resistant cells with a mean number of DMs greater than 100, such as the human lines described by Masters et al. (1982) and our MAZ/A/MQ60 cells (Biedler et al., 1980a). In these instances the cells had correspondingly high DHFR levels indicative of a high degree of gene amplification. Whether particularly high numbers of DMs such as observed in SMS-KAN and SMS-MSN connote high

TABLE IV

Frequency of DMs and Homogeneously Staining Ring Chromosomes in Human Neuroblastoma Cells[a]

Cell line	Frequency of DM-positive cells (%)	Mean no. of DMs per cell ± SD	Frequency of cells with rings (%)
SK-N-MC	70	17 ± 21	0
SK-N-BE(1)	100	19 ± 16	0
NAP	99	50 ± 56	5
LA-N-2	100	48 ± 46	2
CHP-212	100	43 ± 39	ND[b]
CHP-234	100	44 ± 46	ND
SMS-KAN	100	162 ± 45	0
SMS-MSN	100	123 ± 125	ND
SMS-SAN	100	54 ± 80	ND
SMS-KCN	82	14 ± 13	ND
SMS-KCNR	100	22 ± 24	ND

[a] Adapted from Biedler et al. (1980c, submitted).
[b] ND, not determined.

levels of DNA sequence amplification or high numbers of active genes is not known at this time.

Neuroblastoma cells of several of the lines have been seen to contain ring chromosomes which, like the DMs, stain homogeneously and with an intermediate stain intensity (Fig. 3c and Biedler et al., 1979, 1980c). These structures resemble the homogeneously staining rings (or ring HSRs) often found in association with DMs in the highly methotrexate-resistant mouse lines described by Bostock and Tyler-Smith (1981) (see Section II,A).

Because of our observation of ABRs in antifolate-resistant Chinese hamster lines with low levels of DHFR overproduction (Biedler et al., 1980c), and the recent demonstration that these sublines have small numbers of amplified DHFR genes situated within these abnormally banding regions, we are attempting to detect possibly analogous regions in G-banded human neuroblastoma cells. Most (13/16) of the cell lines under study in our laboratory have modal chromosome numbers in the diploid range; in addition, some have only a few chromosomal translocations (Biedler et al., 1980c, 1983b). Thus it should be feasible to identify such anomalous regions in these cells. Eight of the lines have been found to have usually one or occasionally multiple regions with a clearly abnormal banding pattern (Table III). As illustrated in Fig. 3d and e, these putative ABRs are short as compared to most of those observed in antifolate-resistant CHL cells (Biedler et al., 1980c) and are not preferential in their chromosomal location.

However, HSRs of human neuroblastoma, unlike those of the drug-resistant hamster cells, are also not localized to one or even a few chromosomes (see Section III,B). Of possible significance is the finding that SMS-KANR cells (Fig. 3e) have several ABR-like regions. SMS-KAN cells, characterized by the presence of large numbers of DMs (Table IV), represent the first isolate from a patient before initiation of therapy; SMS-KANR cells, isolated from the same patient in clinical relapse after drug treatment, lack both DMs and HSRs. The presence of apparently identical structurally abnormal marker chromosomes indicates that both lines were derived from a common cell precursor. Since it is unusual for human neuroblastoma cells to have neither HSRs nor DMs, the question is whether the putative ABRs of SMS-KANR cells indeed signify chromosomally integrated, amplified DNA sequences.

B. Chromosomal Location of HSRs in Neuroblastoma Cells

As discussed in Section II,B, our studies of antifolate-resistant Chinese hamster cells have revealed that HSRs, and ABRs as well, are preferentially located on the long arm of Chinese hamster chromosome 2 (Biedler *et al.*, 1980b) and that amplified DHFR genes are localized to these abnormal regions (Biedler, 1982; Lewis *et al.*, 1982; Biedler *et al.*, 1983a). Thus it has been of interest to determine the chromosomal location of the HSRs of human neuroblastoma lines. A survey of lines maintained in our laboratory and/or described in the literature has not uncovered a preferential involvement of one or more chromosomes or chromosome arms (Table V). Several interpretations are possible. One is that the

TABLE V

Chromosomal Location of HSRs in Human Neuroblastoma Cells[a]

Cell line	Chromosome number and arm of HSR location	Reference
SK-N-BE(2)	4q; 6p; 10p; 19q	Biedler *et al.* (1980c)
SK-N-MC	19q	Biedler *et al.* (1980c)
IMR-32	1p	Biedler *et al.* (1980c)
NAP	7p	Biedler *et al.* (1980c)
LA-N-1	1p; 2p; 16q; 19p	Biedler *et al.* (1980c)
CHP-126	5q	Balaban-Malenbaum and Gilbert (1977)
CHP-134	6q; 7p	Balaban-Malenbaum and Gilbert (1977)
NMB	13p	Balaban-Malenbaum and Gilbert (1977)
NGP	4p; 13q	Brodeur *et al.* (1977)
NCG	16p	Brodeur *et al.* (1981)

[a] Found in 10% or more of cells examined.

HSRs of the ten different lines contain differing sets of DNA sequences or (putative) structural genes. Another is that only one or a small number of "basic" sequence sets of coding genes are amplified in the various lines and their chromosomal location is trivial. The latter situation is exemplified by the antifolate-resistant CHL lines that we have described (Section II,B) where HSRs and ABRs are occasionally located on chromosomes other than a 2q (Biedler *et al.*, 1980c). Furthermore, if amplified DNA sequences do undergo initially an extrachromosomal phase, as suggested by the results described in Sections II,B and C, and this phase is prolonged in the human cells, as suggested by the presence of DMs in many lines, then the amplified sequences of these human neuroblastoma cells may not be prone to reintegration at or near their original chromosomal site.

C. Molecular Evidence of DNA Sequence Amplification

The compelling evidence relating the occurrence of ABRs, HSRs, and DMs with the amplification of DNA sequences has spurred efforts to determine the nature of these putative sequences in human neuroblastoma cells that carry these chromosomal abnormalities. In attempts to identify HSR- and DM-associated gene products, we have extensively characterized human neuroblastoma cells for expression of neurotransmitter-synthesizing enzyme activities in several collaborative investigations (Biedler *et al.*, 1978; Ross *et al.*, 1980, 1981). All of the cell lines listed in Table III contain enzyme activities of adrenergic and/or cholinergic neurons; six of the lines expressed activities of both neuronal types (Ross *et al.*, 1981; Biedler *et al.*, 1983b). Moreover, the neurological phenotype was stable over a period of several years, as was the presence of HSRs or DMs. Nonetheless we have found no specific correlations between HSRs and DMs and amount or kind of neurotransmitter enzyme activity (Biedler *et al.*, 1979, 1980c).

In a different investigative approach we have utilized techniques of SDS–polyacrylamide and two-dimensional gel electrophoresis to look for putative protein products correlated with presence and/or number of HSRs and DMs in neuroblastoma and other types of cells (Biedler *et al.*, 1980c, 1983b), based on the observation that our DHFR-overproducing Chinese hamster and mouse cells display on gels a highly prominent band or spot corresponding in molecular weight and pI to DHFR (Biedler *et al.*, 1980a; Melera *et al.*, 1982). However, to date we have not discerned candidate proteins (Biedler *et al.*, 1980c, 1983b).

Since attempts to identify in these human tumor cells quantitative or qualitative changes in protein patterns that might indicate the amplification of a specific gene or set of genes have been unsuccessful, it has not been possible to purify specific mRNAs and clone their cDNAs for use as probes to carry out genomic analysis. As an alternative to this approach, we have prepared probes directly from genomic DNA that will eventually allow isolation of amplified DNA sequences from cloned libraries of neuroblastoma DNA and carried out some preliminary genomic analysis. The preparation of these probes (Montgomery *et al.*, 1983) relies on the kinetic properties of genomic DNA and assumes that sequences present in low or single copy amounts in nonneuroblastoma cells, if amplified in neuroblastoma cells, will be associated with the middle repetitive DNA fraction of those cells. Middle repetitive DNA ($C_o t$ 10–300) was therefore prepared via hydroxylapatite chromatography and, after removal of residual highly repetitive DNA by exhaustive hybridization against cellulose-bound total genomic DNA from control fibroblasts (Brison *et al.*, 1982), was nick-translated (Rigby *et al.*, 1977) and used to probe Southern transfers of neuroblastoma and nonneuroblastoma DNAs. The results of such an experiment are shown in Fig. 5. Middle repetitive DNA from the control human fibroblast line WI-38 was used to probe *Eco*RI digests of DNA from neuroblastoma lines CHP-234, NAP, and BE(2)-C as well as human placental and WI-38 DNA itself (Fig. 4a). Multiple bands ranging in size from 4 to 20 kb are evident in these blots, with no apparent

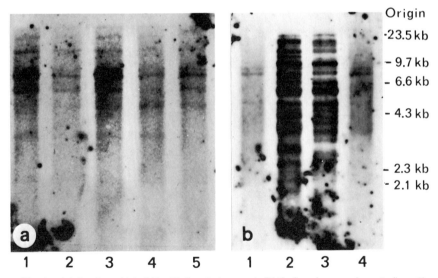

Fig. 4. (a) Southern blot of *Eco*RI digested genomic DNAs from human placenta (lane 1), CHP-234 (lane 2), NAP (lane 3) and BE(2)-C (lane 4) human neuroblastoma cells, and WI-38 human diploid fibroblasts (lane 5), probed with middle repetitive ($C_o t$ 10–300) DNA from WI-38 cells. (b) Southern blot of *Eco*RI digested genomic DNAs from WI-38 fibroblasts (lane 1), CHP-234 (lane 2), BE(2)-C (lane 3) neuroblastoma cells, and human placenta (lane 4), probed with CHP-234 neuroblastoma DNA ($C_o t$ 10–300). (From Montgomery *et al.*, 1983).

differences between the restriction patterns of the neuroblastoma and non-neuroblastoma cell lines. The approximately equal intensity of the bands between each line indicates that sequences reactive with the middle repetitive probe from control cells are present in similar concentrations in all cell types tested. When middle repetitive DNA from the neuroblastoma line CHP-234 is used to probe *Eco*RI digests of human placental and WI-38 DNA (Fig. 4b, lanes 1 and 4), the hybridization patterns appear generally as they do when control cell probe is used, although slight differences in specific band intensities suggest that the neuroblastoma probe may contain somewhat different sequence concentrations than those present in the control probe. That a remarkable difference in the sequence composition of the neuroblastoma probe does indeed exist is illustrated in Fig. 4b, lanes 2 and 3, in which *Eco*RI-digested neuroblastoma DNAs were hybridized with the middle repetitive neuroblastoma probe. The results show that neuroblastoma DNA contains a large number of *Eco*RI fragments whose concentration is much greater than in nonneuroblastoma DNA, indicating that DNA sequence amplification has occurred in these human tumor cells. A survey of several other neuroblastoma lines, as well as other nonneuroblastoma tumors, shows that amplification can be demonstrated in nearly all neuroblastoma cells that contain HSRs or DMs, whereas SK-N-SH cells, without these chromosomal aberrations, and nonneuroblastoma tumor cells, including the HSR containing COLO 321 line (Quinn *et al.,* 1979), do not show evidence of amplified sequences reactive with the middle repetitive probes from neuroblastoma cells (Montgomery *et al.,* 1983). Although the significance of these amplified neuroblastoma-specific sequences remains obscure, our ability to partially purify them should facilitate their further analysis via recombinant DNA methodology.

IV. Discussion

We have described the many cytological similarities between the gene amplification-associated abnormal chromosome structures of DHFR-overproducing antifolate-resistant Chinese hamster mouse and human cells and those found in human neuroblastoma cells. Although it is clear that the presence of HSRs and often large numbers of DMs is a widely prevalent feature of this type of human tumor, as represented by a large number of tumor lines in cell culture, the biological significance of DNA sequence amplification in human neuroblastoma is not yet known. Continuation of molecular approaches such as we have initiated and described for our system and such as those undertaken with other tumor systems (e.g., George and Powers, 1981, 1982; Atitalo *et al.,* 1983) should ultimately provide an understanding of the role of these amplification-associated abnormal chromosome structures in tumor cells.

Acknowledgments

These studies were supported by the NCI Core Grant CA-08748, NCI Grants CA-28679 and CA-31553, the Kleberg Foundation, and the Special Projects Committee of the Society of the Memorial Sloan-Kettering Cancer Center.

References

Alitalo, K., Schwab, M., Lin, S. C., Varmus, H. E.. and Bishop, J. M. (1983). *Proc. Natl. Acad. Sci. U.S.A.* **80**, 1707–1711.
Alt, F., Kellems, R. E., Bertino, J. R., and Schimke, R. T. (1978). *J. Biol. Chem.* **253**, 1357–1370.
Balaban-Malenbaum, G., and Gilbert, F. (1977). *Science* **198**, 379–741.
Balaban-Malenbaum, G., and Gilbert, F. (1980). *In* "Advances in Neuroblastoma Research" (A. E. Evans, ed.), pp. 97–107. Raven, New York.
Berenson, R. J., Francke, U., Dolnick, B. J., and Bertino, J. R. (1981). *Cytogenet. Cell Genet.* **29**, 143–152.
Biedler, J. L. (1982). *In* "Gene Amplification" (R. T. Schimke, ed.), pp. 39–45. Cold Spring Harbor Lab., Cold Spring Harbor, New York.
Biedler, J. L., and Spengler, B. A. (1976a). *Science* **191**, 185–187.
Biedler, J. L., and Spengler, B. A. (1976b). *J. Natl. Cancer Inst.* **57**, 683–695.
Biedler, J. L., Albrecht, A. M., Hutchison, D. J., and Spengler, B. A. (1972). *Cancer Res.* **32**, 153–161.
Biedler, J. L., Helson, L., and Spengler, B. A. (1973). *Cancer Res.* **33**, 2643–2652.
Biedler, J. L., Albrecht, A. M., and Spengler, B. A. (1974). *Genetics* **77**, s4–5.
Biedler, J. L., Roffler-Tarlov, S., Schachner, M., and Freedman, L. (1978). *Cancer Res.* **38**, 3751–3757.
Biedler, J. L., Spengler, B. A., and Ross, R. A. (1979). *Gaslini (Genoa)* **11**, 128–139.
Biedler, J. L., Chang, T. D., Meyers, M. B., Melera, P. W., and Spengler, B. A. (1980a). *Eur. J. Cell Biol.* **22**, 106.
Biedler, J. L., Melera, P. W., and Spengler, B. A. (1980b). *Cancer Genet. Cytogenet.* **2**, 47–60.
Biedler, J. L., Ross, R. A., Shanske, S., and Spengler, B. A. (1980c). *In* "Advancces in Neuroblastoma Research" (A. E. Evans, ed.), pp. 81–96. Raven, New York.
Biedler, J. L., Chang, T. D., Peterson, R. H. F., Melera, P. W., Meyers, M. B., and Spengler, B. A. (1983a). *In* "Rational Basis for Chemotherapy—UCLA Symposia" (B. A. Chabner, ed.), Vol. 4, pp. 71–92. Alan R. Liss, Inc., New York.
Biedler, J. L., Meyers, M. B., and Spengler, B. A. (1983b). *Adv. Cell. Neurobiol.* **4**, 268–307.
Biedler, J. L., Chang, T. D., Ross, R. A., and Spengler, B. A. Submitted.
Bostock, C. J., and Tyler-Smith, C. (1981). *J. Mol. Biol.* **153**, 219–236.
Bostock, C. J., Clark, E. M., Harding, N. G. L., Mounts, P. M., Tyler-Smith, C., van Heyningen, V., and Walker, P. M. B. (1979). *Chromosoma* **74**, 153–177.
Brison, O., Ardeshir, F., and Stark, G. R. (1982). *Mol. Cell. Biol.* **2**, 578–587.
Brodeur, G. M., Sekhon, G. S., and Goldstein, M. N. (1977). *Cancer (Philadelphia)* **40**, 2256–2263.
Brodeur, G. M., Green, A. A., Hayes, A. F., Williams, K. J., Williams, D. L., and Tsiatis, A. A. (1981). *Cancer Res.* **41**, 4678–4686.
Brown, P. C., Beverley, S. M., and Schimke, R. T. (1981). *Mol. Cell. Biol.* **1**, 1077–1083.
Dolnick, B. J., Berenson, R. J., Bertino, J. R., Kaufman, R. J., Nunberg, J. H., and Schimke, R. T. (1979). *J. Cell. Biol.* **83**, 394–402.

George, D. L., and Powers, V. E. (1981). *Cell* **24**, 117–123.

George, D. L., and Powers, V. E. (1982). *Proc. Natl. Acad. Sci. U.S.A.* **79**, 1597–1601.

Goldstein, M. N. (1968). *J. Pediatr. Surg.* **3**, 166–169.

Haber, D. A., and Schimke, R. T. (1981). *Cell* **26**, 355–362.

Kaufman, R. J., Brown, P. C., and Schimke, R. T. (1979). *Proc. Natl. Acad. Sci. U.S.A.* **76**, 5669–5673.

Kaufman, R. J., Brown, P. C., and Schimke, R. T. (1981). *Mol. Cell. Biol.* **1**, 1084–1093.

Lewis, J. A., Kurtz, D. T., and Melera, P. W. (1981). *Nucleic Acids Res.* **9**, 1311–1322.

Lewis, J. A., Biedler, J. L., and Melera, P. W. (1982). *J. Cell. Biol.* **94**, 418–424.

Martinsson, T., Tenning, P., and Levan, G. (1982). *Hereditas* **97**, 123–137.

Masters, J., Keeley, B., Gay, H., and Altardi, G. (1982). *Mol. Cell. Biol.* **2**, 498–507.

Melera, P. W., Lewis, J. A., Biedler, J. L., and Hession, C. (1980). *J. Biol. Chem.* **255**, 7024–7028.

Melera, P. W., Hession, C. A., Davide, J. P., Scotto, K. W., Biedler, J. L., Meyers, M. B., and Shanske, S. (1982). *J. Biol. Chem.* **257**, 12939–12949.

Milbrandt, J. D., Heintz, N. H., White, W. C., Rothman, S. M., and Hamlin, J. L. (1981). *Proc. Natl. Acad. Sci. U.S.A.* **78**, 6043–6047.

Montgomery, K. T., Biedler, J. L., Spengler, B. A., and Melera, P. W. (1983). *Proc. Natl. Acad. Sci. U.S.A.* (in press).

Nunberg, J. H., Kaufman, R. J., Schimke, R. T., Urlaub, G., and Chasin, L. A. (1978). *Proc. Natl. Acad. Sci. U.S.A.* **75**, 5553–5556.

Quinn, L. A., Moore, G. E., Morgan, R. T., and Woods, L. K. (1979). *Cancer Res.* **39**, 4914–4924.

Rigby, P. W. J., Dieckmann, M., Rhodes, C., and Berg, P. (1977). *J. Mol. Biol.* **113**, 237–251.

Roberts, M., Huttner, K. M., Schimke, R. T., and Ruddle, F. H. (1980). *J. Cell Biol.* **87**, 288a.

Ross, R. A., Joh, T. H., Reis, D. J., Spengler, B. A., and Biedler, J. L. (1980). *In* "Advances in Neuroblastoma Research" (A. E. Evans, ed.), pp. 151–160. Raven, New York.

Ross, R. A., Biedler, J. L., Spengler, B. A., and Reis, D. J. (1981). *Cell. Mol. Neurobiol.* **1**, 301–312.

Seeger, R. C., Rayner, S. A., Banerjee, A., Chung, H., Laug, W. E., Neustein, H. B., and Benedict, W. F. (1977). *Cancer Res.* **37**, 1364–1371.

Tumilowicz, J. J., Nichols, W. W., Cholon, J. J., and Green, A. E. (1970). *Cancer Res.* **30**, 2110–2118.

Tyler-Smith, C., and Alderson, T. (1981). *J. Mol. Biol.* **153**, 203–218.

Worton, R., Duff, C., and Flintoff, W. (1981). *Mol. Cell. Biol.* **1**, 330–335.

Chromosome Changes in Leukemic Cells as Indicators of Mutagenic Exposure

JANET D. ROWLEY

Section of Hematology/Oncology
The University of Chicago
Chicago, Illinois

CHROMOSOMES AND CANCER

I. Introduction

Nonrandom chromosome changes have been detected in a variety of human cancers. These changes have been studied in most detail in human acute non-lymphocytic leukemia (ANLL). These data can be used to consider the question of whether there are certain chromosome changes in human acute leukemia that are related to particular etiologic agents. A preliminary analysis of data from three groups of patients suggests that the answer may be yes. These groups are (1) patients who have acute leukemia secondary to therapy with cytotoxic drugs or radiation, (2) leukemic patients who have been occupationally exposed to potentially mutagenic agents, and (3) children who have ANLL. The data available for each of these groups will be reviewed in some detail and conclusions that appear tenable will be presented.

II. Cancers Induced in Experimental Animals

The identification of nonrandom chromosome abnormalities in human tumors has a counterpart in animal tumors. Murine leukemias have been studied extensively in the last few years, and consistent chromosome changes have been observed. Moreover, consistent changes found in lymphoid leukemias generally differ from those in myeloid leukemias, which is precisely the same observation made in human leukemia. The major findings in murine hematologic malignancies are summarized in this section. A more detailed review of cytogenetic studies in various animal cancers has recently been reported by Sasaki (1982).

A. Thymic (T Cell) Leukemia

Dofuku *et al.* (1975) were the first to describe the presence of an extra chromosome No. 15 (+15) in 10 of 11 leukemic AKR mice. This same chromosome abnormality has subsequently been described in the majority of mice with T cell leukemias induced by two different strains of the radiation leukemia virus (RadLV) (Weiner *et al.*, 1978a), by dimethylbenz[*a*]anthracene (DMBA) (Weiner *et al.*, 1978c; Chan, 1976), by benzpyrene (BP) (Chan, 1976), or by X rays (Chan, 1976; Chang, 1977). Trisomy 15 was also seen in all 11 CFW/D mice that developed leukemia after injection of endogenous murine leukemia virus (MuLV) isolated from DMBA-induced thymomas (Chan, 1976). Moreover, trisomy 15 was also noted in thymic cells, but not in cells from bone marrow or spleens obtained from mice injected with DMBA at birth and sacrificed at 80 or 110 days, prior to the development of leukemia (Chan, 1976). Weiner *et al.* (1978b) recently showed that in CBA mice homozygous for the T6 marker chromosome, which is a balanced translocation between Nos. 14 and 15, the distal portion of No. 15 was present in the trisomic state in DMBA-induced T cell leukemias. The selective advantage of leukemic cells with trisomy 15 was further demonstrated by Spira *et al.*(1979) who used mice carrying various Robertsonian translocations involving No. 15. Trisomy 15 was noted in every mouse with a T cell leukemia; of 28 mice heterozygous for the translocation chromosome, the leukemic cells of 12 mice had two translocation chromosomes. These cells were, thus, trisomic not only for No. 15 but also for Nos. 1, 4, 5, or 6 which was the other chromosome involved in the Robertsonian fusion. Except for the series reported by Dofuku *et al.* (1975), a varying percentage (5–25%) of animals with only normal karyotypes was seen in different experiments.

T cell leukemia originates from a minor population of thymic cells that have a low level of theta antigen and a high level of H-2 alloantigen. This particular T cell is the target cell for both RadLV and MuLV (Chazan and Haran-Ghera, 1976).

B. Myelocytic Leukemia

It is significant that consistent chromosome changes were observed in mouse myeloid leukemias that were distinctly different from those just summarized for T cell leukemias. Cells in two studies were obtained directly from mice with radiation-induced myeloid leukemia (Hayata *et al.* (1979) or from cultured cell clones obtained from such animals (Azumi and Sachs, 1977). A deletion of No. 2 was seen in six of seven mice and in cell cultures established from six other mice. A specific portion of No. 2, namely, all of band 2D, was lost in each instance, although the size of the deleted No. 2 segment varied in different mice. Abnormalities of the Y chromosome, either gain or loss, were observed in some cells from all of the male mice studied by Hayata *et al.* (1979).

C. Transplantable Plasmacytomas

A series of chromosome studies on transplantable mouse plasmacytoma, a tumor of B cell origin, have also revealed at least one consistent change in all tumors. Seven of eight tumors were induced independently with mineral oil (Shepard *et al.*, 1974, 1978; Yoshida and Moriwaki, 1975), and one was induced with Abelson virus (Yoshida *et al.*, 1978). In all eight tumors, one chromosome No. 15 was involved in a translocation; in five, the translocation of 15q was to 12q [t(12q+;15q−)], and in the other three, the translocation was to 6q or 10q or was not identified. In every plasmacytoma studied to date, the break in No. 15 has involved band D3. In every tumor, only one normal X chromosome has been identified; this deficiency has occurred through loss of the Y in males or the deletion of the long arm in females.

D. Relationship of Chromosome Abnormalities to Etiologic Agents

The evidence for a relationship between chromosome abnormalities and etiologic agents comes entirely from tumors induced in experimental animals. There is also evidence in animals and in man that some chromosome changes may be closely associated with a particular cell type. Some of the data from analysis of second malignancies in man, particularly acute leukemia, may be relevant to the problem of human chromosome–mutagen associations.

The work of Mitelman et al. (1972) in experimental animals suggested that there was a close association between the type of carcinogen used and the specific chromosome aberration observed. In the rat, sarcomas induced by Rous sarcoma virus have a relatively consistent pattern involving additions of one chromosome No. 7, followed by one No. 13 and one No. 12 (Mitelman, 1971). On the other hand, a different, but consistent karyotypic change was noted in sarcomas (Mitelman and Levan, 1972), carcinomas (Ahlström, 1974), and leukemias (Kurita et al., 1968) induced by DMBA. The change involved either trisomy for chromosome No. 2 or a structural rearrangement that led to trisomy for a variable portion of No. 2 that always includes bands 31 to 33 (Kurita et al., 1698; Levan and Levan, 1975). Similar changes in chromosome No. 2 were observed in leukemias induced with BP, methylcholanthrene (MC) (Levan and Levan, 1975), and with N-nitroso-N-butylurea (Uenaka et al., 1978). The distinct difference in karyotype in the sarcomas produced by virus and in those induced by chemical agents was noted despite the fact that the sarcomas were histologically identical. A similar phenomenon was observed in the Chinese hamster (Kato, 1968).

Even in experimental animals, some chromosome variability was present in tumors induced with a single, known oncogenic agent; however, chromosome variability was less in inbred (20–30%) than in random-bred (about 50%) animals. Levan et al. (1977) have proposed that the more potent the carcinogen, the more selective its action on the chromosomal loci involved in oncogenesis. Strong carcinogens such as DMBA will therefore induce fewer accidental chromosome disturbances than weaker carcinogens, as MC and BP.

III. Acute Leukemia Secondary to Cytotoxic Therapy

The occurrence of acute nonlymphocytic leukemia (ANLL) in patients who have previously received cytotoxic therapy, either radiation and/or chemotherapy, for a prior disease is being recognized with increasing frequency (Rowley et al., 1981). It would appear reasonable to consider most, if not all, of these leukemias as being induced by the therapy. Radiation is well recognized for its leukemogenesis potential, and many of the drugs used to treat patients are alkylating agents that are also known for their mutagenic activity.

During the last decade I have had occasion to study the karyotypes of the leukemic cells of 47 patients who had ANLL following treatment for some other disease (Rowley *et al.*, 1977, 1981, and unpublished observations).

A. Clinical Data

Of the 47 previously treated patients, 21 had Hodgkin's disease (HD), 6 had poorly differentiated lymphocytic lymphoma (PDL), 4 had multiple myeloma (MM), one had hairy cell leukemia (HCL), 13 had various cancers, and two had had a renal transplant. Of the 21 HD patients, 12 had mixed-cell type and 9 had nodular sclerosis; 3 patients were in stage II, 13 in stage III, and 5 in stage IV. Of the 6 PDL patients, 4 had nodular histology and 2 had diffuse type; 3 patients were stage III, and 3 were stage IV.

Twenty-four of the patients had received both radiotherapy and chemotherapy prior to the development of their second malignancy; 15 patients had only chemotherapy; and 8 patients had only radiotherapy. Of the 24 patients who had both types of therapy (16 HD, 3PDL, 2MM, 3 cancer) the time between the original diagnosis and the diagnosis of bone marrow dysfunction ranged from 19 to 132 months; median time was 59 months (Table I).

Of the 15 patients who had only chemotherapy (3 HD, 2 PDL, 2 MM, 1 HCL, 5 cancers, 2 renal transplants), the time from diagnosis of original disease to diagnosis of myelodysplasia was 26 to 192 months, with a median of 47 months. Eight patients received only radiotherapy (2 HD, one PDL, 5 carcinomas); the time to the development of acute leukemia ranged from 9 to 87 months, with a median of 34 months.

Thirty-two patients could be documented as having a preleukemic phase; the duration of the preleukemic phase ranged from 2 to 20 months, with a median time of 6 months.

Of the 33 patients whose leukemia could be accurately classified 23 had acute myelogenous leukemia (AML); 5 were M1, 13 were M2, and 6 were not classified as either M1 or M2. Three had acute promyelocytic leukemia (APL), 4

TABLE I

Type of Therapy and Survival of Patients

	Malignant lymphoma patients[a]	Other patients	Median time to marrow dysfunction (months)
Radiation therapy and chemotherapy	21	3	59 (19–132)
Chemotherapy	8	7	47 (26–192)
Radiation therapy	3	5	34 (9–87)

[a] Includes four multiple myeloma and one hairy cell leukemia patients.

erythroleukemia (EL), and 2 acute myelomonocytic leukemia (AMMoL). In 11 additional patients, a myeloproliferative process, characterized by panhyperplasia with increased numbers of blasts, was present at the time of study; these patients did not have sufficiently high blasts counts to be considered as having overt leukemia (Vardiman *et al.*, 1978). No relationship was observed between the type of leukemia, the type of therapy, and the initial disease.

Eighteen patients who developed acute leukemia or the blast phase of a myeloproliferative disease were treated with combination chemotherapy in an attempt to induce a remission. Thirteen of these did not respond at all; 2 patients had a partial response, but each died 4 months after the initiation of therapy, and 3 patients had a complete response. It may be significant that one patient with a complete response had a normal karyotype and the other had a very small chromosome deletion; the third was +8.

B. Cytogenetic Data

None of the 47 patients had received therapy for leukemia at the time of the first chromosome analysis. A chromosomally abnormal clone of cells was seen in the bone marrow of all patients except 3. A consistent clonal abnormality could be identified in every aneuploid patient, although in some the clone became dominant in subsequent samples. The model chromosome number was 43 to 45 in 26 patients, 46 in 13 patients, only 3 of whom had a normal karyotype, and 47 to 59 in 8 patients (Fig. 1).

One or both of two consistent chromosome changes was noted in 39 of 44 (89%) patients with aneuploidy. Fourteen patients had loss of No. 5, and 6 others were lacking a part of the long arm of No. 5 (5q−). Chromosome No. 7 was missing from cells of 24 patients, and 5 others had loss of part of the long arm of No. 7 (7q−). Twelve patients had a −7 as well as either −5 or 5q−. In four patients this occurred with evolution of the initial −5 or −7 clone with loss of the other chromosome (either 5 or 7) (Fig. 2). These changes were particularly noticeable since losses of other chromosomes occurred at most in 4 patients (9%), and since gains of chromosomes were rarely seen. In general, the karyotype became even more complex as the disease entered the leukemic phase; this evolution affected the original clone in every patient. Patients who had abnormalities other than −5 or −7 are also instructive. Thus only two of our patients had +8; one of these has had a long complete remission. This contrasts with most series of ANLL *de novo* in which +8 is the most frequent chromosome aberration. Of particular interest is the observation that the leukemic cells of one patient with a rare type of ANLL showed the particular karyotype associated with that leukemia; this patient with APL had a t(15;17).

In addition to demonstrating that there are nonrandom karyotypic changes in secondary ANLL, our work suggests that there may be a relationship between (a)

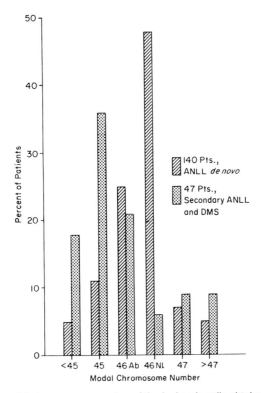

Fig. 1. The modal chromosome number of the leukemic cells obtained from 47 patients with secondary ANLL or dysmyelopoietic syndrome (DMS) compared with that of 140 patients with ANLL *de novo*.

the type of primary disease and the karyotype of the leukemic cells and (b) the therapy used and the karyotype of the leukemic cells. Thus as can be seen in Table II combined losses of both No. 5 and No. 7 were only seen in our patients with malignant lymphoma and other lymphoproliferative diseases. Loss of either No. 5 (which was a 5q− in 3 cancer patients) or No. 7 was seen in patients with various diseases.

However, as can be seen in Table III, these abnormalities also seem to occur with different frequencies depending on the type of therapy used. Thus 9 of 24 (38%) patients who had received both radiotherapy and chemotherapy had loss of both chromosomes compared with 2 of 8 who had received only radiotherapy and 2 of 15 patients who received chemotherapy alone. Of the 23 patients who received only one type of treatment, six had loss of only No. 5 or 5q and seven had loss of only No. 7 or 7q.

Several of our patients with secondary ANLL have deletions of the long arm of No. 5 or No. 7. We have 5 patients with a 7q− chromosome; 3 had a del(7)(q11);

TABLE II

Relationship of Initial Disease and Karyotype of Leukemic Cells

| Disease | Patients | Chromosome change[a] | | | | Normal chromosome |
		-5/5q-	-7/7q-	Both -5 and -7	Other[b]	
Malignant Lymphoma	32	3(0)	12(3)[c]	13[d]	2	2
Other	15	4(3)	7(1)	0	3	1

[a] Numbers in parentheses are those that were q-.
[b] None of these changes.
[c] Includes karyotypic evolution in one.
[d] Includes karyotypic evolution in four.

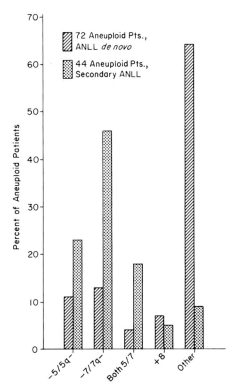

Fig. 2. The types of chromosome aberrations detected in leukemic bone marrow cells of 44 patients with secondary ANLL whose cells were abnormal compared with aberrations seen in 72 aneuploid patients with ANLL *de novo.*

TABLE III

Correlation of Karyotype and Therapy

Therapy	Patients	−5/5q−	−7/7q−	−5 and −7	Other	Normal
Radiotherapy and chemotherapy	24	1	12	9	1	1
Chemotherapy	15	3	5	2	3	2
Radiotherapy	8	3[a]	2	2	1	

[a] All 5q−.

the fourth had a deletion of 7q22 to 7qter; and the fifth had a deletion of 7q34 to 7qter. Of four patients with 7q− reported by others, three are del(7)(q22), and one is similar to the patient just described with a deletion 7(q34) (Mitelman *et al.*, 1981). These deletions can be analyzed to determine whether certain segments are consistently lost, and if so whether there is a particular segment that is lost in all patients. An analysis of abnormalities of chromosome No. 7 from four patients is represented in Fig. 3. Because the only consistent segment of the genome that appears to be missing is that on 7q34 to 7qter, the genes related to malignant transformation are likely to be located on this portion of No. 7. We are in the process of analyzing deletions of chromosome No. 5 to provide a similar map.

Our data indicate that the hallmark of secondary leukemia is (1) aneuploidy, (2) loss of part or all of No. 5 and/or No. 7, and (3) an excess of patients with AML (M1 and M2) and EL (M6). These observations have been confirmed by other investigators.

Deletions of Chromosome No. 7
in Human Acute Leukemia

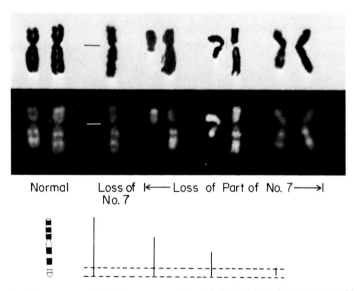

Normal   Loss of |◄──── Loss of Part of No. 7 ────►|
              No. 7

Fig. 3. Chromosome No. 7 from a normal cell (left) and from four patients with abnormalities of No. 7. Upper row, Giemsa stain, and middle row, quinacrine fluorescence of same chromosome pair. Lower row, the diagrammatic representation of the part of No. 7 that is missing. The portion consistently missing from all cells is within the horizontal dashed lines.

C. Summary of Data from Other Laboratories

Forty-two patients with secondary ANLL or a myelodysplastic syndrome studied with banding have been reported by others (Oshimura et al., 1976; Cavallin-Stahl et al., 1977; Swolin et al., 1978; Secker-Walker and Sandler, 1978; Ellerton et al., 1979; Papa et al., 1979; Whang-Peng et al., 1979; Harris et al., 1979; Kapadia et al., 1980; Patil, et al., 1980; Pederson-Bjergaard et al., 1981). The prior disease was HD in 16, other lymphomas in 12, MM, various cancers, and nonneoplastic conditions each in 4, and acute lymphoblastic leukemia, chronic lymphocytic leukemia, and postrenal transplant each in 1 patient. Where the therapy was described, 3 patients had received primarily radiotherapy, 20 had received only chemotherapy, and 17 had received a combination of radiotherapy and chemotherapy. A diagnosis of AML was made in 20 patients; 6 patients had EL, 4 had AMMoL, and 1 had acute monocytic leukemia (AMoL). Where adequate clinical data were provided, a preleukemic phase was seen in almost every patient. The median time from diagnosis of the initial disease to marrow dysplasia was 45 months (range, 13–102 months). As in our series, these patients failed to respond to treatment of the leukemic phase; the median survival was 2 months (range, >1 to 9 months).

These patients had a clone of chromosomally abnormal cells comprising 50 to 100% of the cells in division. Twenty-seven of the 42 patients (64%) had clones with a hypodiploid modal number. Moreover, 30 of the 42 (71%) had loss of part or all of chromosome No. 5 and/or No. 7. These observations are similar to those that we have reported.

IV. Correlation of Karyotype and Occupation in Adult Patients with Acute Leukemia

The observations on our patients with ANLL secondary to cytotoxic therapy suggest that it might be possible to identify patients with ANLL de novo who may have their disease as a result of occupational exposure to potentially mutagenic agents. It must be emphasized that the data to be presented in this section are preliminary and are based on a relatively few patients. Three centers (Lund, Rome, and Chicago) have been gathering information on the occupation of adult patients with ANLL using hospital charts for a retrospective study and patient interviews for a prospective study. The data obtained from our study at the University of Chicago (Golomb et al., 1982) will be presented first and then an analysis of the combined study of all three centers will follow.

A. Data from the University of Chicago

1. *Age, Sex, and Occupation of Patients*

We studied the karyotype of 74 adult patients with ANLL *de novo* for whom we had sufficient information to determine their occupation (Golomb *et al.*, 1982). The patients were divided into two groups either exposed or nonexposed; the exposed group was then subdivided according to the type of exposure to insecticides, chemicals, metals, or petroleum products (Table IV). Data on hobbies that exposed patients to potentially mutagenic agents were also documented. The information was collected from hospital records and also, whenever possible, by interviews with the patient's relatives. The classification as exposed or nonexposed done by hematologists without knowledge of the karyotype was confirmed by Dr. P. G. Nilsson (Lund) who also classified all patients in the Lund/Rome study (Mitelman *et al.*, 1981).

The 74 patients included 26 males and 48 females, ranging in age from 17 to 83 years, with a median of 43 years for all, of 42 years for men, and of 44 years for women. The median age of the exposed patients was 54 years, and that of the nonexposed patients was 42.5 years. Forty-three patients were less than 50 years old (35 in the nonexposed and 8 in the exposed group). Almost all females were in the nonexposed group (46 of 48). The males were distributed almost equally between exposed and nonexposed groups (14 and 12).

2. *Cytogenetic Pattern*

Chromosome abnormalities were present in 37 of the 74 patients (50%). When the exposed and nonexposed patients were subdivided according to karyotype as having leukemic cells that are only normal (NN), a mixture of normal and

TABLE IV

Distribution of Exposure to Potential Mutagenic/Carcinogenic Agents of 74 Patients (Chicago) and 162 Patients (Lund and Rome)[a]

Type of exposure	Number of patients			
	Chicago	Lund	Rome	Total
Insecticides	1	5	6	13
Chemicals, solvents, metals	7	18	9	34
Petroleum	8	12	2	22
Total exposed	16	35	17	68
Total nonexposed	58	58	52	168
Total exposed and nonexposed	74	93	69	236

[a] Reprinted from *Blood*, Golomb *et al.*, 1982, with permission.

abnormal (AN), or only abnormal (AA) (Table V), a marked difference in the distribution of the chromosome patterns between the two groups of patients became evident; 12 of the 16 (75%) exposed patients had an abnormal karyotype (AA or AN), whereas only 25 of the 58 (43%) nonexposed patients had an abnormal karyotype. The difference is significant ($p=0.02$).

When the exposed patients were classified according to type of exposure, no differences in the incidence of aneuploidy were noted among the three groups: 5 of 7 patients (71%) exposed to chemicals and 6 of 8 (75%) patients exposed to petroleum products had an abnormal karyotype. The only patient exposed to insecticides was AN.

The frequency of involvement of particular chromosomes in the present series of patients is listed in Table VI. The chromosomes most frequently involved in any type of abnormality were Nos. 5 (24.5%), 7 (32.7%), 8 (37.8%), 17 (35.1%), and 21 (24.3%). When specific abnormalities were considered, those most commonly detected were partial or complete monosomy of chromosomes Nos. 5 and 7, which were observed in 8 (21.6%) and 12 (32.4%), respectively, of the patients (Fig. 4). However, the distribution of such aberrations appeared to differ consistently in the two groups of patients: the $-5/5q-$ anomaly was observed in 4 of the 12 (33.3%) exposed and in 4 of the 25 (16%) nonexposed

TABLE V

Chromosomal Pattern and Occupational Exposure of 168 Patients with ANLL (Chicago + Lund + Rome Series)[a]

Center	Cytogenetic pattern			No. of patients
	NN	AN	AA	
Chicago				
Exposed	4(25)	7(43.8)	5(31.2)	16
Nonexposed	33(56.9)	16(27.6)	3(15.5)	58
Lund				
Exposed	11(31.4)[b]	13(37.1)	11(31.4)	35
Nonexposed	43(74.1)[c]	6(10.3)	9(15.5)	58
Rome				
Exposed	2(11.8)[b]	7(41.2)	8(47.1)	17
Nonexposed	32(61.5)[c]	12(23.1)	8(15.4)	52
Total				
Exposed	17(25)	27(39.7)	24(35.3)	68
Nonexposed	108(64.3)	34(20.2)	26(15.5)	168

[a] Reprinted from *Blood*, Golomb *et al.*, 1982 with permission.
[b] Mean = 25.0%.
[c] Mean = 68.2%.

TABLE VI

Incidence of Specific Aberrations in 12 Exposed and 25 Nonexposed Patients (18 without Hobbies and 7 with Hobbies) With Chromosome Aberrations[a]

Occupation	Number of patients with specific type of chromosome aberration						
	−5/5q−	−7/7q−	+8	+21	t(8;21)	t(15;17)	Others
Exposed							
Insecticides (1)[b]	—	—	—	—	—	—	1
Chemicals–solvents–metals (5)	3(60)[c]	2(40)	—	—	—	1(20)	1(20)
Petroleum products (6)	1(17)	5(83)	—	—	1(17)	—	—
Total	4(33)	7(58)			1(8)	1(8)	2(17)
Nonexposed							
No hobbies (18)	2(11)	3(17)	3(17)	1(6)	3(17)	4(22)	7(39)
Hobbies (7)	2(29)	2(29)	1(14)	—	—	—	3(43)
Total	4(16)	5(20)	4(16)	1(4)	3(12)	4(16)	10(40)
Total exposed and nonexposed	8(22)	12(32)	4(12)	1(3)	4(12)	5(13.5)	12(32)

[a] Reprinted from *Blood*, Golomb et al., 1982, with permission.
[b] Numbers in parentheses are numbers of patients.
[c] Percent of patients.

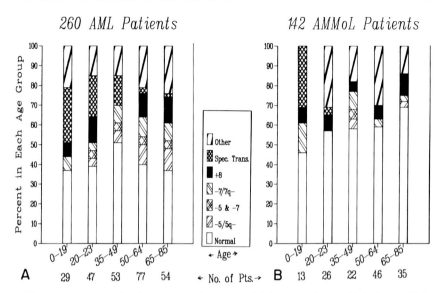

Fig. 4. Incidence of various karyotypic patterns (A) in 260 patients with AML and (B) in 142 patients with AMMoL, according to age of patients. The total number of patients in each age group is listed below the appropriate bar. Reprinted by permission from Rowley *et al., Blood* **59**, 1013–1022, 1982.

abnormal patients. The $-7/7q-$ was detected in 7 of the 12 (58.3%) abnormal exposed patients and in 5 of the 25 (20%) abnormal nonexposed patients. Both of these differences are significant ($p<0.05$). At least one of these two changes was present in 8 of the 12 (66.7%) exposed patients, but only in 7 of the 25 (28%) nonexposed patients (Table VI). When the abnormal nonexposed patients were subdivided into groups "without hobbies" and "with hobbies," 3 of 18 patients (16.7%) in the first group versus 3 of 7 patients (43%) in the second group displayed one or both of these aberrations. When the type of exposure is considered, it can be seen that 5 of the 6 abnormal patients exposed to petroleum products (83.3%) had monosomy for chromosome 7, and 3 of the 5 abnormal patients exposed to chemicals (60%) had monosomy of chromosome 5. A gain of chromosome No. 8 or No. 21 was seen only in nonexposed patients who had no hobby-related exposure. The specific translocations were also detected primarily in the nonexposed group. Of the four patients who had a t(8;21) and the five who had a t(15;17), three and four, respectively, were nonexposed.

B. Combined Data of Lund, Rome, and Chicago

The data from all three studies are summarized in Tables IV, V, and VII. The results are concordant especially with regard to the frequency of an abnormal

TABLE VII

Relationship of Karyotype and Occupation[a]

	No. of patients	Percent abnormal	Number of patients with abnormalities			
			$-5,5q-,-7,7q-$	$+8$	Specific translocations	All others
Exposed	68	75	25(37%)	11(16%)	4(6%)	11(16%)
Nonexposed	168	36	20(12%)	9(5%)	10(6%)	21(13%)

[a] Data from Mitelman et al. (1981) and Golomb et al. (1982).

karyotype in the different groups (Table V). Thus 64% of the nonexposed patients had a normal karyotype compared with only 25% of exposed patients. This agreement is especially remarkable because individuals in the United States tend to have a number of different jobs, whereas those in Europe have a much more stable occupational history.

With regard to specific chromosome changes, the incidence of certain karyotypic patterns differs somewhat between the European and American patients. Thus, in Chicago, $-7/7q-$ occurred in 58% of exposed and in 20% of nonexposed patients, compared with 36 and 25% of exposed and nonexposed patients, respectively, in the European group. As to the $-5/5q-$ anomaly, it was present in 33% of exposed and in 16% of nonexposed patients in Chicago; in the European study the percentages were 28 and 14. One of these two changes ($-5/5q-$ and $-7/7q-$) were present in 67% of exposed and in 28% of nonexposed American patients and in 57% of exposed and in 30% of nonexposed European patients. Although the frequency of $+8$ was comparable in the nonexposed patients in all three series (about 15%), none of the exposed patients in Chicago compared with 31% of European patients had a $+8$ karyotype. The same relationship was observed for $+21$.

In the Chicago series, the specific translocations t(8;21) and t(15;17) were more frequent in the nonexposed (12%) than in the exposed group (8%); in the European study, the t(8;21) occurred equally (5%) in both, and the t(15;17) was not observed. The t(9;22) was present in 5% of the exposed European patients, but was not detected in any American patients. Taken together, these data indicate that the occurrence of these translocations is independent of exposure to mutagenic agents. This interpretation is compatible with the fact that both the t(8;21) and the t(15;17) are more common in children and in younger adults than in older adults (Rowley et al., 1982). Of the 9 patients in our series who had one of these two translocations, all were between 21 and 38 years of age.

In summary, these data indicate that the incidence of obvious chromosome aberrations is higher in exposed rather than nonexposed patients. Moreover, the

TABLE VIII

Chromosome Abnormalities in Children According to Age and Type of Leukemia[a]

Type of leukemia	Number of patients in each age group														
	0 to 2.5 years			2.5 to 9 years			10 to 14 years			15 to 19 years			Total	
	NI[b]	Abn[b]	(type)	NI	Abn	(type)	NI	Abn	(type)	NI	Abn	(type)	NI	Abn
AML	3	5	1:+8[c] 1:t(11q) 3:other[c]	4	12	6:t(8;21) 1:+8[c] 4:other 1:Ph1	0	4	4:t(8;21)	5	8	1:t(8;21) 2:+8[d] 1:−7 1:+8,7q 3:other	12	29
AMMol	1	5	3:t(11q) 1:+8 1:other	3	2	1:t(11q) 1:−7,+8	4	1	1:7q−	1	0		9	8
AMol	1	5	3:t(11q) 2:+8 1:other	0	2	1:Ph1 1:other	0	0		0	2	1:t(11q) 1:+8	1	9
EL	0	2[c]	1:+8 1:other	0	1	1:other	2[c]	0		0	0		2	3
APL	1	0		0	2	2:t(15;17)	0	2	2:t(15;17)	0	1	1:t(15;17)	1	5
Total	6	17		7	19		6	7		6	11		25 (32%)	53 (68%)

[a] Modified from Rowley et al. (1982), Kaneko et al. (1982), and Kondo et al. (1982).

[b] NI, normal karyotype; Abn, abnormal karyotype.

[c] One patient had Down's syndrome.

[d] One also t(11q).

specific types of chromosome aberrations that are more common in the exposed populations, namely, $-5/5q-$, $-7/7q-$, and $+8$, are those frequently increased in patients with secondary ANLL. Other aberrations, notably specific translocations, do not show an increase in exposed compared with nonexposed populations.

V. Chromosome Pattern in Children with ANLL Compared with Adults

One way to approach the question of the influence of occupational exposure to toxic agents on the chromosome pattern in leukemic cells is to examine the karyotype seen in children. Although ANLL is less common in children than is ALL, a sufficient number of children have been examined to provide data for a comparison. The results of the analysis of the karyotype in 78 patients under the age of 19, 61 of whom were under the age of 15 years are summarized in Table VIII (Rowley *et al.*, 1982; Kaneko *et al.*, 1982; Kondo *et al.*, 1982). The frequency of aberrations is highest in the two youngest age groups, and is 74% in all children under the age of 10 years. The most common chromosome aberrations in children under 15 years are t(8;21) in 10, t(11q) in 8, $+8$ in 6, t(15;17) in 4, Ph[1] in 2, and $-7+8$ or 7q$-$ each in 1 patient (Table IX). It should be noted that not a single child had a -5 or a 5q$-$. It is also important that 7 of the 8 children with a translocation involving 11q23 were under 2.5 years of age; where

TABLE IX

Relationship of Karyotype and Age

| Karyotype | Number of patients in each age group | | | |
	0 to 2.5 years	2.5 to 9 years	10 to 14 years	Total
Total	23	26	13	62
Normal	6	7	6	19
Abnormal	17	19	7	43
$+8$	(5)[a]	(1)		(6)
$-5/5q-$				(0)
$-7/7q-$		(1)	(1)	(2)
t(8;21)		(6)	(4)	(10)
t(15;17)		(2)	(2)	(4)
t(11q)	(7)	(1)		(8)
Others	(5)	(8)		(13)

[a] Numbers in parentheses indicates number of patients with a particular type of chromosome aberration. Together they equal the total number of patients with abnormal karyotypes.

the FAB subtype was noted 3 each were M4 or M5 and one was M2. This close association between monocytic leukemia, particularly of the immature type, and aberrations of the long arm of No. 11 was first noted by Berger and his associates (1982).

Fifty-six of the children just described were part of a collaborative study (Rowley *et al.*, 1982) of 503 patients whose karyotype was correlated with the FAB subtype of the leukemic cell and with the age of the patient. Data for the 260 patients with AML (M1 and M2) and for the 142 patients with AMMoL (M4) were sufficient for analysis both by karyotype abnormality and by age groups (Fig. 4) (Rowley *et al.*, 1982). Of the 260 AML patients, 107 (41%) were considered to have a normal karyotype; a normal karyotype was seen in a slightly larger proportion of patients below the age of 50 years (43%) than in those over 50 years (39%). On the other hand, except for the t(8;21) the frequency of all other nonrandom chromosome changes increased with increasing age. The most common abnormalities, other than the t(8;21), were −5/5q− and/or −7/7q−. Nineteen patients had −5/5q−, 22 patients had −7/7q−, and 9 patients had loss of both No. 5 and No. 7. These two aberrations showed a distinct difference in incidence with age and they occurred more often in older (25% of AML patients) compared with younger (14%) patients as illustrated in Fig. 4. A gain of chromosome No. 8 was also common and increased with age; it occurred in 6% of patients under 50 compared with 12% of those over 50 years of age.

When these data were compared to 142 patients with AMMoL, it was observed that the frequency of patients with a normal karyotype was higher, 60%, than in AML. Moreover, older patients had a higher percentage of normal karyotypes (63%) compared with those under 50 years of age (56%). Aberrations of Nos. 5 and 7 were less common, occurring in only 10 and 5%, respectively, of those under and over 50 years of age. A gain of No. 8 occurred in 6% of patients under 50 and in 9% of those over 50 years of age.

VI. Conclusions

Analysis of unselected patients with ANLL *de novo* indicates that the incidence of specific chromosome aberrations varies with the age of the patient. In general, consistent translocations occur in younger patients. On the other hand, other aberrations, such as −5/5q−, −7/7q−, and +8, generally are more common in older (>50 years) patients compared with younger (<50 years) patients. These three aberrations are more common in occupationally exposed compared with nonexposed patients. Losses of Nos. 5 and/or 7 occur in up to almost 90% of aneuploid patients with ANLL secondary to cytotoxic therapy. These data suggest that −5/5q− and −7/7q− may be chromosome markers that indicate that the leukemia may be induced by exposure to mutagenic agents.

In the future, the use of recombinant DNA technology will allow the precise identification of the genes on chromosomes 5, 7, and 8 that are associated with the differential growth potential of cells that have aberrations of these chromosomes. The genes at the sites of consistent translocations will also be defined. For all of these aberrations it will then be possible to determine the changes in gene function that are associated with these numerical and structural karyotypic changes. Ultimately, it will be possible to capitalize on the changes in gene function observed in particular malignant cells to tailor therapy to specifically eliminate that particular malignant cell.

Acknowledgments

The investigations summarized in this chapter were supported by the United States Department of Energy Contract DE-AC02-80EV10360, and USPHS Grants CA-16910, CA-23954, and CA-25568 awarded by the National Cancer Institute, Department of Health and Human Services.

References

Ahlström, U. (1974). *Hereditas* **78**, 235–244.
Azumi, J.-I., and Sachs, L. (1977). *Proc. Natl. Acad. Sci. U.S.A.* **74**, 253–257.
Berger, R., Bernheim, A., Sigaux, F., Daniel, M.-T., Valensi, F., and Flandrin, G. (1982). *Leuk. Res.* **6**, 17–26.
Cavallin-Stahl, E., Landberg, T., Ottow, Z., and Mitelman, F. (1977). *Scand. J. Haematol.* **19**, 273–280.
Chan, F. P. H. (1976). Ph.D. Thesis, Univ. of Western Ontario, London, Canada.
Chang, T. D., Biedler, J. L., Stockert, E., and Old, J. L. (1977). *AACR Abstr.* p. 898.
Chazan, R., and Haran-Ghera, N. (1976). *Cell Immunol.* **23**, 356–362.
Dofuku, R., Biedler, J. L., Spengler, B. A., and Old, L. J. (1975). *Proc. Natl. Acad. Sci. U.S.A.* **72**, 1515–1517.
Ellerton, J. A., deVeber, G. A., and Baker, M. A. (1979). *Cancer (Philadelphia)* **43**, 1924–1926.
Golomb, H. M., Alimena, G., Rowley, J. D., Vardiman, J. W., Testa, J. R., and Sovik C. (1982). *Blood* **60**, 404–411.
Harris, R. E., Seo, I. S., Provisor, D., Otter, M., and Baehner, R. L. (1979). *Med. Pediatr. Oncol.* **7**, 303–308.
Hayata, I., Ishihara, T., Hirashima, K., Sado, T., and Yamagiwa, J. (1979). *J. Natl. Cancer Inst.* **63**, 843–848.
Kaneko, Y., Rowley, J. D., Maurer, H. S., Variakojis, D., and Moohr, J. W. (1982). *Blood* **60**, 389–399.
Kapadia, S. B., Krause, J. R., Ellis, L. D., Pan, S. F., and Wald, N. (1980). *Cancer (Philadelphia)* **45**, 1315–1321.
Kato, R. (1968). *Heraditas* **59**, 63–119.
Kondo, K., Larson, R. A., Vardiman, J. W., Golomb, H. M., and Rowley, J. D. (1982). *Abstr., Am. Soc. Hum. Genet,* 72A.
Kurita, Y., Sugiyama, T., and Nishizuka, Y. (1968). *Cancer Res.* **28**, 1738–1752.
Levan, G., and Levan, A. (1975). *Hereditas* **79**, 161–198.

Levan, A., Levan, G., and Mitelman, F. (1977). *Hereditas* **86**, 15–30.

Mitelman, F. (1971). *Hereditas* **69**, 155–186.

Mitelman, F., and Levan, G. (1972). *Hereditas* **71**, 325–334.

Mitelman, F., Mark, J., Levan, G., and Levan, A. (1972). *Science* **176**, 1340–1341.

Mitelman, F., Nilsson, P. G., Brandt, L., Alimena, G, Gastaldi, R., and Dallapiccola, B. (1981). *Cancer Genet. Cytogenet.* **4**, 197–214.

Oshimura, M., Hayato, I., Kakati, S., and Sandberg, A. A. (1976). *Cancer (Philadelphia)* **38**, 748–761.

Papa, G., Alimena, G., Annino, L., Anselmo, A. P., Ciccone, F., DeLuca, A. M., Granati, L., Petti, N., and Mandelli, F. (1979). *Scand. J. Haematol.* **23**, 339–347.

Patil, S. R., Corder, M. P., Jochimson, P. R., and Dick, F. R. (1980). *Cancer Res.* **40**, 4076–4080.

Pederson-Bjergaard, J., Philip, P., Martensen, B. T., Ersboll, J. Jensen, G., Panduro, J., and Thomsen, M. (1981). *Blood* **57**, 712–723.

Rowley, J. D., Golomb, H. M., and Vardiman, J. W. (1977). *Blood* **50**, 759–770.

Rowley, J. D., Golomb, H. M., and Vardiman, J. W. (1981). *Blood* **58**, 759–767.

Rowley, J. D., Alimena, G., Garson, O. M., Hagemeijer, A., Mitelman, F., and Prigogina, E. L. (1982). *Blood* **59**, 1013–1022.

Sasaki, M. (1982). *Cancer Genet. Cytogenet.* **5**, 153–172.

Secker-Walker, L. M., and Sandler, R. M. (1978). *Br. J. Haematol.* **38**, 359–366.

Shepard, J. S., Wurster-Hill, D. H., Pettengill, O. S., and Sorenson, G. D. (1974). *Cytogenet. Cell Genet.* **13**, 279–309.

Shepard, J. S., Pettengill, O. S., Wurster-Hill, D. H., and Sorenson, G. D. (1978). *J. Natl. Cancer Inst.* **61**, 255–258.

Spira, J., Wiener, F., Ohno, S., Klein, G. (1979). *Proc. Natl. Acad. Sci. U.S.A.* **76**, 6619–6621.

Swolin, B., Ridell, B., Waldenstrom, J., Weinfeld, A., and Westin, J. (1978). *Int. Soc. Hematol. Proc. Congr., 17th* p. 971a.

Uenaka, H., Ueda, N., Maeda, S., and Sugiyama, T. (1978). *J. Natl. Cancer Inst.* **60**, 1399–1404.

Vardiman, J. W., Golomb, H. M., Rowley, J. D., and Variakojis, D. (1978). *Cancer (Philadelphia)* **42**, 229–242.

Whang-Peng, J., Knutsen, T., O'Donnell, J. F., and Brereton, H. D. (1979). *Cancer (Philadelphia)* **44**, 1592–1600.

Wiener, F., Ohno, S., Spira, J., Haran-Ghera, N., and Klein, G. (1978a). *J. Natl. Cancer Inst.* **61**, 227–238.

Wiener, F., Ohno, S., Spira, J., Haran-Ghera, N., and Klein, G. (1978b). *Nature (London)* **275**, 658–660.

Wiener, F., Spira, J., Ohno, S., Haran-Ghera, N., and Klein, G. (1978c). *Int. J. Cancer* **22**, 447–453.

Yoshida, M., and Moriwaki, K. (1975). *Proc. Jpn. Acad.* **51**, 588–592.

Yoshida, M. C., Moriwaki, K., and Migita, S. (1978). *J. Natl. Cancer Inst.* **60**, 235–238.

PART III

New Approaches to Correlating
Location of Chromosome
Abnormalities with
Specific Genes

Introduction

JANET D. ROWLEY

Section of Hematology/Oncology
The University of Chicago
Chicago, Illinois

This part of the Symposium was to have been chaired by Dr. Frank Ruddle; he was unfortunately unable to attend. He had given a great deal of thought to the problem considered in this part, namely, what techniques are available to bridge the gap between those chromosome changes that we can identify with the light microscope, which are on the order of 10^6 nucleotide pairs, and those changes in the DNA at the level of specific base pairs? At the International Congress in Human Genetics held in Jerusalem in 1981, Dr. Ruddle outlined some strategies for "jogging the genome" as he called it. A number of the techniques that he described are presented in this part of the book.

The choice of topics reflects my perceptions and my biases; because of Symposium time limitations only some of the pertinent strategies could be discussed. Given some of the recurring chromosome aberrations that were described in Part II, how do we obtain the specific DNA of interest? As will become apparent in this part, scientists who have investigated some of the lymphoid tumors have had a substantial advantage. If you are interested in isolating the DNA of the 15;17 translocation in acute promyelocytic leukemia, for example, or the deleted DNA of chromosome 13 in patients with retinoblastoma, how do you proceed? It is clear that our increasing knowledge of the human gene map will be of great help, because there are genetic markers in the vicinity of many of the chromosomes that are consistently abnormal in human tumors. Except for chromosome 8, almost every chromosome that is involved in aberrations in cancer cells carries a number of identified genes, some of which have been cloned, and these probes will be useful in the isolation of specific DNA segments.

The emphasis in Part III will be on some of the techniques that can help identify the critical segments of DNA. Techniques that lead to a better definition of the chromosome regions that are affected by structural rearrangements are

163

considered first. The use of somatic cell hybrids to isolate those chromosomes or chromosome segments that are of particular interest in a specific study will be discussed.

Chromosome sorting and *in situ* chromosome hybridization are both means to isolate and precisely locate the DNA of interest. The reason to define the DNA at the sites of chromosome rearrangements is to identify the affected genes and then to analyze the modifications of gene function that occur because of these rearrangements. Two chapters will describe the use of new techniques to study protein synthesis and transcriptional activation in malignant cells.

It is apparent that these are complementary rather than isolated techniques. Used together to study the same tumor type, they can provide the information that is essential to a more sophisticated understanding of malignant transformation.

Chromosome Translocations, Immunoglobulin Genes, and Neoplasia

P. NOWELL,* R. DALLA-FAVERA,† J. FINAN,* J. ERIKSON,‡
AND C. CROCE‡

I. Introduction

The widespread use of modern banding techniques has led, in recent years, to increasing recognition of chromosomal translocations that occur nonrandomly in a variety of human tumors, particularly leukemias and lymphomas (Rowley, 1980a; Mitelman and Levan, 1981). Because all of the cells in a tumor typically have the same chromosome rearrangement, it is believed that these alterations confer a selective advantage on the neoplastic cells. Further, it has been suggested that these translocations indicate sites in the human genome where genes

*Department of Pathology and Laboratory Medicine, University of Pennsylvania School of Medicine, Philadelphia, Pennsylvania.

†Laboratory of Tumor Cell Biology, National Cancer Institute, Bethesda, Maryland.

‡The Wistar Institute, Philadelphia, Pennsylvania.

CHROMOSOMES AND CANCER
165

important in neoplastic development are located, although there is very little information concerning how gene function is altered and what the key gene products may be (Klein, 1981).

Several interesting possibilities have been indicated by the recent recognition that certain translocations in human *lymphoid* tumors involve chromosome segments where immunoglobulin genes are located. The genes for human immunoglobulin (Ig) heavy chains have been mapped to the terminal portion of the long arm of chromosome 14 (Croce *et al.*, 1979; Kirsch *et al.*, 1982). The genes for the κ and λ light chains have been mapped to the short arm of chromosome 2 (2p) and the long arm of chromosome 22 (22q), respectively (Erikson *et al.*, 1981; McBride *et al.*, 1982; Malcolm *et al.*, 1982).

At the same time, studies of chromosome changes in the Burkitt's lymphoma have demonstrated that in approximately 90% of the cases the neoplastic cells have a characteristic translocation involving the terminal portions of 8q and 14q. In those few cases that do not have the 8;14 translocation; there is in nearly every instance a translocation between 8q and 2p or between 8q and 22q (Sandberg, 1981; Bernheim *et al.*, 1981).

In other lymphomas, translocations involving the terminal portion of 14q and another chromosome (often 11q or 18q) have also been observed to occur with nonrandom frequency (Rowley, 1980a; Mitelman and Levan, 1981; Sandberg, 1981). Such translocations, producing a 14q+ marker chromosome, have also been reported in multiple myeloma and in chronic lymphocytic leukemia of both the B cell and T cell variety (Gahrton and Robert, 1982; Nowell *et al.*, 1981; Finan *et al.*, 1978) as well as in the adult T cell leukemia (ATL) endemic in Japan (Ueshima *et al.*, 1981). Although less common, translocations involving 2p and 22q also occur in human lymphoid neoplasms other than the Burkitt tumor (Rowley, 1980a; Mitelman and Levan, 1981; Sandberg, 1981; Nowell *et al.*, 1981).

These observations, and similar findings in murine leukemias (Klein, 1981), have led to the suggestion by several workers (Klein, 1981; Cairns, 1981) that chromosome translocations involving Ig gene segments might bring "promoter" sequences of these genes (transcriptionally active in a lymphoid cell) into juxtaposition with other DNA sequences (on chromosome 8 and elsewhere) that when thus activated might play an important role in cellular transformation and the development of neoplasia.

Additional support for such concepts has come from recent studies of both viral and human oncogenes and mechanisms for their activation. It now appears that there are DNA sequences in the human genome analogous to known retrovirus oncogenes, and that such sequences may be expressed in some human tumors and have the capacity, in transfection experiments, to transform other cells (Murray *et al.*, 1981; Shih *et al.*, 1981). Furthermore, at least one mechanism by which such an oncogene may be activated is the insertion of "promoter'' DNA adjacent to it (Hayward *et al.*, 1981; Oskarsson *et al.*, 1980). This ''promoter-insertion'' phenomenon for oncogene activation has thus far been demonstrated only in the avian myelocytomatosis system, involving the *myc* oncogene (Hayward *et al.*, 1981), but it adds credence to the possibility that a similar promoter mechanism might be mediated by translocations in mammalian lymphoid cells that involve Ig genes.

In order to begin testing directly these concepts of human leukemogenesis, we have undertaken studies of several Burkitt tumor cell lines. Using techniques of mouse–human cell hybridization, we have been able to demonstrate the following:

1. The breakpoint on chromosome 14 in the Burkitt tumor does involve the Ig heavy chain locus, with a portion of the locus translocated to chromosome 8 (Erikson *et al.*, 1982).

2. The human analog of the the viral *myc* gene (*c-myc*) is located on the terminal portion of 8q and is translocated to chromosome 14, adjacent to Ig gene sequences, in the Burkitt tumor (Dalla-Favera *et al.*, 1982b).

The details of these findings, and their possible implications, are discussed in the following sections.

II. Translocation of Immunoglobulin Genes in Burkitt's Lymphoma

To obtain clones in which the human chromosomes involved in the 8;14 translocation in Burkitt's lymphoma would segregate, we produced somatic cell hybrids between mouse myeloma cells and lymphocytes of the Daudi Burkitt's lymphoma cell line. The resultant hybrid clones were then studied by isozyme and cytogenetic methods, including trypsin–Giemsa and G-11 banding, for the presence of the normal and translocated human 8 and 14 chromosomes (Erikson *et al.*, 1982). We also analyzed the DNA derived from the parental Daudi and myeloma (NP3) cells and from the hybrid cells for the presence of the genes for the variable region (V_{HIII}) of human heavy chains and for the μ and γ constant (C) regions by Southern blotting procedures (Southern, 1975). As shown in Table I, we detected the human μ and γ constant region genes in all hybrids containing either the normal chromosome 14 or the 14q+. Hybrids that did not contain either the normal or translocated chromosome 14, but did retain the 8q− chromosome, had lost the genes for the μ and γ constant regions.

The filters were then rehybridized with a probe specific for the human variable region gene (V_{HIII}). This human chromosome 14-specific probe has been used to demonstrate the synteny of the V_H and C_H genes in man by Rabbitts and his associates (Matthyssens and Rabbitts, 1980; Robart *et al.*, 1981). As shown in

TABLE I

Human Immunoglobulin Genes in NP3–Daudi Cell Hybrids[a]

Cell line	Human chromosomes[b]				Human isozymes[c]		Expression of human μ chains	Human immunoglobulin genes		
	8	8q−	14	14q+	Glutathione reductase	Nucleoside phosphorylase		V_H	C_μ	C_γ
Daudi	++	++	++	++	+	+	+	+	+	+
NP3	−	−	−	−	−	−	−	−	−	−
3E5 Cl 1	+	−	+	+	+	+	+	+	+	+
3E5 Cl 3	+	+	++	−	+	+	+	+	+	+
3F2	++	++	−	+	+	+	−	+	+	+
1D8	++	−	−	++	+	+	−	+	+	+
1E8 Cl 2	++	+	−	−	+	−	−	+	−	−
2B8 Cl 22	++	±	−	−	+	−	−	±	−	−

[a] From Erikson et al. (1982).

[b] Frequency of metaphases with relevant chromosome: − = none; ± = <10%; + = 10–30%; and ++ = >30%.

[c] Glutathione reductase is a marker for human chromosome 8; nucleoside phosphorylase is a marker for human chromosome 14.

Fig. 1 and Table I, the two hybrids (1E8 Cl 2 and 2B8 Cl 22) that contained human chromosome 8q− and had lost both the normal chromosome 14 and the 14q+ chromosome contained human V_{HIII} gene sequences. This result indicated that in the Daudi cells some of the variable region genes were translocated to chromosome 8. Because the 14q+ chromosome in clone 1D8, which lacked the 8q− and the normal 14, had retained the V_{HIII} gene sequences (Fig. 2 and Table I), we further concluded that the chromosomal breakpoint in the Daudi cells occurred in a region of chromosome 14 containing V_H genes.

Because the genes for the μ and γ constant regions were all present in the hybrids 1D8 and 3F2, which contained the 14q+ chromosome, and were not present in the hybrids containing only the 8q− (1B8 Cl 2 and 2B8 Cl 22) (Figs. 2 and 3 and Table I), we also concluded that these heavy chain genes were

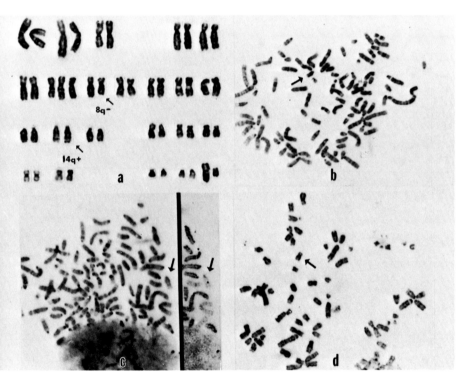

Fig. 1. (a) Karyotype of parental Daudi cell line with t(8;14)(q24;q32) (arrows) and small interstitial deletion in 15q. Trisomy 7 was present in a minority of the cells. (b) Trypsin–Giemsa banded metaphase from hybrid 3E5 Cl 3 containing normal 14 (arrow) and no 14q+. (c) Trypsin–Giemsa banded metaphase from hybrid 3F2 with 14q+ (arrow) and no normal 14. G-11 staining of the same metaphase (inset) indicates the human origin of 14q+. (d) Trypsin–Giemsa banded metaphase from hybrid 1E8 Cl 2 containing human 8q− (arrow) and no 14 or 14q+. (From Erikson *et al.*, 1982.)

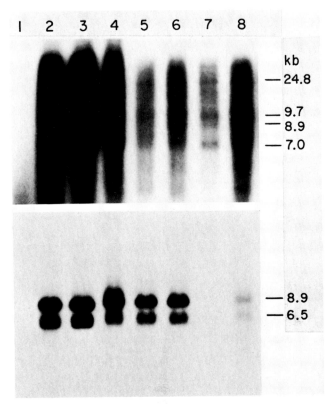

Fig. 2. Hybridization of *Hind*III-digested cellular DNA with the V_{HIII} probe (upper) and the same filter rehybridized with the γ cDNA probe (lower). In lane 1 is DNA from the mouse myeloma parent NP3, which shows no hybridization to either probe. Lane 2 is Daudi DNA, which hybridizes to both probes, as does DNA from 6M54VA, a simian virus 40 (SV40)-transformed human cell line, in lane 3. In lane 4 is the hybrid clone 3E5, which produces human μ chain. Lanes 5 and 6 are DNAs from two clones that are nucleoside phosphorylase positive. Lane 7 is DNA from the 1E8 Cl 2 clone, which is nucleoside phosphorylase negative and has the 8q− chromosome. This DNA hybridizes to the variable region probe (upper) but not the (γ) constant region probe. In lane 8 is DNA from the 1D8 clone, which has the 14q+ chromosome but not the 8q− chromosome. DNA from this clone hybridizes to both probes. (From Erikson *et al.*, 1982.)

proximal to the breakpoint observed in Daudi cells, and that the variable region genes are distal to the constant region genes on human chromosome 14 (Fig. 4).

The cellular DNA from the parental line was also cleaved with *Bam*HI and, after agarose gel electrophoresis and Southern transfer, it was hybridized with μ-specific cDNA. As shown in Fig. 5, Daudi cells appeared to have the μ chains on both number 14 chromosomes rearranged. The results from the hybrids, in

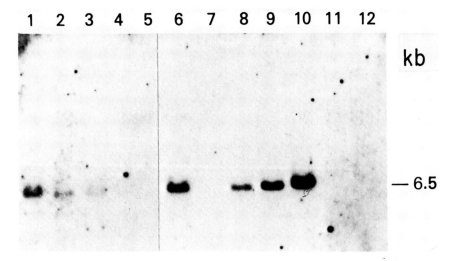

Fig. 3. Hybridization of XbaI-digested cellular DNA with the μ cDNA probe, demonstrating the presence or absence of μ gene sequences in Daudi hybrids. Lanes 1 and 2 (clones 3E5 and 3A9) are DNAs from hybrid clones that produce μ chain. In lane 3 is DNA from clone 3F2, which is nucleoside phosphorylase positive. In lanes 4 and 5 are DNAs from two nucleoside phosphorylase-negative clones. In lanes 6–10 are human DNAs: lane 6 is Daudi; lane 7 is an IgA-expressing lymphoblastoid line; line 8 is an IgM-expressing lymphoblastoid line; and lanes 9 and 10 are two SV40-transformed human cell lines (Croce, 1977) (GM54VA and GM637). In lane 11 is DNA from NP3, and in lane 12 is DNA from a SV40-transformed mouse cell line, neither of which hybridizes to the human μ cDNA probe. (From Erikson et al., 1982.)

conjunction with the data in Table I, indicated that the 14q+ chromosome in these cells contained the *Bam*HI μ chain-specific fragment (18.0 kb), whereas the normal chromosome 14 carried the smaller fragment (12.5 kb). Germ line DNA gave a single band at 16.0 kb. We had previously shown that hybrids between Daudi cells and mouse myeloma cells secrete human IgM when the chromosomes carrying the active gene for light and heavy chains are present in the hybrids (Erikson and Croce, 1982). Therefore, we screened the hybrids described in Table I for the expression of secreted and cytoplasmic μ chains, and found that the presence of human cytoplasmic μ chains correlated with the presence of the normal chromosome 14 and not with the 14q+ chromosome. There was no secretion of IgM because the hybrids did not produce light chains. These findings strongly suggested that in Daudi cells the μ chain genes on both number 14 chromsomes had undergone rearrangement, but that only the rearranged gene on the normal chromosome 14 was expressed.

Recently, these studies have been extended to the P3HR-1 Burkitt tumor line (Erikson *et al.*, 1983). Using similar techniques, we demonstrated that in this

P. NOWELL, R. DALLA-FAVERA, J. FINAN, J. ERIKSON, AND C. CROCE

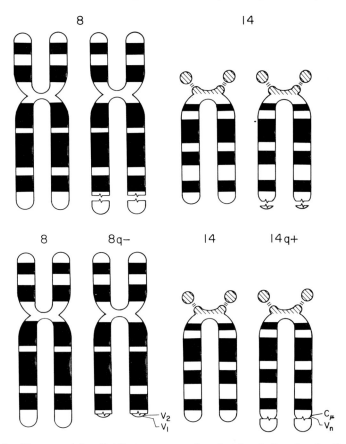

Fig. 4. Diagram of the (8;14) chromosome translocation in Daudi cells. Upper: The breakpoint on chromosome 8 and 14; lower: the t(8;14) reciprocal translocation. The figure also shows the postulated position of the genes for variable regions ($V_1 \rightarrow V_n$) and constant regions of immunoglobulin heavy chains on the involved chromosomes as indicated by our data. (From Erikson *et al.*, 1982.)

cell line, which also has the 8;14 translocation, the breakpoint on chromosome 14 is between C_μ and V_H, with V_H genes again translocated to the 8q− chromosome, but none remaining on the 14q+ (Fig. 6). Thus, the breakpoint on chromosome 14 may differ in different Burkitt tumors, but in both instances, Daudi and P3HR-1, expression of immunoglobulin heavy chains was coded for by the nontranslocated chromosome 14 (Erikson *et al.*, 1982, 1983).

These various findings with the Daudi cell line and derived hybrids, as well as from additional Burkitt lymphoma cell lines (CA46, JD38IV) (see below), were consistent with the hypothesis that the 8;14 chromosome translocation in the

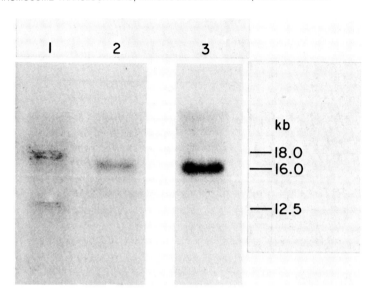

Fig. 5. Hybridization of *Bam*HI-digested cellular DNA with the μ-specific cDNA probe. In lane 1 is Daudi DNA with two bands. In lane 2 is DNA from an adenovirus-transformed human cell line (FC Cl 3), and in lane 3 is GM54VA, a SV40-transformed fibroblastic human cell line (Croce, 1977); both lanes 2 and 3 show a single band that does not comigrate with either of the Daudi bands. (From Erikson *et al.*, 1982.)

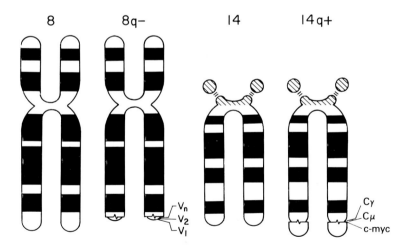

Fig. 6. Diagram of the t(8;14) chromosome translocation in P3HR-1 cells. The C_μ and C_γ genes are proximal to the breakpoint on chromosome 14, while the V_H gene translocates to the 8q− chromosome. The human *c-myc* gene on the broken chromosome 8 translocates to the heavy chain locus. (From Erikson *et al.*, 1983.)

Burkitt tumor involved the Ig heavy chain locus, and that expression of malignancy might result from activation of a gene located on the long arm of chromosome 8, brought into association with the translocated V_H gene on the 8q− chromosome or with retained Ig sequences proximal to the breakpoint on the 14q+ chromosome.

The possibility that the critical gene on chromosome 8 might be the human analog of the viral oncogene of avian myelocytomatosis (*c-myc*) was suggested by parallel studies which indicated the location of *c-myc* on human chromosome 8 (Dalla-Favera *et al.*, 1982b). The details of this work follow.

III. Human *c-myc* Oncogene on the Region of Chromosome 8 Translocated in Burkitt's Lymphoma Cells

This study was also carried out with mouse–human cell hybrids as well as with a hybrid between Chinese hamster and human cells that had retained only human chromosome 8. The human *c-myc* probe used for Southern blotting studies was a recombinant pBR322 plasmid (clone pMC41RC) that contains the entire 3′ *c-myc* exon (Dalla-Favera *et al.*, 1982a). Initial studies with human and mouse cellular DNA, using this probe, indicated that it was possible to distinguish between the human and the mouse *c-myc* DNA sequences (Fig. 7). Following digestion with ScT-1, the human *c-myc* DNA migrates as a 2.8 kb band, while the mouse homolog migrates as a 17.0 kb band.

We then studied the segregation of the human-specific 2.8 kb band in a panel of mouse–human hybrids to establish the chromosomal location of the human *c-myc* homolog. Table II shows the results of the analysis of a panel of hybrid clones that were studied for the expression of isozyme markers assigned to each of the human chromosomes and for the presence of the human *c-myc* homolog. Only human chromosome 8 segregated concordantly with the presence of the human *c-myc* gene.

To confirm this indication that the human *c-myc* gene was located on chromosome 8, we also studied a somatic cell hybrid between Chinese hamster and human cells that had retained only human chromosome 8 (Fig. 8). This hybrid (706B6-40 Cl 17) also contained the human *c-myc* homolog (Table II).

For regional mapping of the *c-myc* gene, mouse–human hybrids were utilized from both the Daudi and the P3HR-1 Burkitt's lymphoma cell lines. As indicated in Table III, hybrids M44 Cl 2S5 and M44 Cl 2S9, from the P3HR-1 line and retaining only the human 14q+ chromosome (Dalla-Favera *et al.*, 1982b; Erikson *et al.*, 1983) also retained the human *c-myc* gene. Hybrid 3F1, from the Daudi line, which had the 14q+ chromosome and neither the normal nor the 8q− chromosome, also contained the human *c-myc* gene (Table III). These

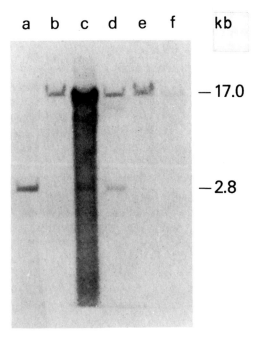

Fig. 7. Segregation of the human *c-myc* homolog in mouse–human hybrids. Lane a, normal human DNA. Lane f, normal mouse DNA. Lanes b–e, DNAs derived from four mouse–human hybrids. (From Erikson *et al.*, 1983.)

results indicated that the human *c-myc* gene was located on region q24→qter of human chromosome 8, the segment translocated to the 14q+ chromosome. Furthermore, since the human *c-myc* gene was present on the 14q+ chromosome of both the Daudi and P3HR1 cell lines, we concluded that it must be distal to the breakpoint on human chromosome 8 in both of these tumors. Interestingly, no obvious rearrangement of the 3′ exon of the human *c-myc* DNA segment was detected in its new location on the 14q+ chromosome of these two cell lines.

The results of this study thus not only further supported the involvement of an Ig gene locus in a consistently observed translocation in a human lymphoid tumor, but also provided a possible candidate, the human *c-myc* gene, for an "oncogene" which might be activated by its new association with promoter regions of the Ig gene following translocation.

This hypothesis has been strengthened by our recent evidence that the human *c-myc* gene translocation lies in close proximity to the human heavy chain locus in a number of Burkitt's lymphomas with the 8;14 chromosome translocation. We have digested the DNA of five different Burkitt lymphoma cell lines with *Bam*HI, a restriction enzyme that cuts outside the human μ gene (Erikson *et al.*,

TABLE II

Presence of the Human c-myc Homolog in a Panel of Rodent–Human Hybrid Clones[a]

Hybrids	Human Chromosomes

Hybrids	1	2	3	4	5	6	7	8	9	10	11	12	13	14	15	16	17	18	19	20	21	22	X	Human c-myc
DSK1B2A5 Cl2			■				■							■	■		■			■				+
DSK1B2A5 Cl20														■	■		■		■		■			−
Nu 9				■																				−
PAFxBalbIV Cl5	■			■					■									■						+
GMxLM Cl3			■													■								−
GMxLM Cl4			■				■																	+
GMxLM Cl5											■	■												+
GMxLM Cl6											■	■				■								−
706B6-40 Cl17		■						■																+
77-B10 Cl5	■							■						■			■							+
77-B10 Cl8			■					■							■			■						+
77-B10 Cl25	■											■					■							−
77-B10 Cl26			■					■			■					■								+
77-B10 Cl28	■											■					■							−
77-B10 Cl30											■						■							−
77-B10 Cl31	■					■											■							+

[a] A black square indicates that the hybrid clone named in the left column contains the chromosome named in the upper row. An empty square indicates that the hybrid clone has lost the human chromosome indicated in the upper row. (From Dalla-Favera *et al.*, 1982b.)

TABLE III

Presence of the Human c-myc Homolog in Hybrids with the Burkitt's Lymphoma 14q+ Chromosome[a]

	Isozymes[b]		Chromosomes				
Hybrids	NP	GSR	8	8q−	14	14q+	Human c-myc
M44 Cl 2S5	+	−	−	−	−	+	+
M44 Cl 2S9	+	−	−	−	−	+	+
3F1	+	−	−	−	−	+	+

[a] From Dalla-Favera *et al.* (1982b).
[b] NP, nucleoside phosphorylase; GSR, glutathione reductase.

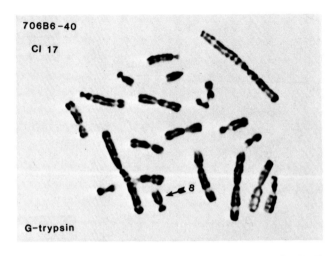

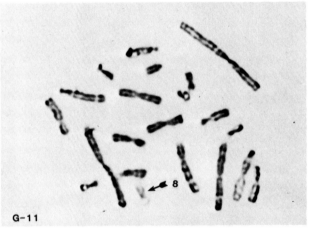

Fig. 8. Metaphase of Chinese hamster–human hybrid 706B6-40 Cl 17, which has re-tained human chromosome 8 and no other human chromosome, stained by the tryp-sin–Giemsa method (upper) and the G-11 method (lower). (From Erikson *et al.*, 1983.)

1982) and the *c-myc* gene (Marcu *et al.*, 1982). After agarose gel electrophoresis and Southern transfer, we have hybridized the nitrocellulose filter first with the µ-specific probe (Fig. 9a) and then with the human *c-myc* cDNA probe (Fig. 9b). As shown in Fig. 9, the same 22 kb band hybridized with both the *c-myc* and the µ probes, indicating that these two genes are contained in the same restriction fragment in some (CA46 and JD38-IV) of the Burkitt's lymphomas with the 8;14

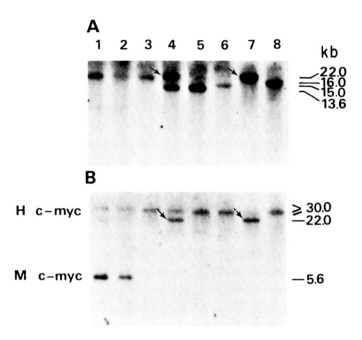

Fig. 9.   Southern blotting analysis of *Bam*HI-digested DNA derived from different Bur-kitt's lymphoma cell lines. Lanes 1 and 2, two independent somatic cell hybrids between mouse myeloma cells and P3HR-1 Burkitt's lymphoma cells. Lane 3, P3HR-1 Burkitt cell line. Lanes 4–7, Burkitt's lymphomas Ca46, AD876, EW36, and JD38-IV cell lines, respectively. Lane 8, PAF (an SV40-transformed human fibroblastic cell line). (A) was hybridized with a C_μ probe. The probe was washed and the filter rehybridized to the human *c-myc* probe (B). Arrows indicate the bands that cross hybridize with the *c-myc* and the C_μ probe. (From Marcu *et al.,* 1982.)

chromosomal translocation. Figure 6 describes the organization of the *c-myc* gene and of the heavy chain gene in the P3HR-1, CA46, and JD38-IV cell lines.

We have detected a similar rearrangement of the *c-myc* gene with the Ig heavy chain locus in mouse plasmacytoma cells carrying the 12;15 chromosome trans-location (Marcu *et al.,* 1982). Interestingly, expression of high levels of *myc* transcription was detected in mouse plasmacytomas (Marcu *et al.,* 1982).

IV. Implications of Translocation Model of Oncogene Activation

The results of the studies just described are consistent with the view that one mechanism of human leukemogenesis in lymphoid cells might involve chro-

mosomal translocations that bring segments of Ig genes adjacent to human oncogenes, leading to their activation. Similar results have now been reported from
several other laboratories (Taub et al., 1982; Neel, et al., 1982), also involving
the Burkitt tumor.

Although the critical gene product involved in these leukemogenic phenomena
has not been identified, presumably a human or mouse lymphocyte with such a
chromosome translocation acquires a selective growth advantage as the result of
oncogene activation, and its progeny expand as a neoplastic clone. It has been
generally assumed that the translocations themselves are random events, with
only those cytogenetic changes that confer a selective growth advantage becom-
ing apparent, but it is interesting to speculate on whether the chromosome breakage itself may be nonrandom. It is possible that Ig gene sequences engaged in
physiological rearrangements are unusually susceptible to breakage and thus, in
developing lymphoid cells, become fragile "hot spots." Our data on the Daudi
and P3HR-1 lines indicate that the translocated chromosome is not the one
expressing gene function (this activity resides with the rearranged gene of the
normal chromosome 14), but the critical translocation could take place during an
abortive attempt at physiological rearrangement.

As one attempts to extend these translocation–activation concepts to human
lymphoid tumors other than the Burkitt's lymphoma, it will be necessary to
suggest other candidates for the activated oncogene. Although translocations
involving the terminal portion of 14q are present in a variety of lymphoid leukemias and lymphomas, it is rare for chromosome 8 to be the "donor" except in
the Burkitt tumor (and leukemic equivalent) (Rowley, 1980a; Mitelman and
Levan, 1981; Sandberg, 1981). As noted above, translocations between 14q and
either 11q or 18q appear to be the two most common findings in the non-
Burkitt's lymphoid neoplasms. Mapping of a number of the human analogs of
known oncogenes (other than c-myc) to specific human chromosomes is currently under way in several laboratories, including ours. A summary of recent
assignments is incorporated elsewhere in this volume (see Chapter 18 by Evans).
Obviously, those human "oncogenes" identified through their homology with
viral oncogenes will not constitute the entire spectrum of genes importantly
involved in human leukemogenesis, but the tools are currently available for the
analysis of both structure and function of these DNA sequences in human tumors, and so they represent a fruitful area for immediate study.

It is also interesting to speculate as to whether certain of the nonrandom
translocations observed in nonlymphoid human leukemias might also involve Ig
gene sequences and/or oncogenes. For instance, the Philadelphia (Ph[1]) chromosome in chronic granulocytic leukemia typically involves a translocation between
the long arms of chromosome 22 and chromosome 9. The breakpoint in chromosome 22 (q11) is consistent with possible involvement of the λ-light chain locus
(Erikson et al., 1981), as well as the c-sis oncogene (Dalla-Favera et al., 1982c).

Similar translocations involving 22q are also present in some disorders which present *de novo* as acute leukemia classified as myeloid, undifferentiated, or lymphoid (Rowley, 1980b; Mitelman and Levan, 1981). Although translocations involving 2p are much less common, and a 14q+ chromosome is extremely rare in nonlymphoid tumors (Sandberg, 1980; Mitelman, 1981), the wide occurrence of the Ph[1] chromosome at least suggests the possibility that Ig gene involvement, and also oncogene involvement, may play important roles in tumors arising at the hematopoietic stem cell level as well as in those already differentiated along a lymphoid pathway.

In addition to speculations concerning the type of tumors in which these genes may be significant, there are also considerations of the nature of the ''activation'' process when oncogenes are involved in such chromosome translocations. The limited data available suggest that the transforming ability for 3T3 cells of oncogenes may result in some instances from point mutations within the gene, producing an altered gene product, and in other instances from an increased production of abnormal gene product (R. Weinberg and M. Barbacid, personal communication). The possibility that point mutations are involved, however, requires additional careful investigation to exclude differences due to genetic polymorphisms. It is also not yet clear whether the ability to transform 3T3 cells reflects the role of the oncogene in the pathogenesis of the original tumor. In any event, there may be variation not only in different types of tumors but even in different individual cases of the same neoplasm. The numerous Burkitt cell lines available for detailed study as described above may provide some indication of the spectrum of changes in oncogene structure and expression associated with tumorigenesis, at least for this one tumor and one gene (*c-myc*).

It must be recognized, however, that even the elucidation of these questions, and the characterization of oncogene products, may still leave us some distance from complete understanding of the full development of a clinical tumor. In this regard, it is interesting to recall the recent history of our thinking about the Burkitt lymphoma. Its geographical distribution initially suggested the possibility of horizontal transmission of a causative agent by an insect vector. It now seems likely that these geographical patterns reflect a poorly explained influence of various infectious diseases, particularly malaria, on the development of the tumor, perhaps through distortion of the patient's immune system. Subsequently, the association of the Epstein-Barr virus (EBV) with the Burkitt tumor led to speculation as to its etiologic role. Again, our thinking has been modified since it has become apparent that EBV is frequently absent in non-African Burkitt tumors, appears not to integrate at consistent sites within the host cell genome, and does not have direct damaging effect on host chromosomes. It now seems likely that EBV acts to ''freeze'' the infected B cells in an actively proliferating state (analogous to its role in maintaining proliferation of normal B cells in tissue culture) (Klein, 1980), and thus increases the probability that when a carcinogenic event occurs in a lymphocyte (the 8;14 translocation?), that cell will be actively proliferating and hence expand as a lymphoma. Subsequent progression of the tumor may be further promoted by additional genetic and cytogenetic changes within the neoplastic clone (Nowell, 1983).

The specific translocation events that we have been discussing may thus represent only one essential step in a sequence necessary to produce the clinical disease. This does not reduce the significance of the findings, and the need to further elucidate the specific genes and gene products involved. It simply indicates the complexity of carcinogenesis, and the probability that we will need to dissect carefully a series of events if reasonably complete understanding is to be attained of the factors and mechanisms involved in the development of any human cancer.

References

Bernheim, A., Berger, R., and Lenoir, G. (1981). *Cancer Genet. Cytogenet.* **3,** 307.

Cairns, J. (1981). *Nature (London)* **289,** 353.

Croce, C. M. (1977). *Proc. Natl. Acad. Sci. U.S.A.* **74,** 315.

Croce, C. M., Shander, M., Martinis, J., Cicurel, L., D'Ancona, G. G., Dolby, T. W., and Koprowski, H. (1979). *Proc. Natl. Acad. Sci. U.S.A.* **76,** 3416.

Dalla-Favera, R., Wong-Staal, F., and Gallo, R. C. (1982a). *Nature (London)* **299,** 61.

Dalla-Favera, R., Bregni, M., Erikson, J., Patterson, D., Gallo, R. C., and Croce, C. M. (1982b). *Proc. Natl. Acad. Sci. U.S.A.* **79,** 7824.

Dalla-Favera, R., Gallo, R. C., Giallongo, A., and Croce, C. M. (1982c). *Science* **218,** 686.

Erikson, J., and Croce, C. M. (1982). *Eur. J. Immunol.* **12,** 697.

Erikson, J., Martinis, J., and Croce, C. M. (1981). *Nature (London)* **294,** 173.

Erikson, J., Finan, J., Nowell, P. C., and Croce, C. M. (1982). *Proc. Natl. Acad. Sci. U.S.A.* **79,** 5611.

Erikson, J., ar-Rushdi, A., Drwinga, H., Nowell, P., and Croce, C. M. (1983). *Proc. Natl. Acad. Sci. U.S.A.* **80,** 820.

Finan, J., Daniele, R., Rowlands, D., and Nowell, P. (1978). *Virchow Arch. B* **29,** 121.

Gahrton, G., and Robert, K.-H. (1982). *Cancer Genet. Cytogenet.* **6,** 171.

Hayward, W. S., Neel, B. G., and Astrin, S. M. (1981). *Nature (London)* **290,** 475.

Littlefield, J. W. (1964). *Science* **145,** 709.

Kirsch, I. R., Morton, C. C., Nakahara, K., and Leder, P. (1982). *Science* **216,** 301.

Klein, G. (1980). *Cancer (Philadelphia)* **45,** 2486.

Klein, G. (1981). *Nature (London)* **294,** 313.

McBride, O. W., Hieter, P. A., Hollis, G. F., Swan, D., Otey, M. C., and Leder, P. (1982). *J. Exp. Med.* **155,** 1680.

Malcolm, S., Barton, P., Murphy, C., Ferguson-Smith, M. A., Bentley, D. L., and Rabbits, T. H. (1982). *Proc. Natl. Acad. Sci. U.S.A.* **79,** 4957.

Marcu, K., Harris, L., Stanton, L., Erikson, J., Watt, R., and Croce, C. M. (1983). *Proc. Natl. Acad. Sci. U.S.A.* **80,** 519.

Matthyssens, G., and Rabbits, T. (1980). *Proc. Natl. Acad. Sci. U.S.A.* **77,** 6561.

Mitelman, F. (1981). *Adv. Cancer Res.* **34,** 141.

Mitelman, F., and Levan, G. 1981). *Hereditas* **95,** 79.

Murray, M. J., Shilo, B. Z., Shih, C., Corning, D., Hsu, H. W., and Weinberg, R. A. (1981). *Cell* **25,** 355.

Neel, B., Jhanwar, S., Chaganti, R., and Hayward, W. (1982). *Proc. Natl. Acad. Sci. U.S.A.* **79,** 7842.

Nowell, P. (1983). *In* "Chromosome Breakage and Neoplasia," (J. German, ed.), p. 413, Wiley, New York.

Nowell, P., Shankey, T., Finan, J., Guerry, D., and Besa, E. (1981). *Blood* **57,** 444.

Oskarsson, M., McClements, W. E., Blair, D. G., Maizel, J. V., and Vaude Woude, G. F. (1980). *Science* **207,** 1222.

Robart, M. J., Rabbitts, T. H., Goodfellow, P. N., Solomon, E., Chambers, S., Spurr, N., and Povey, S. (1981). *Ann. Hum. Genet.* **45,** 331.

Rowley, J. (1980a). *Cancer Genet. Cytogenet.* **2,** 175.

Rowley, J. (1980b). *Clin. Haematol.* **9,** 55.

Sandberg, A. (1980). "The Chromosome in Human Cancer and Leukemia." Elsevier/North-Holland, New York.

Sandberg, A. (1981). *Hum. Pathol.* **12,** 531.

Shih, C., Padhy, L. C., Murray, M., and Weinberg, R. A. (1981). *Nature (London)* **290,** 261.

Southern, E. (1975). *J. Mol. Biol.* **98,** 503.

Taub, R., Kirsch, L., Morton, C., *et al.* (1982). *Proc. Natl. Acad. Sci. U.S.A.* **79,** 7837.

Ueshima, Y., Fukuhara, S., Hattori, T., Uchiyama, T., Takatsuki, K., and Uchino, H. (1981). *Blood* **58,** 420.

10

Genetic Mapping of the 15;17 Chromosome Translocation Associated with Acute Promyelocytic Leukemia

DENISE SHEER,* LYNNE R. HIORNS,* DALLAS M. SWALLOW, †
SUSAN POVEY, † PETER N. GOODFELLOW,* NORA HEISTERKAMP,‡
JOHN GROFFEN, ‡ JOHN R. STEPHENSON, ‡ AND ELLEN SOLOMON*

*Imperial Cancer Research Fund, London, England.

†MRC Human Biochemical Genetics Unit, The Galton Laboratory, University College, London, England.

‡Laboratory of Viral Carcinogenesis, National Cancer Institute—Frederick Cancer Research Facility, Frederick, Maryland.

I. Introduction

Conversion of a cell to the malignant state may result from increased or inappropriate expression of a normal cellular gene, which could be caused by the gene coming under the influence of a highly active promoter (Klein, 1981). For example, the cloned human *c-Ha-ras*1 gene, which is the cellular homolog of the Harvey murine sarcoma virus (HaMSV), cannot alone transform NIH-3T3 cells. However, the *in vitro* linking of *c-Ha-ras*1 to the long terminal repeat sequence of HaMSV results in an actively transforming gene (Chang *et al.*, 1982). Since chromosome translocations alter the relative positions of genes, their significance in the malignant process can only be understood if those genes involved in the translocations are identified. We have used the techniques of somatic cell genetics to localize several genetic markers, including the *c-fes* oncogene, around the breakpoints in the 15q+;17q− chromosome translocation found in acute promyelocytic leukemia.

II. Acute Promyelocytic Leukemia (APL)

Patients with the typical "M3" form of APL have an abundance of heavily granulated promyelocytes (Bennett *et al.*, 1976). The nuclei of the promyelocytes vary greatly in size and shape, and are often bilobed or reniform. Bundles of Auer rods are found in the cytoplasm (Bennett *et al.*, 1976). In the "M3 variant" form there is a relative scarcity of cells with heavy granulation and Auer rods (Bennett *et al.*, 1980).

III. 15q+;17q− Chromosome Translocation

The 15q+;17q− chromosome translocation is specific for APL and has never been seen in any other tumor (Second International Workshop on Chromosomes in Leukemia, 1980). The breakpoints are difficult to localize cytologically, and have been placed in various positions by different groups of workers, e.g., 15q23 and 17q12 (Kondo and Sasaki, 1979) and 15q25–26 and 17q22? (Second International Workshop on Chromosomes in Leukemia, 1980). More recently, Rowley has placed the breakpoints at 15q22.2 and 17q12–21.1 using elongated chromosome preparations from several patients with APL (J. D. Rowley, personal communication).

The t(15q+;17q−) occurs in APL in an apparently uneven geographical distribution. For example, in Chicago, Illinois, the translocation was seen in 25/25 patients with APL (J. D. Rowley, personal communication), in Buffalo, New York, 1/18, in Belgium 16/18, and in Finland 0/9 (Second International Workshop on Chromosomes in Leukemia, 1980). The reasons for this distribution are unclear, and methodological factors may play a role, i.e., normal karyotypes found in direct preparations, but the translocation found in preparations of cells cultured for longer than 24 hours (Berger *et al.*, 1980). It is obviously necessary to standardize karyotypic findings according to the technique used.

IV. Somatic Cell Genetics

When human primary cells are fused with established mouse cell lines, human chromosomes are preferentially lost from the resulting hybrids (Weiss and Green, 1967). Correlation of the presence of particular human markers with the human chromosomes present in different hybrids has enabled the localization of over 200 human genes (Human Gene Mapping 6, 1982). Many genes have been localized to particular regions of human chromosomes using chromosome translocations (Ferguson-Smith and Aitken, 1982).

The human *thymidine kinase* (*TK*) gene has been mapped to 17q210–220 (Human Gene Mapping 5, 1979). According to the position of the breakpoint in chromosome 17 in the t(15q+;17q−), the *TK* gene would either remain on the 17q− translocation chromosome or move to the 15q+ chromosome. Blood leukocytes from a patient with APL who had the t(15q+;17q−) (Fig. 1) were fused, using polyethylene glycol (Galfre *et al.*, 1977), with a subclone of the 3T3

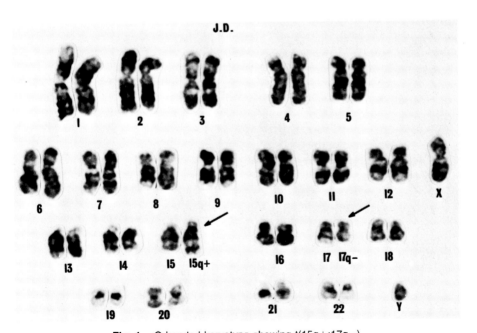

Fig. 1. G-banded karyotype showing t(15q I ;17q−).

mouse cell line (Todaro and Green, 1963) which is deficient for TK activity. Hybrids were grown in RPMI 1640, 20% fetal calf serum, 10^{-4} M hypoxanthine, 10^{-5} M methotrexate, and 1.6×10^{-5} M thymidine (HAT medium) (Szybalski et al., 1962; Littlefield, 1964). Cells require TK to survive in this medium. Thus hybrids containing the normal human chromosome 17 could be selected, as well as hybrids containing either the 15q+ or 17q− translocation chromosome, according to the relative positions of the TK gene and the breakpoint on chromosome 17. The unfused 3T3 mouse cells die in HAT medium as they lack TK activity, and the unfused human leukocytes cannot grow in culture without mitogenic stimulation.

V. Chromosome Analyses

Human chromosomes were identified in the hybrids by the sequential use of the G-11 (Bobrow and Cross, 1974) and Q banding (Caspersson et al., 1971) techniques. G banding (Seabright, 1972) was also used.

VI. Hybrids

Seven hybrids contained the normal chromosome 17, and no 15q+ or 17q− translocation chromosomes. Four hybrids contained the normal chromosome 17, both the 15q+ and 17q− chromosomes, and 16–30 other human chromosomes. One hybrid, designated PJT_2/A_1, contained the 15q+ chromosome in 37/40 cells, chromosome 21 in 9/40 cells, and a marker chromosome which does not appear to be related to chromosomes 15 or 17 in 5/40 cells (Fig. 2).

VII. Markers Present on the 15q+ Translocation Chromosome

The hybrid PJT_2/A_1 was tested for the following markers mapped to chromosome 15: β_2-Microglobulin (B2M); hexosaminidase α (HEXA); mannosephosphate isomerase (MPI); pyruvate kinase-3 (PKM2); and a cell surface antigen of apparent molecular weight 95,000 encoded by the gene $MIC7$ (Blaineau et al., 1983). PJT_2/A_1 was also tested for the presence of c-fes (Heisterkamp et al., 1982), the human cellular homolog of the feline sarcoma virus.

PJT_2/A_1 was also tested for the following markers mapped to chromosome 17: Galactokinase (GALK); acid α-glucosidase (GAA); the $\alpha1(I)$ chain of Type I collagen encoded by the gene $COL1A1;$ and a cell surface antigen of apparent molecular weight 125,000 encoded by the gene $MIC6$ (Bai et al., 1982).

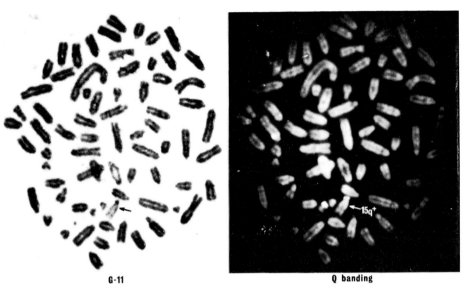

G-11   Q banding

Fig. 2. Metaphase spread of hybrid PJT$_2$/A$_1$ showing 15q+ translocation chromosome. Left: G-11 staining. Right: Q banding.

The chromosomal localization of each marker tested is shown in Table I. Methods of detection are shown in Table II.

The following genes were present in PJT$_2$/A$_1$: *B2M, GAA, GALK, MIC7, MIC6,* and *COL1A1.* The presence of the *TK* gene is assumed from growth of the hybrid in HAT medium. The *c-fes* gene is not present in this hybrid (Tables III and IV). Analysis of HEXA gave ambiguous results.

TABLE I

Regional Localization of Genes on Chromosomes 15 and 17

Gene	Location	Reference
c-fes	15q11–qter	Heisterkamp *et al.* (1982)
B2M	15q21–qter	Pajunen *et al.* (1978)
MIC7	15q11–qter	Blaineau *et al.* (1983)
HEXA	15q22–q25.1	Magenis *et al.* (1979)
MPI	15q22–qter	Chern *et al.* (1977)
PKM2	15q22–qter	Chern *et al.* (1977)
MIC6	17p11–qter	Bai *et al.* (1982)
GALK	17q210–q220	Elsevier *et al.* (1974)
TK	17q210–q220	Human Gene Mapping 5 (1979)
GAA	17q21–q25	Nickel *et al.* (1982)
COL1A1	17q21–q22	Church *et al.* (1980), Huerre *et al.* (1982)

TABLE II

Methods for Detection of Markers

Marker	Method of detection	Reference
c-fes	DNA Southern blots with human genomic probe	Heisterkamp et al. (1982)
B2M	Indirect radioimmunoassay	Brodsky et al. (1979), Goodfellow et al. (1980)
MIC7	Indirect radioimmunoassay	Goodfellow et al. (1980), Blaineau et al. (1983)
HEXA	Immunodiffusion	Swallow et al. (1977)
MPI	Starch gel electrophoresis and enzyme staining	van Heyningen et al. (1975)
PKM2	Starch gel electrophoresis and enzyme staining	van Heyningen et al. (1975)
MIC6	Indirect radioimmunoassay	Goodfellow et al. (1980), Bai et al. (1982)
GALK	Starch gel electrophoresis and autoradiography	Solomon et al. (1979)
TK	Growth in HAT medium	Weiss and Green (1967)
GAA	Starch gel electrophoresis, thermostability, and enzyme staining	Solomon et al. (1979)
COL1A1	DNA Southern blots with human genomic probe	Solomon et al. (1983)

PJT_2/A_1 was grown in 60 μg/ml bromodeoxyuridine (BrdU) to confirm that the *TK* gene is present on the 15q+ chromosome. Cells containing the *TK* gene can incorporate BrdU and therefore die in this medium (Kit *et al.*, 1963; Weiss and Green, 1967). The back-selected hybrid, designated PJT_2/A_1R, lost the 15q+ chromosome and also *B2M, MIC7, GAA,* and *MIC6* expression (Table III). These results indicate that the 15q+ translocation chromosome carries the gene for these markers and for TK.

VIII. Regional Localization of c-fes on Chromosome 15

The availability of PJT_2/A_1 hybrid cells has also enabled a more precise localization of *c-fes*, previously mapped to chromosome 15 (Heisterkamp *et al.*, 1982; Dalla-Favera *et al.*, 1982). As shown in Fig. 3, using an 0.5 kb *c-fes* specific molecular probe (*c-fes* $K_{0.5}$), the human cellular homolog of *v-fes* (lane B), seen as *SstI* restriction fragments of around 4.0 and 7.0 kb, was readily distinguishable from the mouse *c-fes* gene (lane A). Human *c-fes* sequences were present in hybrid Horl-I (Heisterkamp *et al.*, 1982), which contains chromosome 15 and a fragment of chromosome 11 as its only karyotypically detectable human

TABLE III

Genes Present in Hybrids PJT$_2$/A$_1$ and PJT$_2$/A$_1$R

Hybrid	15q+ chromosome	Chromosome 15 markers		Chromosome 17 markers	
PJT$_2$/A$_1$	+	c-fes	−		
		MIC7	+	MIC6	+
		B2M	+	TK	+
		HEXA	±	GALK	+
		MPI	−	COL1A1	+
		PKM2	−	GAA	+
PJT$_2$/A$_1$R	−	MIC7	−	MIC6	−
		B2M	−	TK	−
				GAA	−

material (lane C), and in DT2.12 (Swallow *et al.*, 1977) containing a translocation between the long arms of chromosomes 15 and X (lane E). The absence of detectable human *c-fes* specific sequences in hybrid DT2.1R3 (lane F), a derivative of DT2.1R (Swallow *et al.*, 1977) lacking the 15/X translocation chromosome, confirms the earlier assignment of *c-fes* to chromosome 15 (Heisterkamp *et al.*, 1982; Dalla-Favera *et al.*, 1982). Finally, the absence of human *c-fes* sequences in hybrid PJT$_2$/A$_1$ (lane D) establishes that *c-fes* is not present within the 15q+ translocation chromosome and thus strongly suggests that *c-fes* maps within the region of chromosome 15 which is translocated to chromosome 17.

TABLE IV

DNA Southern Blot Analysis of PJT$_2$/A$_1$ and Appropriate Controls Using COL1A1 Genomic Probe

Cells	Reference[a]	Human chromosomes	COL1A1 Human bands	COL1A1 Mouse bands
PJT$_2$/A$_1$	—	15q+	+	+
PCTB/A$_1$.8	1	17	+	+
P7A/2.7	2	3pter−3p11::17p11−17qter	+	+
Clone 21	3	7	−	+
LNSV	4	Human fibroblast line	+	−
3T3	5	Mouse fibroblast line	−	+

[a] Key to references: 1, Bai *et al.* (1982); 2, Voss *et al.* (1980); 3, Croce *et al.* (1973a); 4, Croce *et al.* (1973b); 5, Todaro and Green (1963).

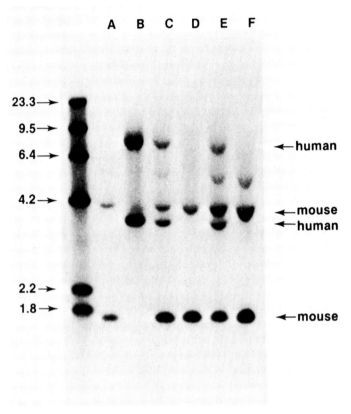

Fig. 3. Localization of *c-fes* relative to the translocation breakpoint on human chromosome 15. *Sst*I digested cellular DNAs (25 μg/lane) were electrophoresed on 0.7% agarose gels, blotted to nitrocellulose and hybridized to *c-fes* $K_{0.5}$. Cell lines are (A) mouse, 1R (Nabholz *et al.*, 1969); (B) human, LNSV (Croce *et al.*, 1973b); (C) HorI-I (Heisterkamp *et al.*, 1982); (D) PJT$_2$/A$_1$; (E) DT2.12 (Swallow *et al.*, 1977); and (F) DT2.1R3 (Swallow *et al.*, 1977). The positions of mouse and human specific restriction fragments are as indicated. *Hind*III digested λ DNA, included as a size marker in kb, is shown on the left side of the figure.

IX. Localization of Breakpoints in the t(15q+;17q−)

As regional gene localizations are often made using chromosome translocations where it is difficult to define precisely the breakpoints, caution should be exercised in drawing conclusions from these data. However, the localization of the *TK* gene to 17q210–220 is probably one of the most secure. Since the *TK* gene is present on the 15q+ translocation chromosome, the breakpoint in chromosome 17 appears to be within or above band 17q210–220. This information combined with a karyotypic analysis of the translocation chromosomes suggests that the breakpoint in chromosome 15 is within 15q22. These breakpoints are consistent with those proposed most recently by Rowley (J. D. Rowley, personal communication), i.e., 15q22.2 and 17q12–21. Figure 4 shows a diagram of the rearranged chromosomes with these breakpoints. Experiments are in progress to confirm that *c-fes, MPI,* and *PKM2* have moved to the 17q− chromosome.

Our results have also enabled an ordering of genes on chromosome 15, i.e., *B2M* and *MIC7* are located above *c-fes, MPI,* and *PKM2.*

X. Conclusion

We have used somatic cell hybridization to isolate the 15q+ translocation chromosome, to localize more precisely the breakpoints involved in the t(15q+;17q−) found in APL, and to map c-fes within the region of chromosome 15 which is translocated to chromosome 17. Erikson *et al.* (1982) have shown that in the t(8q−;14q+) found in Burkitt's lymphoma, the break in chromosome 14 occurs within the V region of the immunoglobulin heavy chain genes so that some of the V_H genes move to the 8q− translocation chromosome. Furthermore, Nowell *et al.* (see Chapter 9) have shown that in this translocation, the *c-myc* gene from chromosome 8 has become associated with the C_μ gene on the 14q+ translocation chromosome. The availability of somatic cell hybrids containing

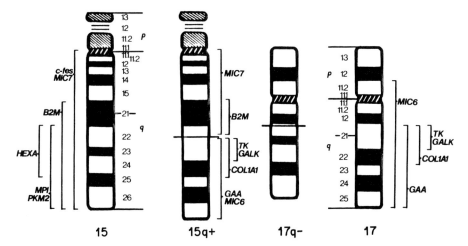

Fig. 4. Schematic representation of the t(15q+;17q−) with breakpoints in bands 15q22 and 17q21. Localizations of genes tested in the hybrid PJT$_2$/A$_1$ are shown on the normal chromosomes 15 and 17. Those genes present in the hybrid PJT$_2$/A$_1$ are shown on the 15q+ translocation chromosome.

the 15q+ and 17q− translocation chromosomes should enable a similar study of DNA sequences at the breakpoints in the t(15q+;17q−).

Acknowledgments

We wish to thank the Imperial Cancer Research Fund Medical Oncology Unit, St. Bartholomew's Hospital, London, for their generosity in providing us with cells from APL patients. We are also grateful to Dr. Janet Rowley for interesting discussion, to Mrs. Karina F. Stanley and Mr. Mohamed Parkar for technical assistance, and to Miss Christine Furse for typing.

References

Bai, Y., Sheer, D., Hiorns, L., Knowles, R. W., and Tunnacliffe, A. (1982). *Ann. Hum. Genet.* **46,** 337–347.

Bennett, J. M., Catovsky, D., Daniel, M.-T., Flandrin, G., Galton, D. A. G., Gralnick, H. R., and Sultan, C. [French-American-British (FAB) Co-operative Group] (1976). *Br. J. Haematol.* **33,** 451–458.

Bennett, J. M., Catovsky, D., Daniel, M.-T., Flandrin, G., Galton, D. A. G., Gralnick, H. R., and Sultan, C. [French-American-British (FAB) Co-operative Group] (1980). *Br. J. Haematol.* **44,** 169–170.

Berger, R., Bernheim, A., and Flandrin, G. (1980). *C. R. Hebd. Seances Acad. Sci., Ser. D* **290D,** 1557–1559.

Blaineau, C., Avner, P., Tunnacliffe, A., and Goodfellow, P. N. (1983). *EMBO J.* (in press).

Bobrow, M., and Cross, J. (1974). *Nature (London)* **251,** 77–79.

Brodsky, F. M., Bodmer, W. F., and Parham, P. (1979). *Eur. J. Immunol.* **9,** 536–545.

Caspersson, T., Lomakka, G., and Zech, L. (1971). *Hereditas* **67,** 89–102.

Chang, E. H., Furth, M. E., Scolnick, E. M., and Lowy, D. R. (1982). *Nature (London)* **297,** 479–483.

Chern, C. J., Kennett, R., Engel, E., Mellman, W. J., and Croce, C. M. (1977). *Somatic Cell Genet.* **3,** 553–560.

Church, R. L., Sundar Raj, N., and McDougall, J. K. (1980). *Cytogenet. Cell Genet.* **27,** 24–30.

Croce, C. M., Girardi, A. J., and Koprowski, H. (1973a). *Proc. Natl. Acad. Sci. U.S.A.* **70,** 3617–3620.

Croce, C. M., Knowles, B. B., and Koprowski, H. (1973b). *Exp. Cell Res.* **82,** 457–461.

Dalla-Favera, R., Gallo, R. C., Giallongo, A., and Croce, C. M. (1982). *Science* **218,** 686–688.

Elsevier, S. M., Kucherlapati, R. S., Nichols, E. A., Creagan, R. P., Giles, R. P., Ruddle, F. H., Willecke, K., and McDougall, J. K. (1974). *Nature (London)* **251,** 633–635.

Erikson, J., Finan, J., Nowell, P. C., and Croce, C. M. (1982). *Proc. Natl. Acad. Sci. U.S.A.* **79,** 5611–5615.

Ferguson-Smith, M. A., and Aitken, D. A. (1982). *Cytogenet. Cell Genet.* **32,** 24–42.

Galfre, G., Howe, S. C., Milstein, C., Butcher, G. W., and Howard, J. C. (1977). *Nature (London)* **266,** 550–552.

Goodfellow, P. N., Banting, G., Levy, R., Povey, S., and McMichael, A. (1980). *Somatic Cell Genet.* **6,** 777–787.

Heisterkamp, N., Groffen, J., Stephenson, J. R., Spurr, N., Goodfellow, P. N., Solomon, E., Carritt, B., and Bodmer, W. F. (1982). *Nature (London)* **299,** 747–749.

Heurre, C., Junien, C., Weil, D., Chu, M.-L., Morabito, M., van Cong, N., Myers, J. C., Foubert, C., Gross, M.-S., Prockop, D. J., Boue, A., Kaplan, J. C., de la Chapelle, A., and Ramirez, F. (1982). *Proc. Natl. Acad. Sci. U.S.A.* **79**, 6627–6631.

Human Gene Mapping 5 (1979). *Cytogenet. Cell Genet.* **25**, 59–73.

Human Gene Mapping 6 (1982). *Cytogenet. Cell Genet.* **32**, Nos. 1–4.

Kit, S., Dubbs, D. R., Piekarski, J. R., and Hus, T. C. (1963). *Exp. Cell Res.* **31**, 297–312.

Klein, G. (1981). *Nature (London)* **294**, 313–318.

Kondo, K., and Sasaki, M. (1979). *Cancer Genet. Cytogenet.* **1**, 131–138.

Littlefield, J. (1964). *Science* **145**, 709–710.

Magenis, R. E., Vidgoff, J., Chamberlin, J., and Brown, M. G. (1979). *Cytogenet. Cell Genet.* **25**, 181.

Nabholz, M., Miggiano, V., and Bodmer, W. F. (1969). *Nature (London)* **223**, 358–363.

Nickel, B. E., Chudley, A. E., Pabello, P. D., and McAlpine, P. J. (1982). *Cytogenet. Cell Genet.* **32**, 303.

Pajunen, L., Solomon, E., Burgess, S., Bobrow, M., Povey, S., and Swallow, D. (1978). *Cytogenet. Cell Genet.* **22**, 511–512.

Seabright, M. (1972). *Chromosoma* **36**, 204–210.

Second International Workshop on Chromosomes in Leukemia, 1979 (1980). *Cancer Genet. Cytogenet.* **2**, 103–107.

Solomon, E., Swallow, D., Burgess, S., and Evans, L. (1979). *Ann. Hum. Genet.* **42**, 273–281.

Solomon, E., Hiorns, L., Sheer, D., and Rowe, D. (1983). Submitted for publication.

Swallow, D. M., Solomon, E., and Pajunen, L. (1977). *Cytogenet. Cell Genet.* **18**, 136–148.

Szybalski, W., Szybalski, E., and Rayni, G. (1962). *Natl. Cancer Inst. Monogr.* No. 7, pp. 75–89.

Todaro, G. J., and Green, H. (1963). *J. Cell Biol.* **17**, 299–316.

van Heyningen, V., Bobrow, M., Bodmer, W. F., Gardiner, S. E., Povey, S., and Hopkinson, D. A. (1975). *Ann. Hum. Genet.* **38**, 295–302.

Voss, R., Lerer, I., Solomon, E., and Bobrow, M. (1980). *Ann Hum. Genet.* **44**, 1–9.

Weiss, M. C., and Green, H. (1967). *Proc. Natl. Acad. Sci. U.S.A.* **58**, 1104–1111.

11

Flow Cytogenetics: Methodology and Applications

A. V. CARRANO, J. W. GRAY, R. G. LANGLOIS, AND L.-C. YU

Biomedical Sciences Division
Lawrence Livermore National Laboratory
Livermore, California

I. Introduction

Because knowledge of genetic fine structure is important for understanding gene regulation and aiding in the diagnosis and prevention of human genetic disease, scientists have sought for decades to probe the structure of the mammalian chromosome. This goal has been approached on many levels. At the level of the light microscope, chromosome banding methods have yielded information pertinent to chromosome morphology and chromatin organization. DNA cytophotometry has added to this information by providing precise measurements of inter- and intraspecies chromosomal DNA variation. *In situ* hybridization has further advanced our knowledge of the distribution of repeated DNA sequences among chromosomes and is now at the threshold for detecting the location of unique sequence DNA. Each of these methods continues to furnish excellent data relevant to chromosome structure, but they lack the sensitivity to probe the architecture of the chromosome beyond the limit of optical resolution. Flow cytogenetics is a rapidly developing technology which complements rather than supplants the traditional methods of cytogenetic analysis. As an adjunctive approach to chromosome classification, flow systems measurements of isolated chromosomes give new information relative to the enrichment of A-T or G-C base sequences on specific chromosomes. As a result, chromosomal fluorescence polymorphisms both within and among individuals that are not always associated with banding polymorphisms can be detected. Finally, flow sorting provides bulk quantities of highly purified chromosomes for use in biochemical studies.

II. Methodology

A. Cell Culture and Chromosome Isolation

In order to measure chromosomes using flow systems, a reliable source of growing cells from which chromosomes can be isolated is needed. Diploid fibroblast cultures or established cell lines have been used extensively (Gray *et al.*, 1975; Stubblefield *et al.*, 1975; Carrano *et al.*, 1979b), but it is now possible to culture human lymphocytes to yield adequate mitotic indices for chromosome isolations (Yu *et al.*, 1981; Young *et al.*, 1981; Matsson and Rydberg, 1981). Previously we attempted to isolate chromosomes directly from Chinese hamster bone marrow cells following a prolonged colchicine block *in vivo* or short culture *in vitro*, but this has generally resulted in too few mitotic cells. In such cases, isolated chromosomes could be observed, but the amount of cellular debris from nondividing cells was so great as to mask chromosome resolution in the flow measurements. In general, for any cell type, a higher mitotic index results in more free chromosomes, less cellular or chromatin debris, and therefore a greater signal-to-noise ratio during analysis.

The number of cultures needed for chromosome isolation is dependent upon the experimental design. Accumulation of a chromosome distribution on a flow system for the purpose of determining the presence of abnormal chromosomes or chromosomal polymorphisms or for measuring variability among individuals requires less than 10^6 chromosomes, but our current optimal procedure for chromosome isolation uses 5×10^6 to 8×10^6 mitotic cells as starting material. This number of mitotic cells is easily obtained from one 650 ml roller bottle. Mitotic indices of the shaken-off cell population obtained after 6–14 hours of

Colcemid treatment usually vary from 80 to 95%. If chromosomes are to be sorted additional cell cultures could be necessary. Lymphocyte cultures are established by first separating the white blood cells by gradient centrifugation, stimulating them with mitogen, and culturing for 60–90 hours. As little as 2 ml of whole blood can yield sufficient cells for flow analysis, but, as for fibroblasts, larger quantities will be necessary for chromosome sorting (30–50 ml). Colcemid is added to the cultures for 12–20 hours to obtain mitotic indices from 10 to 40%. The details of the culture methods in use in our laboratory for human cells have been described previously for fibroblasts (Carrano et al., 1979a,b) and lymphocytes (Yu et al., 1981).

Historically, several methods have been used to isolate chromosomes from mitotic cells, and these have been summarized (Carrano et al., 1979a). Today, three buffer systems are commonly used for maintaining the integrity of the isolated chromosomes: (1) a Tris–hexylene glycol buffer (25 mM Tris-HCl, pH 7.5, 0.75 M hexylene glycol, 0.5 mM $CaCl_2$ and 1 mM $MgCl_2$) derived from that originally described by Wray and Stubblefield (1970); (2) a polyamine buffer (15 mM Tris-HCl, 2 mM EDTA, 0.5 mM ethylene glycol bis(β-aminoethyl ether)-N,N,N^1,N^1-tetraacetic acid, 80 mM KCl, 20 mM NaCl, 0.2 mM spermine, 0.5 mM spermidine, 14 mM 2-mercaptoethanol, pH 7.2) described by Young et al. (1981); and (3) a Tris or saline buffer containing the fluorochrome to be used for flow analysis (Otto et al., 1980; Matsson and Rydberg, 1981). Any of these methods could be coupled with appropriate detergents to allow more gentle shear of the mitotic cells, but our experience with the hexylene glycol buffer and fibroblast cells is that the use of either Nonidet P-40 or Triton X-100 is associated with an increase in the debris continuum in the fluorescence distribution. The choice of buffer is ultimately dependent upon the disposition of the isolated chromosomes. Any of the buffers with the appropriate fluorochrome can yield excellent resolution of the chromosome peaks in a flow distribution. We chose to use the hexylene glycol based buffer in our experiments since it maintains the chromosomal proteins unchanged from the interphase and mitotic cell chromatin (as determined by polyacrylamide gel electrophoresis of the histone and major nonhistone proteins), yields high molecular weight DNA ($>10^7$), and enables us to identify the sorted chromosomes either by trypsin–Giemsa or quinacrine banding (Fig. 1). Finally, the mitotic cells are mechanically sheared in the isolation buffer at a high concentration and small volume (approximately 5×10^6 cells in 1 ml) with a Virtis homogenizer or by manually forcing them through a 22–27 gauge needle.

B. Chromosome Staining and Flow Instrumentation

Isolated chromosomes can be stained with either one or two fluorochromes depending on the type of flow instrumentation used and the nature of the experi-

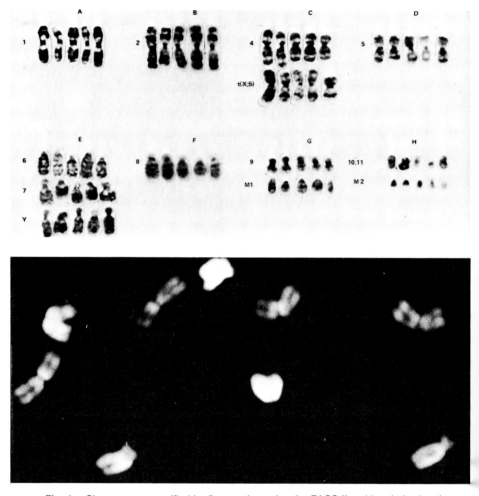

Fig. 1. Chromosomes purified by flow sorting using the FACS II and banded using the trypsin–Giemsa or quinacrine methods. Top: Chinese hamster M3-1 chromosomes sorted on the basis of their relative ethidium bromide fluorescence and arranged according to their karyotype and peak in the flow distribution. Five Giemsa-banded chromosomes of each type are displayed. Bottom: Human chromosomes 3 and 4 sorted on the basis of their relative Hoechst fluorescence.

ment. Our earlier experiments to measure human chromosomal polymorphisms and to sort chromosomes for biochemical studies were performed using a Beckton-Dickinson FACS II cell sorter equipped with a Spectra Physics 171-05 argon ion laser, which delivers 0.7–1.0 W of 351 + 364 nm light. Chromosomes isolated from 5×10^6 mitotic cells and analyzed in this system were stained with 33258 Hoechst at a final concentration of 2–4 μg/ml.

High resolution of the human chromosomes can be achieved if they are stained with two fluorochromes and analyzed in a dual beam flow system. In this case, the chromosome suspension is mixed with a stain solution of 33258 Hoechst and chromomycin A3 in dilute KCl to give a final suspension containing the equivalent of 50 μM DNA, 1.3 μM Hoechst, 18 μM chromomycin A3, 6 mM Tris at pH 7.5, 0.19 M hexylene glycol, 0.1 mM CaCl$_2$, 0.25 mM MgCl$_2$, and 19 mM KCl. Flow cytometry is generally performed within 1 day of staining, but stained chromosomes can be stored up to 7 days at 4°C prior to analysis.

Figure 2 illustrates the principle of dual laser flow cytometry as accomplished using the Lawrence Livermore National Laboratory dual beam flow sorter (Dean and Pinkel, 1978) equipped with two Spectra Physics 171 lasers. Chromosomes in the sample stream first intersect a 458-nm beam from an argon ion laser (1.0 W) to excite the chromomycin A3 and then intersect the ultraviolet beam from a krypton ion laser (337–356 nm, 0.8 W) to excite the Hoechst stain. The fluorescence emissions are independently processed, and the bivariate three-dimensional histogram produced by this method is also shown for human chromosomes 9–22. Chromosomes are normally analyzed at a rate of 1000 per second, and typically $10^5–10^6$ are analyzed per distribution.

III. Single-Parameter Flow Analysis

When human chromosomes are isolated from diploid fibroblast or lymphocyte cultures and stained with 33258 Hoechst, approximately 14 peaks representing the 24 chromosome types are evident in the flow distribution (Carrano *et al.*, 1979b). The identification of the chromosomes associated with each peak in the distribution is determined by first sorting the chromosomes from each peak and

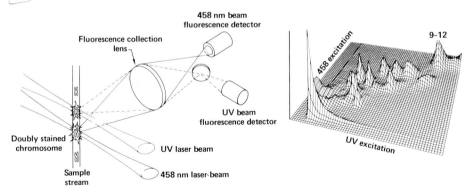

Fig. 2. Schematic representation illustrating the principle of the dual beam flow sorter. Left: Sample flow and fluorescence collection. Right: Bivariate flow distribution of human chromosomes. The distribution shows only chromosomes 9–22.

banding the sorted fractions using quinacrine. To aid in the collection of chromosomes for positive identification, we sort about 20,000 chromosomes on a frozen petri dish (approximately $-32°C$). Upon contact with the frozen dish, the liquid drops containing the chromosomes freeze and form a large bead. This bead is then manually moved with a pair of cold forceps into the well of a modified Leif bucket (Leif *et al.*, 1971), immediately fixed with about 30 μl of fixative (3 : 1, absolute methanol–glacial acetic acid), and spun onto a microscope slide. Only about 15–25% of the sorted chromosomes can be positively identified by banding since they often do not lie flat on the microscope slide or are twisted after sorting. Most of the remaining chromosomes, however, can be identified as to group. We have exploited this single-parameter capability to examine the variation in the fluorescence distribution among individuals and to sort chromosomes for gene mapping.

A. Variability among Individuals

We have demonstrated that the relative position of Hoechst stained human chromosomes in the flow distribution of a single individual can be markedly influenced by the dye to base pair ratio (Langlois *et al.*, 1980). Thus this ratio must be kept invariant when comparing chromosomal polymorphisms among individuals. Univariate Hoechst distributions of chromosomes isolated from diploid fibroblast strains derived from four normal individuals are shown in Fig. 3. Results with individual 592 have been reported previously, and the Hoechst distribution was compared to the chromosomal DNA contents as determined by cytophotometry (Carrano *et al.*, 1979b). For the most part, the relative Hoechst fluorescence parallels the DNA content of each chromosome but some differences are evident. Chromosomes 4, 8, 13, 18, and Y are brighter and chromosomes 16, 17, and 19 are dimmer than expected based upon their DNA amounts. This is in consonance with the increased affinity of 33258 Hoechst for DNA rich in A–T base sequences (Latt and Wohlleb, 1975; Comings and Drets, 1976) and parallels the quinacrine fluorescence intensity observed in metaphase chromosomes from these individuals. The homolog difference in Hoechst fluorescence observed for chromosome 14 in individual 592 is also seen for DNA content.

The most variable chromosome observed among the four individuals is the Y. This chromosome has the same fluorescence intensity as chromosomes 16 and 18 in individual 706 but as chromosomes 19–22 for individual 761. This is also consistent with the A–T rich satellite DNA present in the distal region of the long arm of this chromosome (Jones *et al.*, 1974; Gosden *et al.*, 1975). Other homolog differences can be noted, namely, chromosome 13 in individuals 706 and 761, chromosome 14 in individual 761, and chromosome 15 in individual 759. Again, these same homolog differences are observed for quinacrine polymorphisms in these people. The presence of these polymorphisms creates potential

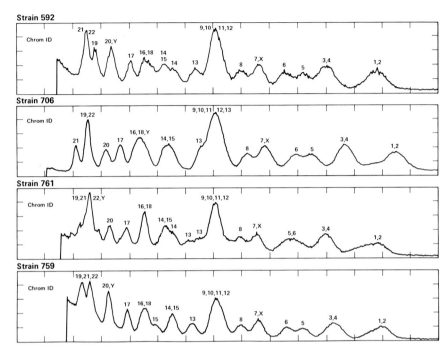

Fig. 3. Univariate flow distributions of human chromosomes stained with 33258 Hoechst. The chromosomes were isolated from four diploid fibroblast strains and analyzed on the FACS II. Chromosomes associated with each peak are indicated above the peak.

problems for chromosome identification based upon the Hoechst distribution alone. Unless all the chromosomes can be uniquely identified and/or the areas under each peak can be precisely quantified, the detection of abnormal chromosomes is difficult. The polymorphisms, however, are interesting from a biochemical viewpoint. It is now possible to sort each of the homologs and determine the biochemical basis for their difference in Hoechst fluorescence.

B. Biochemical Studies

One of the first biochemical experiments on chromosomes purified by a flow sorter was performed on chromosomes from the Chinese hamster M3-1 cell line (Sawin et al., 1979). Since each Chinese hamster chromosome could be sorted to a purity of 80–98%, the question asked was whether the repetitive DNA sequences present on the hamster chromosome 1 were unique to that chromosome. For this experiment approximately 10^6 No. 1 chromosomes were purified (approximately 1 μg of DNA) and the DNA extracted and transcribed with E. coli RNA polymerase to produce a radiolabeled cRNA. The cRNA was then hybridized *in situ* to metaphase spreads from the same cells under conditions such that only the repetitive DNA would hybridize. The results of this experiment showed that the cRNA from chromosome 1 was present on all the metaphase chromosomes. Similar results were obtained for cRNA from sorted chromosome 2. These experiments demonstrated that DNA could be recovered from small numbers of highly purified flow-sorted chromosomes and that the DNA was of sufficient integrity to be used as a template for RNA polymerase to yield a product that could be employed for *in situ* hybridization.

In a collaborative experiment with Dr. Masa Hatanaka (Kyoto University, Kyoto, Japan), it was shown that a murine sarcoma gene fragment could be localized to sorted chromosomes (Table I) (M. Hatanaka and A. V. Carrano, unpublished results). The initial experiments with the Chinese hamster chromosomes suggested that it would be possible to identify the location of single copy DNA sequences on specific chromosomes. In order to verify this, a karyotypically simple mammalian species was used, namely, the Indian muntjac. The female of this species has only six chromosomes, three homolog pairs, each of which is distinguishable in a flow distribution. Chromosome 1 could be sorted to a purity of 97%, while the X and No. 2 chromosomes could be sorted 77 and 89% pure, respectively. Using a female cell line that was transformed with murine sarcoma virus and known to contain two copies of the sarcoma gene, it was possible to identify the chromosomal location of the viral gene. In order to do this, the three chromosome types were sorted from the transformed cells. Approximately 10 μg of DNA were extracted from each of the sorted fractions and hybridized separately *in vitro* to radioactive DNA complementary to the sarcoma viral gene. After hybridization, duplex DNA (i.e., chromosomal DNA bound to sarcoma virus DNA) was purified by hydroxyapatite chromatography and detected by scintillation counting. The sarcoma gene probe hybridized to an equal extent to the DNA from the X and No. 2 chromosomes only suggesting that one copy of the viral gene was integrated into each of these two chromosomes.

The obvious extension of these experiments was to map the location of genes on human chromosomes. Using 33258 Hoechst stained chromosomes purified from diploid human fibroblasts coupled with the techniques of restriction enzyme

TABLE I

Hybridization of a Sarcoma Viral Gene Probe with DNA Extracted from Sorted Indian Muntjac Chromosomes

Chromosome	Purity of sort (%)	Hybrid formed (%)
1	97	0
X	77	22.5
2	89	23.5

analysis of DNA, the human β-globin complex was mapped to the short arm of chromosome 11 (Lebo *et al.*, 1979). The procedure was operationally simple. First, selected chromosomes were purified by sorting, the chromosomal DNA extracted and digested with *Eco*R1 restriction enzyme, and the fragments separated by agarose gel electrophoresis. The restricted DNA was transferred to nitrocellulose filters, hybridized to ^{32}P-labeled cDNA prepared by reverse transcription of human globin mRNA and the filters processed by autoradiography. Positive hybridization between the globin cDNA and the chromosomal DNA would be indicative of the presence of globin genes.

The gene for the β-globin complex was mapped to chromosome 11 by first demonstrating positive hybridization to DNA extracted from the peak containing chromosomes 9–12 and to DNA from a translocation involving chromosome 11 in another cell strain. For this second cell strain, hybridization occurred to DNA from two chromosomal peaks, one that contained the normal chromosome 11 and the other that contained the translocated segment of chromosome 11. More

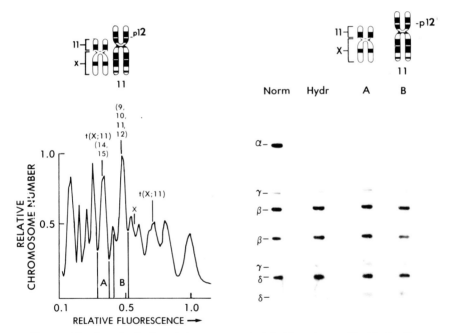

Fig. 4. The flow distribution of chromosomes isolated from human fibroblast cells possessing a translocation between chromosomes X and 11. Hybridization of the globin cDNA to digested DNA from these chromosomes is shown on the gels to the right. Norm, whole cell DNA from a normal individual; Hydr, whole cell DNA from an individual lacking the α-globin gene. A and B refer to the DNA extracted from the chromosomes in the same sorted fractions shown in the flow distribution.

precise localization of the gene was accomplished using chromosomes from a third fibroblast cell strain carrying a translocation between the short arms of chromosomes X and 11 as illustrated in Fig. 4. This translocation moved the bulk of the short arm from one chromosome 11 to a new peak. Chromosomes were sorted from peak B (chromosomes 9, 10, 12, and the normal 11) and peak A (chromosomes 14, 15, and the X;11 translocation containing the short arm of chromosome 11). The results of the hybridization of the globin cDNA to the digested DNA are shown next to the flow distribution. The first gel represents whole cell DNA from a normal individual and demonstrates hybridization to the α-globin as well as β-globin probes. The second gel contains DNA from an individual lacking the α-globin gene. The last two gels, containing DNA from chromosomes sorted from peaks A and B, demonstrate the presence of the β-globin gene complex in both fractions. Since only the short arm of chromosome 11 was present in peak A, the genes must reside in this chromosomal region. In an analogous manner the human insulin gene was mapped to the same region on chromosome 11 (Lebo *et al.*, 1982). Because the two alleles of the insulin gene could be sorted in cells bearing the translocation of chromosome 11, it was also possible to show by restriction enzyme analysis that the insulin gene was polymorphic.

IV. Dual-Parameter Flow Analysis

High-resolution chromosome analysis of Chinese hamster M3-1 and human chromosomes using two fluorochromes has been described previously (Gray *et al.*, 1979). Chromomycin A3 complements Hoechst in this double staining procedure since it binds preferentially to G-C-rich DNA (Behr *et al.*, 1969), while Hoechst binds to A-T-rich DNA. The Hoechst and chromomycin stain content in chromosomes stained with both can be measured almost independently by selectively exciting the Hoechst in the ultraviolet or chromomycin A3 at 458 nm (Langlois *et al.*, 1980). The fluorescence distributions for the chromosomes stained with both stains or with chromomycin A3 alone and excited at 458 nm are not different suggesting that the Hoechst binding has no effect on the measurement of chromomycin binding. There is a small difference between the fluorescence distributions of the doubly stained chromosomes and those stained with Hoechst alone when they are excited in the ultraviolet. The slight differences are probably due to interactions between the two bound stains when they are in close proximity on the same chromosome. To a first approximation,however, the fluorescence of the doubly stained chromosomes when excited in the ultraviolet is a measure of the Hoechst stain content. Using this double staining procedure and dual-parameter flow analysis, we are able to discriminate each of the Chinese hamster M3-1 chromosomes including some homolog differences (Gray *et*

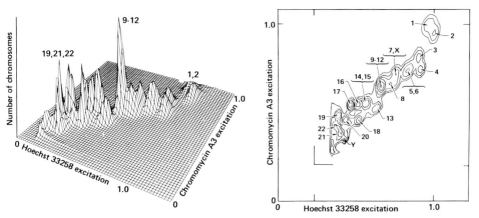

Fig. 5. Bivariate flow distribution of normal human chromosomes stained with both 33258 Hoechst and chromomycin A3. Left: Three-dimensional plot showing the peak heights and relative fluorescence of the chromosomes. Right: Contour plot of the same chromosomes with each peak identified as to chromosome type.

al., 1979). For the human chromosomes, this technique can resolve 18–20 of the different chromosome types as well as homolog differences for some of the chromosomes. Figure 5 illustrates a flow distribution of chromosomes isolated from human diploid fibroblast cells and stained with the two fluorochromes. The three-dimensional histogram on the left is a plot of the accumulated fluorescence signals viewed laterally. The x and y axes show the relative fluorescence for the respective fluorochromes and the z axis the number of chromosomes. Some of the chromosome peaks (1–2, 9–12, and 19, 21, 22) are identified to orient the viewer. The two-dimensional plot on the right results from truncating and collapsing the distribution along the z axis. This contour plot provides information on the mode and the relative separation of peaks. The chromosomes associated with each peak are indicated on the contour plot. Chromosomes that fluoresce equally with chromomycin and Hoechst will lie along the diagonal of the contour plot. Deviations of chromosomes from this diagonal therefore suggest enrichment of either A-T or G-C sequences in that chromosome.

A. Human Chromosome Polymorphisms

As with the single-parameter flow analysis using Hoechst stain, chromosomal polymorphisms are observed both within and among individuals. Figure 6 shows the contour plots for chromosomes isolated from fibroblast cells of four individuals. Only chromosomes 9–22 are shown to illustrate the variability observed within and among individuals. The large unmarked contour at the lower left of each plot represents debris. Chromosome 21, which often lies adjacent to this

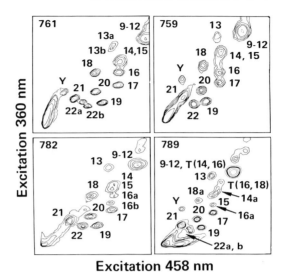

Fig. 6. Contour plots showing the distribution of human chromosomes 9–22 in four individuals: 761, 759, 782, and 789. Chromosomes were isolated from fibroblast cultures and anaylzed on the Lawrence Livermore National Laboratory dual beam sorter.

debris, can be distinguished in all cases. The relative location of the chromosome peaks differs among individuals. As an example, compare the location of chromosomes 14–17 in individuals 761 and 759. Homolog differences in fluorescence intensity are also detected. Individual 761 has a homolog difference in chromosomes 13 and 22, individual 782 has a difference in chromosome 16, and individual 789 a difference in chromosome 22. The contour between the peaks for chromosomes 14–15 and chromosome 16 for individual 759 suggest that one of these chromosomes might be polymorphic. Silver staining shows a polymorphism for the satellite region of chromosome 15 in this individual. Individual 789 possesses a complex translocation involving chromosome 14, 16, and 18. Because of this translocation, it is possible to resolve separately each normal homolog for these three chromosomes (14a, 16a, and 18a in the figure). One derivative chromosome is located with chromosomes 9–12, and the other forms a peak adjacent to chromosome 14a. This increased resolution for individual homologs is ideal for separation of these homologs for biochemical studies such as the identification of polymorphic alleles.

B. Variability among Individuals

We have quantified the extent of variability in the dual-parameter flow distributions of chromosomes isolated from short-term lymphocyte cultures from ten normal individuals (Langlois *et al.*, 1982). The standard deviation in the peak means among individuals is larger than the variability in replicate measurements on the same individual. Thus, the biological variability observed among individuals is the major contribution to the total variability observed in the flow measurements. Those chromosomes that possess polymorphisms by quinacrine banding, in general, have the larger biological variability in Hoechst fluorescence, although this correlation is not absolute. The largest variability in Hoechst fluorescence was observed for the Y chromosome, where the difference in fluorescence between the largest and smallest Y chromosomes measured 37%. Within one individual the difference between the two homologs of chromosome 21 differed in Hoechst fluorescence by 30%. A statistical summary of the combined distributions of all ten individuals is shown in Fig. 7. The mean of each chromosome type is represented by a 95% tolerance region that contains (with a probability of 0.90) 95% of the peak means for normal individuals. In no case did any of the peak means overlap another peak mean. With the exception of chromosomes 9–12 and 14–15, each of the normal chromosome types can be unambiguously classified solely on the basis of its peak position in the bivariate distribution.

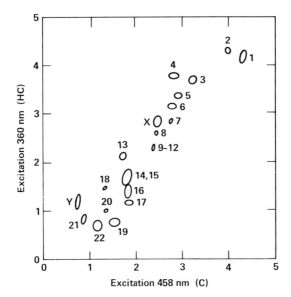

Fig. 7. Statistical summary plot of the peak means for chromosomes isolated from lymphocyte cultures of ten individuals. The ellipses represent the 95% tolerance region of all the peak means for each chromosome type.

V. Prospects for Flow Cytogenetics

Application of the above principles can be made to both the classification of normal and abnormal karyotypes as well as to the molecular biology of chromosomes. Karyotype analysis by flow systems has potential application in clincial diagnosis and would either obviate the need for banding for some disorders or, at least, be an adjunct to it. It would be helpful, for example, in the diagnosis of marker chromosomes such as the Philadelphia chromosome in chronic myelogenous leukemia or translocations observed in other hematologic disorders. It could also be helpful in the cytogenetic characterization of other transformed cell types that have a heterogeneous cell population. In this case, any marker chromosome present in a significant portion of the cells potentially could be identified or sorted for further analysis. Chromosomal DNA libraries have already been established from sorted chromosomes (Davies *et al.*, 1981), lending further support to the credibility and utility of flow sorting in biochemical studies. It should be possible not only to probe the DNA structure of individual chromosomes and alleles but also resolve questions concerning the nature of the chromosomal proteins associated with normal and abnormal chromosomes.

Acknowledgments

This work was conducted under the auspices of the United States Department of Energy by the Lawrence Livermore National Laboratory under Contract W-7405-ENG-48.

References

Behr, W., Honikel, K., and Hartman, G. (1969). *Eur. J. Biochem.* **9**, 82–92.
Carrano, A. V., Van Dilla, M. A., and Gray, J. W. (1979a). *In* "Flow Cytometry and Sorting" (Melamed, M. R., Mullaney, P. F., and Mendelsohn, M. L., eds.), pp. 421–451. Wiley, New York.
Carrano, A. V., Gray, J. W., Langlois, R. G., Burkhart-Schultz, K. J., and Van Dilla, M. A. (1979b). *Proc. Natl. Acad. Sci. U.S.A.* **76**, 1382–1384.
Comings, D. E., and Drets, M. E. (1976). *Chromosoma* **56**, 199–211.
Davies, K. E., Young, B. D., Elles, R. G., Hill, M. E., and Williamson, R. (1981). *Nature (London)* **293**, 374–376.
Dean, P. N., and Pinkel, D. (1978). *J. Histochem. Cytochem.* **26**, 622–627.
Gosden, J. R., Mitchell, A. R., Buckland, R. A., Clayton, R. P., and Evans, H. J. (1975). *Exp. Cell Res.* **92**, 148–158.
Gray, J. W., Carrano, A. V., Steinmetz, L. L., Minkler, J., Mayall, B. H., and Mendelsohn, M. L. (1975). *Proc. Natl. Acad. Sci. U.S.A.* **72**, 1231–1234.
Gray, J. W., Langlois, R. G., Carrano, A. V., Burkhart-Schultz, K., and Van Dilla, M. A. (1979). *Chromosoma* **73**, 9–27.
Jones, K. W., Purdom, I. F., Prosser, J., and Corneo, G. (1974). *Chromosoma* **49**, 161–171.

Langlois, R. G., Carrano, A. V., Gray, J. W., and Van Dilla, M. A. (1980). *Chromosoma* **77,** 229–251.

Langlois, R. G., Yu, L.-C., Gray, J. W., and Carrano, A. V. (1982). *Proc. Natl. Acad. Sci. U.S.A.* **79,** 7876–7880.

Latt, S. A., and Wohlleb, J. C. (1975). *Chromosoma* **52,** 297–316.

Lebo, R. V., Carrano, A. V., Burkhart-Schultz, K., Dozy, A. M., Yu, L.-C., and Kan, Y. W. (1979). *Proc. Natl. Acad. Sci. U.S.A.* **76,** 5804–5808.

Lebo, R. V., Kan, Y. W., Cheung, M. C., Carrano, A. V., Yu, L.-C., Chang, J. C., Cordell, B., and Goodman, H. M. (1982). *Hum. Genet.* **60,** 10–15.

Leif, R. C., Easter, H. N., Waters, R. L., Thomas, R. A., Dunlap, L. A., and Austin, M. F. (1971). *J. Histochem. Cytochem.* **19,** 203–215.

Matsson, P., and Rydberg, B. (1981). *Cytometry* **1,** 369–372.

Otto, F. J., Oldiges, H., Gohde, W., Barlogie, B., and Schumann, J. (1980). *Cytogenet. Cell Genet.* **27,** 52–56.

Sawin, V. L., Rowley, J. D., and Carrano, A. V. (1979). *Chromosoma* **70,** 293–304.

Stubblefield, E., Deaven, L., and Cram, L. S. (1975). *Exp. Cell Res.* **94,** 464–468.

Wray, W., and Stubblefield, E. (1970). *Exp. Cell Res.* **59,** 469–478.

Young, B. D., Ferguson-Smith, M. A., Sillar, R., and Boyd, E. (1981). *Proc. Natl. Acad. Sci. U.S.A.* **78,** 7727–7731.

Yu, L.-C., Aten, J., Gray, J., and Carrano, A. V. (1981). *Nature (London)* **293,** 154–155.

12

Construction and Characterization of Chromosomal DNA Libraries

BRYAN D. YOUNG, MARC JEANPIERRE , MALCOLM H. GOYNS, AND ROBERT KRUMLAUF

Beatson Institute for Cancer Research
Garscube Estate
Glasgow, Scotland

GORDON D. STEWART AND THERESA ELLIOT

Duncan Guthrie Institute of Medical Genetics
Yorkhill Hospital
Glasgow, Scotland

I. Introduction

The availability of cloned genes has rapidly expanded our knowledge of the fine structure, organization, and expression of sequences in the human genome

*Present address: Institut de Pathologie Moleculaire, 24 rue du Faubourg Saint Jacques, Paris, France.

†Present address: Institute for Cancer Research, Fox Chase Cancer Center, Philadelphia, Pennsylvania 19111.

and provided insight into the molecular basis of diseases such as the thalassemia syndromes. In addition, the application of recombinant DNA technology to human genetics has played an important role in attempting to bridge the gap in resolving power between DNA sequence analysis and classic cytological approaches to mapping and gene linkage. Recent studies have shown that highly polymorphic loci can be identified from human genomic libraries (see review, Ruddle, 1981). Using such probes the construction of a fine-structure linkage map would be particularly useful in cases where the chromosomal location of the genetic lesion associated with a disease is known. In this context a general method for rapidly isolating a wide spectrum of DNA probes for specific human chromosomes would be an invaluable aid to human gene mapping. An essential prerequisite for such an approach is the high resolution fractionation of human chromosomes.

There have been many attempts to fractionate metaphase chromosomes using centrifugation (Padgett et al., 1977), countercurrent distribution (Pinaev et al., 1979), and 1 g sedimentation (Collard et al., 1982). While such attempts have achieved some enrichment of different size classes of chromosomes, the similar size of many human chromosomes has prevented the separation of pure fractions of single chromosomes. The construction of human–rodent cell hybrids has allowed the purification of single human chromosomes using selectable markers (McKusick and Ruddle, 1977). Although this approach has the disadvantage of the rodent cell DNA background, it has been used to obtain clones from particular chromosomes (Gusella et al., 1980). However, due to the presence of a larger number of clones containing rodent cell DNA, this approach is useful for obtaining only small numbers of clones. In order to obtain a larger number of clones from a particular chromosome, it is necessary to purify the chromosomes of interest in sufficient quantity to allow direct DNA cloning. We have already reported the sorting of the human chromosomes 22 and 21 flow cytometry in sufficient quantity to allow the construction of DNA libraries (Krumlauf et al., 1982). In this report we extend these observations to include the mapping of more clones on both chromosomes 22 and 21. Chromosomes 22 and 21 were chosen for this study in view of the specific rearrangements of 22 that occur in chronic myeloid leukemia and the association of 21 with Downs syndrome.

II. Results

A. Sorting and Cloning of Chromosomes 21 and 22

The strategy we have adopted for obtaining DNA sequences from human chromosomes 21 and 22 involves directly sorting these chromosomes on a fluorescence-activated cell sorter (FACS II). A high-resolution flow analysis of a

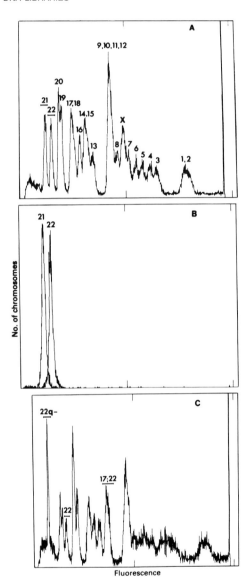

Fig. 1. Flow karyotypes of human chromosomes. Numbers indicate the chromosomes contained in each peak, and the horizontal bars indicate the fluorescent windows used to sort chromosomes. (A) GM1416: 48,XXXX lymphoblastoid cells. (B) Fractions of chromosomes 21 and 22 sorted from (A). (C) GM3197: 46,XX cells bearing the translocation t(17;22) (p13;11).

suspension of metaphase chromosomes prepared (Sillar and Young, 1981) from the lymphoblast cell line GM 1416: 48, XXXX, generates the flow karyotype shown in Fig. 1A. The assignment of chromosomes to each of the distinct peaks was based on their DNA contents (Carrano et al., 1979) and on the results of a study that established correlations between flow karyotypes and conventional G and C banding karyotypes using abnormal human chromosomes and hetero-chromatic polymorphisms (Young et al., 1981). The peaks containing chromosomes 21 and 22 were individually sorted, and a sample of each was reanalyzed on the FACS II to assess the efficiency of sorting (Fig. 1B). Each fluorescence profile showed a sharp single peak suggesting the sorted fractions were pure.

DNA was extracted from each fraction containing 2×10^6 chromosomes (about 90–100 ng DNA) and was used to construct recombinant libraries in λgtWESλB by a modification of the method described by Maniatis et al. (1978). The DNA was completely digested with EcoRI, due to the difficulty in control-ling digestion of such small amounts. A yield of 3×10^5 unamplified recombi-nant phage were obtained for each chromosome, which should be sufficient to ensure that the majority of sequences were represented in the libraries. The inserts of all phage examined to date range in size between 2.5 and 14 kilobase pairs. A background of parental phage (about 10%) was estimated by ligation and packaging of cloning arms alone.

B. Isolation and Assignment of Single Copy Sequences to Chromosome 22

Single copy sequences required for linkage analysis were initially identified by isolating phage DNA from 20 recombinants selected at random. The DNAs were labeled with ^{32}P by nick translation (Rigby et al., 1977) and hybridized to nitrocellulose strips containing EcoRI digested total DNA from GM 1416 cells. All the probes hybridized to the filters, indicating that they contained cloned human sequences. The hybridization from 13 probes produced smears, indicat-ing that they contained sequences repeated with varying frequencies in the human genome (Schmidt and Deininger, 1975). In two cases, complex multiple bands were observed. However, the remaining clones hybridized to discrete DNA fragments identical in size with their human DNA inserts (Fig. 2A). This verifies that the sorting and cloning procedures have not altered the chromosomal DNA. Based on these hybridization data, we initially selected these five recom-binants as single copy probes for further characterization and mapping. The assignment of these sequences to chromosome 22 was determined by hybridiza-tion to DNA from sorted chromosomes. Results for two of the clones are shown in Fig. 2B. DNA from 22-5 and 22-6 was labeled separately by nick translation, mixed, and hybridized to a filter containing DNA from four sorted fractions corresponding to chromosomes 22, 21, 1–8, and 9–20. Both probes hybridize to

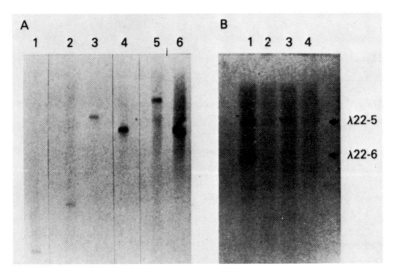

Fig. 2. (A) Hybridization of single copy clones. Nitrocellulose strips containing 20 μg of GM1416 DNA digested with *Eco*RI were hybridized with probes prepared from various recombinant phage. Lane 1 22–1, lane 2 22-2, lane 3 22-3, lane 4 22-4E, lane 5 22-5, lane 6 22-6. (B) Assignment of probes to chromosome 22. Clones 22-5 and 22-6 were labeled separately, mixed, and hybridized to *Eco*RI digested DNA from sorted fractions containing 1 × 10⁶ copies of various chromosomes. Lane 1, chromosome 22, lane 2 chromosome 21, lane 3 chromosomes 1–8, lane 4 chromosomes 9–20.

fragments of the appropriate size only in the fraction containing chromosome 22 (Fig. 2B). This illustrated the high degree of purity of the sorted chromosomes, and allowed us to assign the five clones to chromosome 22. The presence of these sequences on the chromosome has been independently confirmed by hybridization to a series of hybrid cell lines. The probes hybridize to only those lines containing human chromosome 22 (data not shown).

C. Localization of Clones on Chromosome 22

We have utilized three approaches to localize the cloned sequences to specific regions of chromosome 22, based on methods used to map globin genes (Lebo *et al.*, 1979) and noncoding sequences on chromosome 11 (Gusella *et al.*, 1980). First, we have sorted the two respective portions of one homolog of chromosome 22 from the translocated cell line GM 3197: 46, XX, t(17;22)(p13;q11). The flow karyotype of this line showed that the balanced translocation produced derivative chromosomes that were sufficiently different in size from the normal homolog that they could be identified and sorted on the FACS II (Fig. 1C). By hybridizing each of the probes to Southern blots of DNA from the two sorted

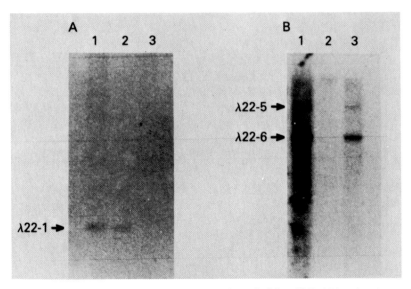

Fig. 3. Mapping probes with sorted translocations. Cell line GM3197 bearing the translocation t(17;22)(p13;q11) was used for sorting 7 × 10⁵ copies of the two portions [22q-(lane
2) and 17;22 (lane 3)] involved in the translocation, and the normal homolog of chromosome
22 (lane 1) as indicated in Fig. 1C. The filter containing *Eco*RI digested DNA from these
fractions was first hybridized with labeled phage DNA from clone 22-1 (A), then melted and
rehybridized with mixed probes from clones 22-5 and 22-6 (B).

portions of chromosome 22, the sequences were localized to a region of the
chromosome. For example, clone 22-1 hybridizes only to total DNA and the
22q− derivative placing it between pter–q11 (Fig. 3A), while clones 22-5 and
22-6 are detected only in the total and 17:22 derivative fractions, mapping them
to q11-qter (Fig. 3B).

In a similar manner, we have used DNA from several human–hamster cell
lines derived from the fibroblasts of a human female carrying a t(X;22)
(q13;q112) reciprocal translocation (Lebo *et al.*, 1979). The hybrid lines contain
either a normal homolog of human chromosome 22 or a segment of one of the
two derivative chromosomes (X/22, 22/X) free of its normal counterpart. Probes
22-5 and 22-6 hybridized to the lane containing X/22 DNA and not 22/X placing
them between q112–qter (Fig. 4A and B). Clone 22-1 again showed the reverse
pattern, localizing it to the pter–q112 region (Fig. 4C). Since the breakpoints of
the X;22 and 17;22 translocations mapped in the same general region of chromosome 22 (q112 versus q11), we expected the results to be similar. They were
identical for each of the five probes, confirming the map assignments made using
the sorted translocations. *In situ* hybridization (Malcolm *et al.*, 1977) was also
used to map clone 22-5 on chromosome 22. The hybridization of this clone to

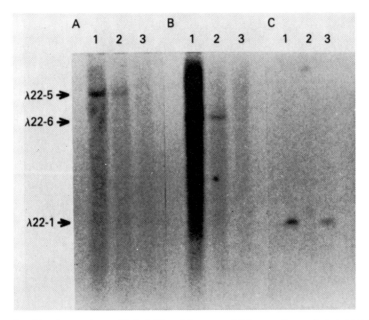

Fig. 4. Mapping probes with hybrid cell lines containing portions of chromosome 22 resulting from the translocation t(X;22)(p13;q112). Filters containing *Eco*RI digests (20 μg/lane) of human DNA (lane 1), and DNA from hybrid lines S and H (lanes 2 and 3, respectively) carrying the X/22 and 22/X portions of the translocation were hybridized to the nick translated phase 22-5 (A), 22-6 (B), and 22-1 (C).

normal human chromosomes is presented in Fig. 5A as a histogram of grain count versus chromosome number, and it can be seen that there is a distinct peak over chromosome 22. This clone was also hybridized against the chromosomes of a cell line that bore the translocation t(11;22)(q25;q13), and it can be seen in Fig. 5B that there is a peak of hybridization over both the normal chromosome 22 and over the chromosome 11/22 but not over 22/11. Thus it can be concluded that clone 22-5 lies distal to the breakpoint in q13 on chromosome 22. Figure 7 summarizes the results and relative map positions of these clones on chromosome 22.

D. Expressed Sequences

We have screened the chromosome 22 library for coding sequences. A cDNA prepared from polyadenylated RNA isolated from the white cells of a patient with chronic myeloid leukemia was used to probe an aliquot of the phage. Recombinants giving strong positive signals with this probe were picked for further analysis. A Northern blot of one of these clones (22-4E) against poly-

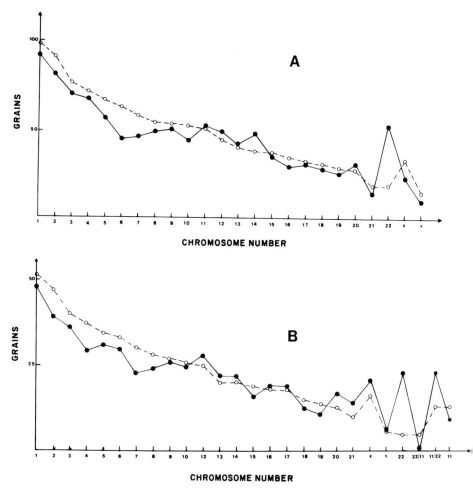

Fig. 5. Results of *in situ* hybridization of nick translated 22-5 phage DNA (10^7dpm/μg) to metaphase chromosomes of normal lymphocytes (A) and to those of a lymphoblastoid cell line (B) bearing the translocation t(11;22)(q25;q13). Grains were counted over 39 normal metaphase lymphocytes (A) and over 15 translocation bearing lymphocytes (B). The solid line represents actual grain counts, and the dashed line represents the expected values if the grains had been randomly distributed according to chromosome length.

adenylated RNA from several types of human cells shows that it is expressed in many cell types and suggests that it codes for an 8 S mRNA (Fig. 6B). The probe hybridizes to a variety of fragments in total human DNA, besides the one corresponding to its insert, suggesting that it maybe encoded by multiple genes. Using DNA from the X/22 somatic hybrid lines we have mapped the sequence corresponding to the 22-4E insert to the q112–qter region of chromosome 22 (Fig.

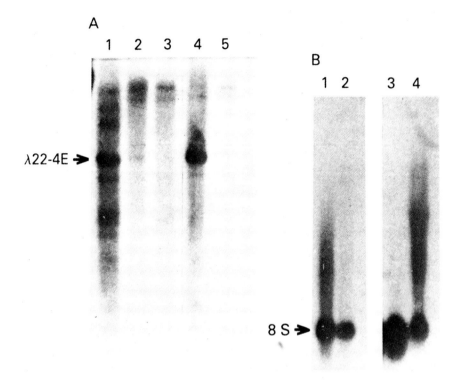

Fig. 6. Characterization of an expressed clone. (A) Clone 122-4E was mapped by hybridization to a filter with *Eco*R1 digests (20 μg/lane) of human DNA (lane 1), Chinese hamster DNA (lane 5), and DNA from the hybrid cell lines M, H, and S containing various portions of chromosome 22 [22, 22/X (lane 2), 22/X (lane 3), X/22 (lane 4)]. (B) The labeled phage, 22-4E, was also hybridized to a filter containing 3 μg of total polyadenylated RNA isolated from a patient with chronic granulyocytic leukemia (lane 1), a patient with chronic lymphatic leukemia (lane 2), cell line K562 (lane 3), and the MRC-5 human fibroblast line (lane 4).

6A). Finally, chromosome 22 has a nucleolar organizer, and we have identified several 18 S and 28 S rRNA clones using a ribosomal probe. One clone in particular, 22-18 S, has been characterized and found to contain a 6.6×10^3 bp fragment from the human ribosomal repeat unit coding for the 18 S rRNA (data not shown).

E. Localization of Clones on Chromosome 21

In a manner similar to that described above for the chromosome 22 library, 96 clones selected at random were screened with nick translated human DNA.

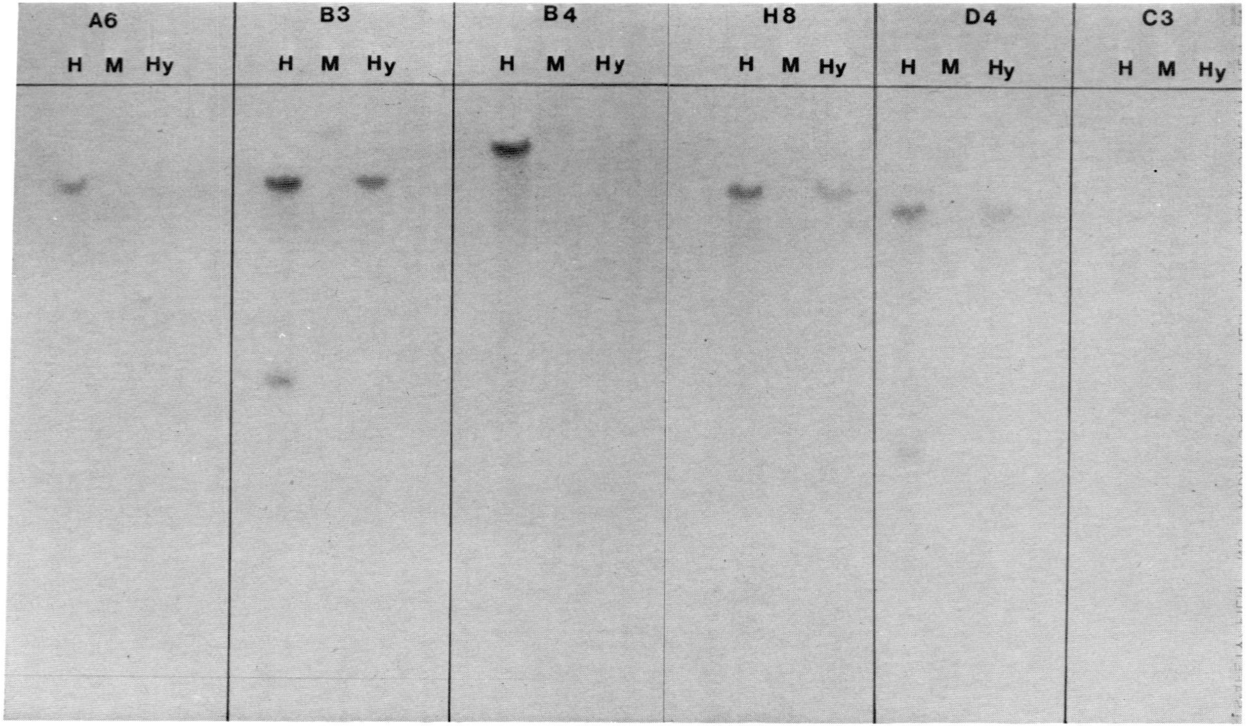

Fig. 7. Mapping probes from the chromosome 21 library with a hybrid cell line containing only chromosome 21. Filters containing *Eco*RI digests of human DNA (H), mouse parent cell line BW5147 (M) and the hybrid cell line Thy B133R (Hy) were hybridized to six different nick-translated phage.

Twenty clones did not hybridize, indicating that they may have had single copy inserts. Six of these 20 clones were found to have single copy inserts and hybridized to *Eco*RI digested human and mouse DNA and also to DNA from a rodent–human cell hybrid that contained only chromosome 21. As shown in Fig. 7 three of these clones (B3, H8, and D4) hybridized to the cell hybrid DNA, thus localizing them to chromosome 21. Of the other three clones, two do not appear to be on chromosome 21 (A6 and B4), and one apparently does not contain human DNA.

III. Discussion

This study on chromosomes 21 and 22, shows that by using the fluorescence-activated cell sorter to isolate purified fractions of specific human metaphase chromosomes, it is possible to construct DNA libraries representing single human chromosomes. The construction of a chromosome 22 library as a total *Eco*RI digest has enabled us rapidly to isolate and localize single copy sequences on the chromosome. Analysis of the chromosome 22 library so far indicates that the background of parental phage is low, since 50 recombinants selected at random have all been found to contain human DNA inserts. Of these, ten single copy clones have been identified and nine have been shown to be on chromo-

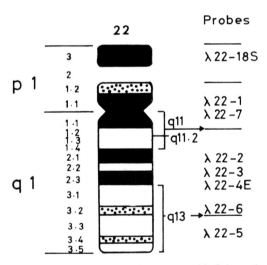

Fig. 8. Summary of mapping results on chromosome 22. Schematic representation of chromosome 22 showing the breakpoint positions of the X/22 (q112), 17/22 (q11), and 11/22 (q13) translocations used for mapping as described in the text. The relative positions of the clones are indicated.

some 22 and one on chromosome 21. The map positions of eight of these sequences is summarized in Fig. 8. This illustrates the purity of chromosomes obtained with the sorting procedure, and suggests that the majority of sequences in this library are derived from chromosome 22.

This approach is simple and direct, offering several advantages over methods utilizing total genomic libraries (Wolf *et al.*, 1980) or libraries prepared from human–rodent hybrid cell lines (Gusella *et al.*, 1980). Relatively small numbers of phage are usually handled, since prescreening steps to identify human clones among a rodent background are not necessary. The level of purity of the sorted chromosomes ensures that most of the clones are derived from the same chromosome. Repetitive sequences can be isolated and characterized regardless of their reiteration frequence or cross-species hybridization. Sequences on chromosomes that exhibit hybrid instability or lack selectable enzyme markers may also be isolated, since hybrid cell lines do not need to be constructed. Furthermore, since this library consists of sequences representing only 1.5% of the genome, relatively few phage (10,000) need to be screened to isolate genes located on the chromosome. Of particular interest are the λ-immunoglobulin light chain genes, located on chromosome 22 (Erikson *et al.*, 1981) which are possibly involved in the translocation between chromosomes 8 and 22 in a variant form of Burkitt's lymphoma (Klein, 1981). A second chromosome 22 library prepared following complete digestion with *Bam*HI will allow us to chromosome walk from any sequences of interest identified from the first library.

The application of our method to all of the human chromosomes should be possible. We have sorted an X chromosome fraction from the human 4X cell line GM 1416, which Davies *et al.* (1981) have also used to construct a recombinant library and characterize several X-specific clones. An essentially identical approach has been used by Kunkel *et al.* (1982) to obtain cloned DNA segments of the human X chromosome and by Disteche *et al.* (1982) to obtain cloned DNA segments of the mouse X chromosome. Further successful extensions of this technique depend upon the sorting and resolution of chromosomes by flow cytometry. A typical flow karyotype can now resolve human chromosomes into about 17 distinct peaks that can be sorted, 13 of which correspond to single human chromosomes (Fig. 1A). The combined use of different types of fluorescent dyes can also provide further separation of some groups of chromosomes (Gray *et al.*, 1979). Many of the remaining chromosomes, for example, chromosomes 1, 2, and 9, are separable from each other on the basis of shifts that have been observed in the fluorescence profiles of chromosomes of similar size, resulting from abnormalities and heterochromatic polymorphisms (Young *et al.*, 1981). It is particularly important that selected specific regions of some chromosomes can also be sorted and cloned using cell lines containing deletions and other derivative chromosomes from rearrangements.

The combination of chromosome sorting and recombinant DNA techniques offers the opportunity for investigating several important areas in human genetics. The relationship of cytologically observed nonrandom chromosome changes to neoplasia and genetic diseases is a significant problem. Consistent chromosomal abnormalities, such as the translocation between chromosomes 22 and 9 producing the Philadelphia (Ph[1]) chromosome associated with chronic myeloid leukemia (Rowley, 1973) and the translocation between 22 and 8 in some cases of Burkitt's lymphoma (Klein, 1981), could be analyzed by this approach to detail specific genomic differences between normal and neoplastic cells. The breakpoint on chromosome 22 is in the same region (q11) for both of these translocations. Questions concerning the nature of the breakpoint and the reciprocity of the translocations could then be tackled at the molecular level by sorting and cloning the translocated derivative chromosomes from several Ph[1]-positive patients, and Burkitt's lymphoma cell lines.

In addition, the large numbers of probes for specific chromosomes isolated and characterized by methods outlined here will eventually help to provide the basis for an extensive human linkage map. The availability of a series of restriction site polymorphisms ordered along the chromosomes serving as linkage markers could allow the detection and antenatal diagnosis of genetic diseases. In view of the potential and simplicity of this approach, the rapidly improving methods for sorting chromosomes by flow cytometry should ensure that chromosome-specific libraries will soon be widely available.

Acknowledgments

We thank Dr. Leanne Wiedemann for providing human leukemic RNA samples and phage cloning arms, Anne Sproul, Rory Sillar, and Jane Kellow for technical assistance and Norma Morrison for assistance in cell culture. We gratefully acknowledge Dr. Marie-Claude Hors-Cayla, Dr. Dominique Veil, and Solange Heurtz for providing X/22 hybrid cells and Dr. Peter Goodfellow and Dr. Chris Bostock for the hybrid cell line Thy B133R. We thank Dr. Kay Davies, Dr. Bob Williamson, Professor M. Ferguson-Smith, and Dr. J. C. Kaplan for encouragement and discussions. This work was supported by the Medical Research Council, Cancer Research Campaign, and the Leukemia Research Fund.

References

Carrano, A. V., Gray, J. W., Langlois, R. G., Burkhart-Schultz, K., and Van Dilla, M. A. (1979). *Proc. Natl. Acad. Sci. U.S.A.* **76**, 1382–1384.

Collard, J. G., Schijven, J., Tulp, A., and Meulenbrock, M. (1982). *Exp. Cell Res.* **137**, 463–469.

Davies, K. E., Young, B. D., Elles, R. G., Hill, M. E., and Williamson, R. (1981). *Nature (London)* **293**, 374–376.

Disteche, C. M., Kunkel, L. M., Lojewski, A., Orkin, S. H., Eisenhard, M., Sahar, E. Travis, B., and Latt, S. A. (1982). *Cytometry* **2**, 282–286.

Erikson, J., Martinis, J., and Croce, C. M. (1981). *Nature (London)* **294**, 173–175.

Gray, J. W., Langlois, R. G., Carrano, A. V., Burkhart-Schultz, K., and Van Dilla, M. A. (1979). *Chromosoma* **73,** 9–27.

Gusella, J., Keys, C., Varsanyi-Breiner, A., Kao, F., Jones, C., Puck, T. T., and Housman, D. (1980). *Proc. Natl. Acad. Sci. U.S.A.* **77,** 2829–2833.

Klein, G. (1981). *Nature (London)* **294,** 313–318.

Krumlauf, R., Jeanpierre, M., and Young, B. D. (1982). *Proc. Natl. Acad. Sci. U.S.A.* **79,** 2971–2975.

Kunkel, L. M., Tantravahi, U., Eisenhard, M., and Latt, S. A. (1982). *Nucleic Acids Res.* **10,** 1557–1578.

Lebo, R. V., Carrano, A. V., Burkhart-Schultz, K., Dozy, A. M., Yu, L. C., and Kan, Y. W. (1979). *Proc. Natl. Acad. Sci. U.S.A.* **76,** 5804–5808.

McKusick, V. A., and Ruddle, F. H. (1977). *Science* **196,** 390–405.

Malcolm, S., Williamson, R., Boyd, E., and Ferguson-Smith, M. A. (1977). *Cytogenet. Cell Genet.* **19,** 256–261.

Maniatis, T., Hardison, R. C., Lowry, E., Lauer, J., O'Connell, C., Quon, D., Sim, G. K., and Efstradiatis, A. (1978). *Cell* **15,** 687–701.

Padgett, T. F., Stubblefield, E., and Varmus, H. E. (1977). *Cell* **10,** 649–657.

Pinaev, G., Bardyopadhyay, D., Glekov, O., Shanbag, V., Johanson, G., and Albertson, P. A. (1979). *Exp. Cell Res.* **124,** 191–203.

Rigby, P. W. J., Dieckmann, M., Rhodes, C., and Berg, P. (1977). *J. Mol. Biol.* **113,** 237–254.

Rowley, J. D. (1973). *Nature (London)* **243,** 290–293.

Ruddle, F. H. (1981). *Nature (London)* **294,** 115–120.

Schmidt, C. W., and Deininger, P. L. (1975). *Cell* **6,** 345–358.

Sillar, R. S., and Young, B. D. (1981). *J. Histochem. Cytochem.* **29,** 74–78.

Wolf, S. F., Mareni, C., and Migeon, B. (1980). *Cell* **21,** 95–102.

Young, B. D., Ferguson-Smith, M. A., Sillar, R. S., and Boyd, E. (1981). *Proc. Natl. Acad. Sci. U.S.A.* **78,** 7727–7731.

13

States of Differentiation in Leukemias: A Two-Dimensional Gel Analysis of Genetic Expression

ERIC P. LESTER

*Section of Hematology/Oncology
and The Cancer Research Center
The University of Chicago
Chicago, Illinois*

PETER F. LEMKIN AND LEWIS E. LIPKIN

*Image Processing Section
National Cancer Institute
Bethesda, Maryland*

CHROMOSOMES AND CANCER

225

I. Introduction

The goals of the work described here are twofold: (1) the practical goal of improved diagnostic and prognostic precision in human leukemias and (2) the fundamental goal of understanding differentiation and the genetic regulation on which it is based. In all of biology, whether one is working at the level of ecology, organ physiology, or molecular biology, a series of complex interrelationships is evident and a global examination of the elements involved (be they species or proteins) is required in order to achieve a full understanding of the subject under study. Cellular differentiation, our subject here, consists of the selective expression of genetic information—not of one or a few genes, but of all the gene products present in the cell in both their qualitative and quantitative aspects. Genetic expression may be considered at a variety of levels in the flow of information from the genome—DNA transcription, RNA processing, mRNA translation, etc.—but the sum of all of the regulatory activity at each of these steps leads to a final set of protein gene products whose various functions largely comprise the differentiated state. Thus, a proper analysis of differentiation will seek a global analysis of the protein constituents of the population of cells under study.

We have initially chosen to focus on the problem of analyzing and comparing states of differentiation in human leukemias. For this purpose, as a first approximation to a global analysis of genetic expression, we have elected to display the pattern of cellular proteins synthesized by leukemic cells using the technique of two-dimensional polyacrylamide gel electrophoresis (2-D gels). This pattern reflects both the underlying differentiation (qualitative and quantitative selection of genetic expression) and the metabolic and growth status of the leukemic cells. To deal with the massive amounts of information provided by such a global approach we have developed the GELLAB computer system capable of analyzing the data implicit in a 2-D gel image.

Fundamental to our analytic approach is the concept of sets of proteins and the implication that the protein members of such a set may share either a common regulatory mechanism governing their synthesis and metabolism, or a common functional goal, or both. In our initial work here we have analyzed the patterns of cellular proteins biosynthetically labeled during a brief incubation of the cells with [³H]leucine. Thus, we are talking about sets of proteins whose relative synthetic rates (relative to total protein synthesis) appear to be somehow linked and to vary in common. Such a set is operationally defined as those proteins whose relative synthetic rates differ significantly when control and experimental 2-D gel patterns, or patterns from differing classes of leukemias, are compared. In the context of the GELLAB computer system, a statistical search of a data base may return a list of spots (proteins) that differ significantly between two classes of gels, such as acute myeloid leukemia (AML) gels versus chronic lymphocytic leukemia (CLL) gels. This "search result list" (SRL) is a set of proteins that are candidates for useful diagnostic markers and also may represent proteins sharing a common regulatory or functional event. Clearly, each protein may belong to multiple sets and may both be regulated by multiple mechanisms and share in multiple functions. The elucidation of these major linkages in the expression of genes will allow us to understand much of the internal economy by which a cell regulates its activities—the ebb and flow of energy and information. Indeed, the definition of such linkages is a first prerequisite to an examination of the mechanisms by which genes are regulated in a coordinated fashion during differentiation. The potential alteration of these linkages may allow us to understand and ultimately overcome the block in differentiation and growth control characteristic of malignant cells.

II. Methods

A. Cell Isolation, Culture, and Protein Labeling

Normal lymphocytes were isolated from the peripheral blood of normal donors by Ficol–Hypaque density gradient centrifugation as previously described (Lester *et al.*, 1981). Leukemic cells were similarly isolated from patients with acute myeloid leukemias [AML—M1, M2, M4, or M5 as defined by the French–American–British (FAB) classification (Bennett *et al.*, 1976)], acute lymphocytic leukemia (ALL), chronic lymphocytic leukemia (CLL), or hairy cell leukemia (HCL), as previously described (Lester *et al.*, 1983). The purity of the leukemic cell populations studied (>95% malignant cells) was verified by examination of Wright-stained cytocentrifuge preparations of aliquots of the isolated cells. After isolation, leukemic cells were immediately biosynthetically pulse-labeled with [^{3}H]leucine for 2 hours in leucine-deficient RPMI-1640 as previously described (Lester *et al.*, 1980, 1983). Normal lymphocytes were cultured in complete RPMI-1640 + 10% fetal calf serum (FCS) in the presence or absence of phytohemagglutinin for varying times and then similarly pulse-labeled as previously described (Lester *et al.*, 1981). The long-term human lymphoblastoid cell lines CCRF-HSB-2 (a T cell line) and CCRF-SB (a B cell line) were cultured for varying periods in RPMI-1640 + 10% FCS and similarly radiolabeled as previously described (Lester *et al.*, 1982). The human acute promyelocytic leukemia (APL) cell line HL-60, a kind gift of Dr. Robert Gallo of the National Cancer Institute, was grown in RPMI-1640 + 15% FCS for varying periods (24–96 hours) with or without the addition of agents capable of inducing differentiation: dimethyl sulfoxide (DMSO) 1.25% (v/v), *cis*-retinoic acid (RA) $10^{-8}M$, or phorbol myristate acetate (PMA), $10^{-6}M$ and then pulse-labeled for 2 hours with [^{3}H]leucine, 133 µCi/ml in leucine-deficient RPMI-1640. Differentiation of HL-60 cells was verified cytologically by examination of Wright-stained cytocentrifuge preparations. After labeling, cells were suspended in 200 μliters of lysis buffer (9 M urea, 2% ampholytes, pH 3.5–10, 5% mercap-toethanol, 2% NP-40, 0.1 mM phenylmethylsulfonylfluoride, alkalinized to pH >9.5) as previously reported (Lester *et al.*, 1983) and stored at −80°C.

B. Electrophoresis and Fluorography

Aliqouts of 40 μl of extracted cellular proteins in lysis buffer were subjected to 2-D gel electrophoresis using the Iso-Dalt apparatus as previously described (Lester *et al.*, 1980, 1982). Gels were stained, prepared for fluorography with 4% diphenyloxazole in glacial acetic acid, and exposed to Kodak XAR-5 film for varying periods as previously described (Lester *et al.*, 1980, 1982, 1983).

C. Computer Analysis with GELLAB

Fluorographic 2-D gel images on X-ray film were digitized into 512 × 512 arrays of pixels (gray values) using a Vidicon television camera system as previously described (Lester *et al.*, 1980). The GELLAB system of programs (Lemkin and Lipkin, 1981a,b,c, 1983; Lipkin and Lemkin, 1980; Lemkin *et al.*, 1982) running on the DEC-20 computer at the Image Processing Section (IPS) at the National Cancer Institute or the DEC-20 at the University of Chicago was then used to analyze the digitized images. The initial program in the GELLAB system, SG2DRV, was used to locate and quantify each spot in each image (representing the synthetic rate of a single polypeptide) and produce a list of spots in each image (a ''.GSF file''). Each image (spot list) was then matched to a reference, or master image (the Rgel) by the gel comparison program CMPGEL to produce a series of gel comparison files (''.GCF files''). The top level GELLAB program, CGELP, was then used to construct a unified data base (a ''.PCG file'') consisting of data from a series of gels (multiple ''.GCF files''). The central concept in data base construction is that of an ''Rspot set'' (Fig. 1) which consists of a given spot in the Rgel and all of the corresponding spots in other gel images in the data base. Included within each Rspot set is data regarding the absolute density (corrected for background), the normalized density, the optical density range within each spot, the x,y coordinates of the spot centroid, and the gel number and class (e.g., AML) from which it was derived. After data base construction, the CGELP program permits extensive interactive analysis. ''Pre-fiters'' which provide ways of removing from consideration certain gel images (e.g., CLL images) or certain Rspot sets (e.g., low density spots likely to represent noise) may be used as well as an extensive series of statistical procedures [e.g., t-test, F-test, or Wilcoxon rank sum (WRS) test]. Using such statistical searches one may find Rspot sets that differ qualitatively or quantitatively between classes of samples. Each such search produces a ''search results list'' (SRL), and multiple SRLs may be retained in memory and compared using standard set operations (union, intersection, subtraction, etc.). After analysis one may examine the resulting list of spots as an ''Rmap'' using the MARKGEL program that will mark and label each spot in a

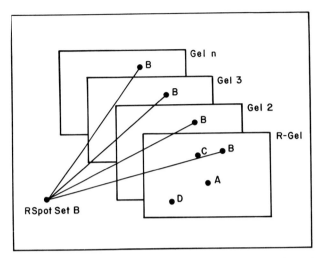

Fig. 1. The Definition of an Rspot set. Rspot set B consists of the information regarding the polypeptide labeled "B" in each gel image in the data base.

SRL on any image in the data base and display the result as a video image. Alternatively, a mosaic image may be created on the video display showing a particular spot and the area immediately around it from each image in the data base.

III. Results

A. Cell Cycle Related Changes in Protein Synthetic Rates

In our initial studies (Lester *et al.*, 1981), we attempted to define alterations in the 2-D gel protein synthetic patterns that may occur in relation to the cell cycle and growth. We chose mitogen activation of normal lymphocytes as our model system since we expected considerable homology in protein composition between normal lymphocytes and leukemic cells, particularly lymphoid leukemias, and we could activate growth and follow the cell population through the cell cycle in a relatively defined fashion using mitogens such as phytohemagglutinin (PHA). We found no qualitative changes in the population of proteins visualized. However, quantitative changes in the relative synthetic rates of a number of proteins were quite apparent (e.g., the spots arbitrarily labeled E and U in Fig. 2 that are relatively increased after 48 hours of PHA stimulation). The set of proteins whose relative synthetic rates showed the greatest change at an early time point in growth activation (4 hours) differed from those that showed the greatest relative change at later time points (e.g., 48 hours). Furthermore, at least two of the proteins showing the greatest increase at 48 hours were also synthe-

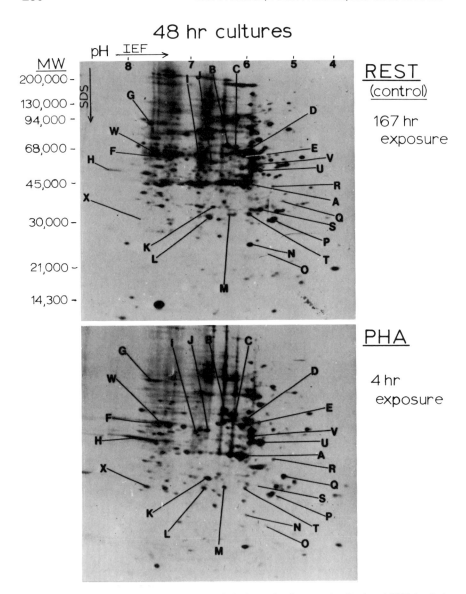

Fig. 2. Fluorographs of 4-hour pulse-labeled proteins from resting (top) and PHA-treated (bottom) human peripheral blood lymphocyte cultures. Relative molecular masses were determined by coelectrophoresis of a mixture of proteins of known molecular weight and are indicated on the left of the top panel. A replicate isoelectric focusing (IEF) gel was divided into 1-cm sections, each of which was eluted with 1 ml of distilled water for determination of the pH scale shown on the top panel. The same set of 24 spots is marked on each gel (A–X).

sized at high rates in both the T cell line MOLT-4 and the B cell line NAMALVA when examined in the log phase of growth. Thus, these changes in normal lymphocytes appeared not to be a reflection of alterations in the quantities of lymphocyte subpopulations but rather were an aspect of growth stimulation per se. Many of these changes in relative protein synthetic rates were confirmed using an early version of GELLAB (Lester *et al.*, 1980).

B. Distinguishing States of Differentiation in Lymphoblastoid Cell Lines

In our next project, we sought to determine whether the patterns of protein synthesis seen in 2-D gel images could be used to distinguish between differing states of differentiation. In particular, we wanted to test the capacity of the GELLAB system to help us in making such a distinction. For this purpose we chose to examine the 2-D gel patterns of an autologous pair of cell lines (Fig. 3) (Lester *et al.*, 1982). The CCRF-HSB-2 line is of T cell origin and the CCRF-SB line is of B cell origin. Since both were derived from the same individual suffering from a T cell acute lymphoblastic leukemia (Kaplan *et al.*, 1974), any differences between them could not be due to genetic heterozygosity. Analysis of the protein synthetic patterns of these cell lines both visually and with GELLAB revealed a small number of qualitative differences (presence or absence of a particular spot within the limits of sensitivity of the technique). A larger number of polypeptides (approximately 10%) showed statistically significant quantitative differences when the patterns of the two cell lines were compared using GELLAB. By examining cells of both lines in both the log and the plateau phase of culture growth, we were able to see growth-related changes in the relative synthetic rates of many of the polypeptides including some that had shown such changes in normal lymphocytes. Furthermore, these changes did not obscure our ability to distinguish between the T cell and the B cell patterns. When we compared the patterns of these cell lines with that of freshly isolated cells from a patient with acute lymphocytic leukemia we found that many of the homologous proteins could be easily identified, and an even larger number of qualitative and quantitative differences were apparent. Thus, our system of analysis seemed to hold the promise of being able to distinguish various states of differentiation in clinically available specimens of human leukemia cel's.

C. Differentiation in the HL-60 Promyelocytic Leukemia Cell Line *in Vitro*

Before proceeding to attempt to characterize the differences in protein synthetic patterns between the major classes of leukemia, we elected to examine a second model system of hematologic differentiation, the HL-60 line. This cell

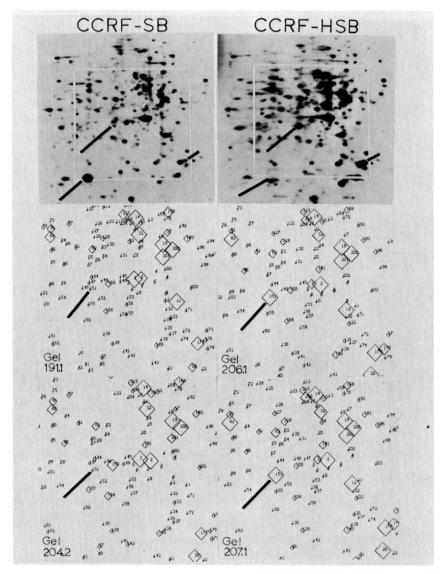

Fig. 3. Comparisons of CCRF-SB (B cell) and CCRF-HSB-2 (T cell) 2-D gel protein synthesis patterns. Top shows the original fluorographic images, and the bottom shows computer graphics plots created at The University of Chicago. Plots of two images of replicate cultures are shown, with SB images on the left and HSB images on the right. The plotted areas are approximately outlined in white in the upper panels, and a few polypeptides varying quantitatively in their synthetic rates between the SB and HSB lines are marked.

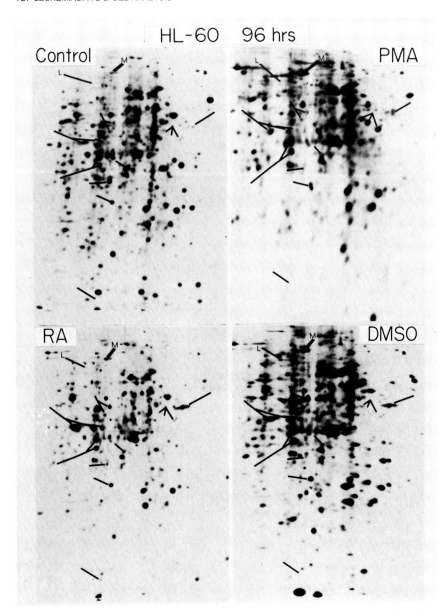

Fig. 4. HL-60 differentiation. Fluorographs of 2-D gels of proteins biosynthetically pulse-labeled for 2 hours after 96 hours of culture with no added agents (control), phorbol ester (PMA) to induce monocyte/macrophage differentiation, or retinoic acid (RA) or DMSO to induce granulocyte differentiation. All lines point centrally to polypeptides whose relative synthetic rates serve to distinguish control (undifferentiated) versus macrophage versus granulocyte differentation. The acid end of each gel is to the right.

line, derived from a patient with acute promyelocytic leukemia but lacking the typical 15–17 chromosomal translocation, had previously been clearly shown by other investigators to be capable of undergoing differentiation *in vitro* (Gallagher *et al.*, 1979; Collins *et al.*, 1980). Under the influence of certain polar solvents such as DMSO it acquires functional and morphologic characteristics typical of mature granulocytes, although it retains abnormalities often seen in the granulocytes of patients with ''preleukemia,'' such as a ''pseudo-Pelger-Huet'' nuclear morphology. *cis*-Retinoic acid produces a very similar differentiation *in vitro* (Breitman *et al.*, 1980). Phorbol esters, however, produce differentiation along a different myeloid pathway with acquisition by the HL-60 cells of functional and morphologic characteristics typical of the monocyte/macrophage lineage (Lotem and Sachs, 1979; Rovera *et al.*, 1979). We thus hoped to be able to use the protein synthetic patterns seen in 2-D gels to distinguish between these pathways and to follow the course of the major changes in genetic expression occurring in these two types of differentiation over 96 hours. We expected to find sets of proteins which, by their presence or absence or by their relative synthetic rates, would delineate both the direction and the stage of myeloid differentiation in these cells. We hypothesized that such protein sets might serve to distinguish between lymphoid and myeloid differentiation in human leukemias and also permit subclassification of the myeloid samples.

Figure 4 shows the 2-D gel patterns of proteins synthesized by HL-60 cells after 96 hours in culture with or without differentiation inducing agents. By 96 hours morphologic changes are well developed and, at the same time, a number of alterations in protein synthetic patterns are apparent. Very few qualitative changes are seen, but a large number of quantitative changes in relative synthetic rates are apparent. The changes produced by each of the agents tested (phorbol ester, retinoic acid, or DMSO) share a number of features in common as well as showing significant differences between each other. The changes produced by retinoic acid and DMSO, both of which produce granulocytic differentiation, are relatively similar when compared to those of monocyte/macrophage differentiation induced by the phorbol ester. Furthermore, each of these agents can be seen to induce a sequence of changes in HL-60 cells. Figure 5 provides an example in which a relatively small number of quantitative changes are seen in cells treated with retinoic acid for 24 hours. By 48 hours a larger set of changes can be seen. Clearly, the data in such images is too complex for complete analysis visually, and a more detailed examination of these issues is underway using the GELLAB system.

D. Protein Synthetic Patterns of Freshly Isolated Human Leukemic Cells

While this work was in progress, we began to explore the application of this approach to leukemic cells directly isolated from patients. We started with a

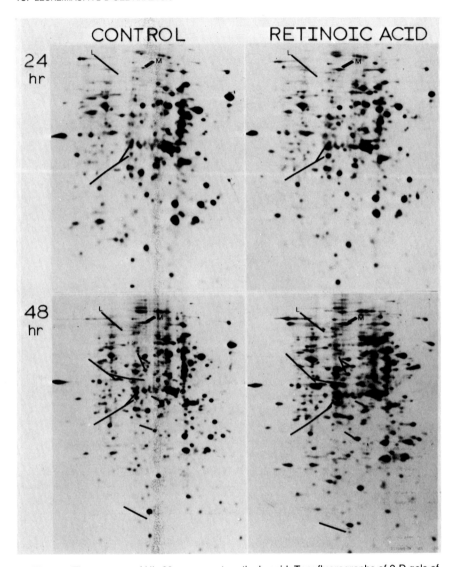

Fig. 5. Time course of HL-60 response to retinoic acid. Top: fluorographs of 2-D gels of HL-60 proteins biosynthetically labeled for 2 hours after 24 hours of culture with or without retinoic acid. Bottom: proteins labeled after 48 hours of culture. The lines point centrally to mark some of the polypeptides whose relative synthetic rates are altered during the course of differentiation.

small number of samples with the initial intention of defining sets of proteins characteristic of the major classes of leukemia—AML, ALL, CLL, and HCL. Images from different patients were sufficiently similar to permit accurate comparison. However, it rapidly became apparent that the variation in protein synthetic patterns betewen patients was often, but not always, considerably greater than the kinds of differences we had seen previously in normal lymphocytes or in the experiments with long-term cell lines. Since this was true even for patients within a single major class of leukemia, it gave us additional reason to believe that the technique would be useful for creating new subclassifications of leukemias. However, it also meant that visual analysis was far more difficult. We therefore built an initial data base (termed JUN27A.PCG) consisting of patterns from 8 patients (3 AML, 1 ALL, 2 CLL, and 2 HCL) using the GELLAB system and explored a variety of methods of analysis within GELLAB. Issues that first needed to be addressed in order to evaluate the differences between classes of leukemia included the method of normalization of relative spot density values and the choice of statistical procedures. The results of our analysis are detailed in Lester *et al.* (1983). In summary, we found that the method of normalization had relatively little effect on our ability to identify sets of proteins with significantly different relative synthetic rates in classes of leukemia. A number of qualitative differences (presence or absence of a protein) were found in comparing AML with either CLL or HCL and, of course, were unaffected by normalization procedures. In our analysis of quantitative changes we are dealing with relative spot density and a nonlinear response curve of film to radiation. Thus nonparametric statistical methods may be preferable. However, even the most sophisticated anlaysis requires visual confirmation of both qualitative and quantitative changes since "noise" may be introduced into the computer analysis at a number of levels (artifactual marks on film, electrical noise in image digitization, and potential inaccuracies by the spot detection and pairing algorithms). Visual confirmation may be achieved with either computer-generated "hard copy" plots of gel images with proteins of interest labeled or, preferably, by examination of a gel image on a video display in which spots of interest have been indicated. Such "marked images," or "Rmaps" are easily produced by GELLAB and may be compared with the original fluorographs. Figure 6 shows an example of such Rmaps in which the visually verified proteins showing quantitative differences in relative synthetic rates in AML versus CLL or AML versus HCL comparisons in this initial data base are marked. Another approach to visual confirmation involves the use of mosaic images synthesized on the video display and showing a particular spot of interest, with the immediately surrounding gel region, from each image in the data base. Figure 7 shows an example of such an image.

While analysis of a small initial data base was very useful in allowing us to develop methods of manipulating such data and creating search strategies, the

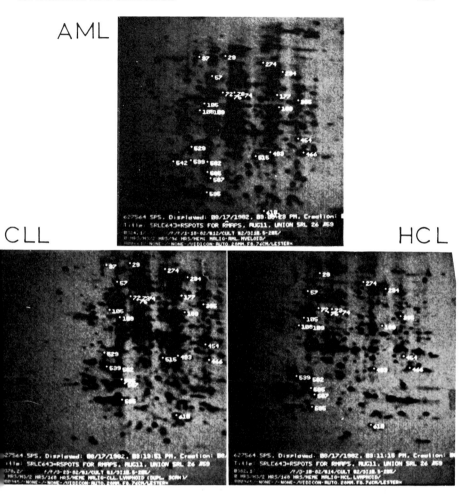

Fig. 6. Candidate spots for quantitative markers serving to distinguish AML from CLL or HCL. Each of the panels is a photograph of a computer-generated video display showing the polypeptides (search result list) obtained by statistical analysis of the JUN27A.PCG data base and subsequently verified by visual checking of the original fluorographs of each of the AML, CLL, and HCL images. The acid end of each gel is to the left.

number of patient samples was clearly inadequate. Thus, we have recently created a new, expanded GELLAB data base (HM3PCG.PCG) using 58 gel images derived from one or more samples from 26 patients (7 AML, 2 ALL, 5 CLL, and 12 HCL). This data base contains measurements of 23,828 individual spots that are segregated into 1434 Rspot sets, each of which contains the values for a given protein in each of the images in which it was identified. We have used a variety

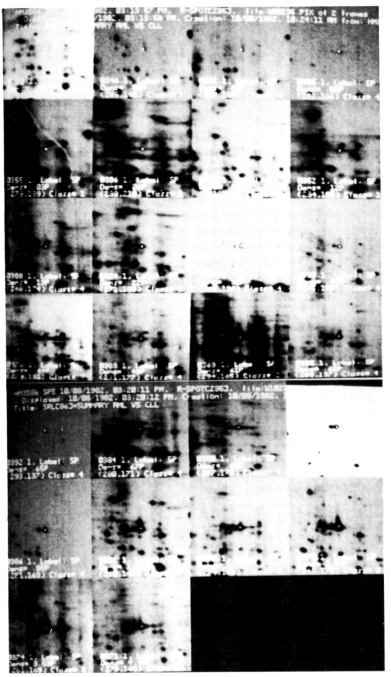

Fig. 7.

of statistical procedures and normalization methods to search the data base for proteins (Rspot sets) showing significant differences between classes of leuke-mias (although we have omitted the ALL samples from consideration because of their small number). The result of each search has returned a set of proteins (Rspot sets) that is termed a search result list. These search result lists have then been interactively compared using set operations. Seventy-nine searches have thus far been undertaken and will be reported in greater detail elsewhere. Figure 8 shows an example of the type of result achieved by comparing AML versus CLL images using four different normalization methods and taking the intersec-tion of the sets found to vary with a $p \leq 0.05$ using a Wilcoxon rank sum test. The intersection of these four sets contained 54 Rspot sets, representing proteins whose relative synthetic rates show significant differences (larger or smaller) in AML versus CLL samples. To further evaluate such a result, mosaic video images showing a given spot and its surrounding context in one image from each of the 26 patients have been created. Figure 7 is an example of one such mosaic showing clearly that Rspot 235 is relative larger in CLL and most HCL samples than in AML.

In addition to finding individual proteins and groups of proteins showing significant differences between types of leukemias, we would like to be able to create some form of "summary" statistic expressing the relatedness of two or more leukemic samples to each other. One approach is to use the correlation coefficient of the spot densities in each Rspot set in each possible pair of gel images (a "density/density" plot). The densities of spots in replicate images show correlation coefficients in the range of 0.90–0.99, whereas correlation of images from different AML patients shows values of 0.53–0.76 (mean 0.63). Comparison of AML versus CLL images gives correlation coefficients of 0.29–0.53 (mean 0.39). As would be expected, we can improve the ability of this approach to achieve a diagnostic distinction between AML and CLL by confining the calculation of a correlation coefficient to those Rspot sets identified as significantly different in our statistical searches. If we use only the 54 Rspot sets displayed in Fig. 8 the correlation coefficients of CLL images with each other rises from a mean of 0.64 to a mean of 0.86. AML versus AML values rise from a mean of 0.63 to 0.66, whereas AML versus CLL values fall from a mean of 0.39 to 0.18. By extending such an approach to include Rspot sets differing significantly between other classes of leukemias, we will ultimately be able to create a powerful series of discriminant functions for the diagnostic sub-classification of human leukemias.

Fig. 7. Computer-generated video display mosaic image of Rspot 235. Each section shows Rspot 235 and the surrounding region from one of the 26 images from 26 different leukemic samples in the HM3PCG.PCG data base. This polypeptide shows a low relative synthetic rate in AML samples (class 1) and higher rates in ALL (class 2), CLL (class 3), or HCL (class 4) samples. Two video display images were photographed and combined in this figure.

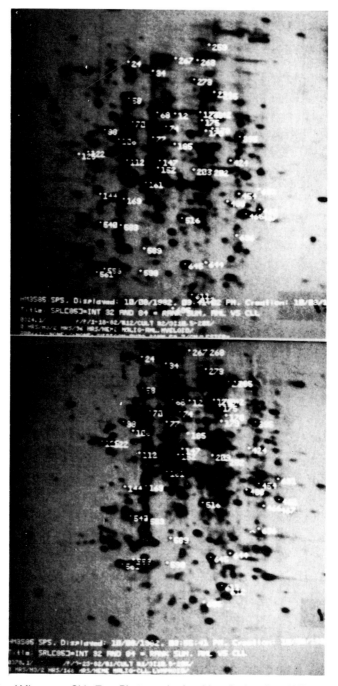

Fig. 8. AML versus CLL. Top: Photograph of a video display of an AML image in which GELLAB has marked the polypeptides differing significantly ($p<0.05$ by Wilcoxon rank sum) when the seven AML samples were compared with the five CLL samples in the HM3PCG.PCG data base. Bottom: The same search result list marked on a CLL image.

IV. Discussion

It is our belief that we are not far from the time when we can utilize a computer analysis of the 2-D gel pattern of proteins synthesized by a given patient's leukemic cells to classify precisely the state of differentiation of that leukemia and place it in a diagnostic category. More importantly, we, and others working in this field (Hanash *et al.*, 1982), hope to be able to improve on current classification schemes. The 2-D gel approach has an important theoretical advantage for this purpose. If one wishes to differentiate between leukemias, one should optimally use a method that examines all the differences, not just a few. While many technical problems have only been partially addressed, the relatively global analysis of genetic expression achieved using 2-D gels gives them a unique diagnostic potential.

The preclinical studies discussed here using normal lymphocytes, T and B lymphoblastoid cell lines, and the myeloid cell line HL-60 have shown clearly that this technique is quite capable of analyzing alternative states of growth and differentiation. Indeed, these early studies have allowed us to focus our attention on certain proteins in leukemic cells while simultaneously pursuing a global analysis. Proteins whose relative synthetic rates are low in normal resting lymphocytes and increase with growth activation show, in general, lower relative synthetic rates in chronic leukemias than in acute leukemias. Rspots 106 and 77 are examples in Fig. 8 and suggest that the cell cycle kinetics of leukemic cells may be predicted, at least in part, from the 2-D gel patterns. Proteins showing an increase in relative synthetic rates during the differentiation of HL-60 cells may mark myeloid differentiation. An example is Rspot 273 in Fig. 8 (labeled "M" in Figs. 4 and 5, and "274" in the earlier data base shown in Fig. 6). Indeed the relative density of Rspots 273 and 235 alone serve to distinguish the myeloid from the lymphoid patterns in all cases so far examined ($273/235 \geq 1$ in myeloid and <1 in lymphoid). Clearly expansion of our data bases to larger numbers of samples should greatly increase the diagnostic power of the 2-D gel approach, particularly when coupled with the use of appropriate "summary" statistics, such as correlation coefficients based on a large number of diagnostically useful proteins.

While expanding our studies numerically, we must continue to address a number of technical points. First, it may be wise to enunciate some of the underlying assumptions of the 2-D gel approach:

1. The method of sample preparation with a denaturing lysis buffer effectively solubilizes the majority of cellular proteins. Clearly, the composition of such buffers may alter their efficacy, but such effects are generally small (Garrels, 1979).

2. The mobility of each structural species of polypeptide in the gels is unique. While a mutation in amino acid sequence may or may not alter protein charge or

apparent size in a 2-D gel matrix, O'Farrell (1975) has presented evidence that different proteins of nearly identical mobility act to exclude each other from local regions of the gel rather than overlapping more extensively.

3. The detection of each species of protein in a gel is stoichiometric. This may well not be the case depending upon the method of detection used—autoradiography, fluorography, or staining with Coomassie blue or silver. Nonetheless, the crucial issue if one is to use the 2-D approach for clinical diagnostic purposes is that the method used, whatever its details, produces a highly reproducible pattern. Proper integration of data between disparate techniques, such as autoradiography and silver staining, will of course require a much more sophisticated analysis of such issues.

Other technical issues to be addressed in the future include the need to increase the number of gene products examined in the gel system. Our current system fails to resolve basic proteins adequately, although it could be readily combined with systems that have been reported to adequately visualize such polypeptides (O'Farrell et al., 1977; Willard et al., 1979). The total number of gene products currently seen in our gels (500–1000) is clearly less than the total number of protein genes expressed in a given cell type and is heavily dominated by the cytoskeletal elements. Options to increase the sensitivity of the technique include the use of purified subcellular fractions from larger numbers of cells or alterations in gel technique (e.g., ampholyte pH range, second dimension acrylamide concentrations, or electrophoresis duration) to, in effect, expand the "magnification" of the pattern visualized. In addition, it would be very desirable to measure protein synthetic rates in terms of absolute radioactivity incorporated into each protein species (cpm or dpm) rather than relative spot density as estimated via the nonlinear intermediary of film. An instrument capable of directly measuring radioactivity in gels has recently been described and may well be ideal (Davidson and Case, 1982).

Another major goal must be the development of continued improvements in our computer software. Other workers have published a variety of algorithms analogous to ours for spot detection and gel comparison (Garrels, 1979; Bossinger et al., 1979; Taylor et al., 1982; Miller et al., 1982; Skolnick et al., 1982), and certain features of these might be advantageously incorporated into GELLAB. More important will be the application of the concept of a "canonical" gel, or theoretical gel image summarizing the data in many images, which we have previously discussed (Lemkin et al., 1982). Such a concept may be used to guide spot detection and pairing algorithms to more efficient and accurate results. It may also permit construction of data bases containing a theoretically unlimited number of gel images in summary form, thus permitting far more robust statistical analyses. We hope, in addition, to add to GELLAB in the near future the capacity to relate the data statistically in the 2-D gel patterns to other quantitative data exogenous to, but related to, the gels such as enzyme activities, growth rates (or DNA synthetic rates), clinical data (e.g., survival times), and karyotypic data.

A variety of considerations of a more fundamental nature may be addressed using our quantitative 2-D gel approach. Prime among these will be the correlations of specific karyotypic abnormalities with specific features of the gel patterns. Other workers have already begun to use the technique to map the genes coding for specific proteins to specific chromosomes (Klose *et al.*, 1982). It will be of even greater interest to discover the proteins whose expression is altered as a result of the karyotypic abnormalities found in human leukemic cells. It has long been argued that the chromosomal alterations seen in human malignancies are a mere epiphenomenon occurring concomitantly with, but not central to, malignant transformation, growth promotion, and clonal evolution along a pathway of increasingly malignant behavior. The identification of specific karyotypic abnormalities that are characteristic of certain malignancies expressing a particular phenotypic differentiation [e.g., t(15;17) in human acute promyelocytic leukemia (Golomb *et al.*, 1976)] makes it very unlikely that such chromosomal changes are totally irrelevant to the events of malignant transformation and progression. Indeed, the recent finding of examples of cellular oncogenes that appear to be situated in or near the sites of chromosomal breakpoints (Taub *et al.*, 1982) strongly suggests that these chromosomal rearrangements may be a central event, and yet they must produce their effects by altering DNA transcription and, ultimately, the population of proteins expressed, either quantitatively or qualitatively. Genetic changes may consist of balanced rearrangements, deletions, or reduplications of genetic material, but the effects of any of these may be to increase or decrease the expression of specific genes or sets of genes.

These genetic alterations and their attendant changes in gene expression may be considered to have three classes of effects on the phenomenon of malignancy: (1) No effect—the rearrangement is either functionally silent or resultant changes in genetic expression are irrelevant to cell growth and differentiation. Such events are indeed "epiphenomena." (2) Tumor initiation—an example may occur in radiation or chemical carcinogenesis in which a primary alteration in the structure (sequence) of DNA may lead, for example, to an increased expression of a cellular oncogene and resultant malignant transformation. (3) Tumor promotion—a genetic alteration occurring in a cell that has already undergone malignant transformation but that still retains some normal growth control mechanisms might inactivate an inhibitory control or activate a positive mechanism to increase growth. Daughter cells possessing the same alterations would grow with increased success, and clonal evolution within the malignancy would result. Conversely, genetic alterations inhibiting the success of cells possessing them might be expected to be difficult if not impossible to identify, since cells possessing them would be overgrown by more successful clones. The finding of a specific karyotypic abnormality (e.g., t15/17) in malignant cells displaying a specific state of phenotypic differentiation (e.g., APL) occurs in many but not in all cases of a leukemia. Thus, such a translocation is not necessary for the development of malignancy, although it might be sufficient, and it may most likely represent an event that has a positive effect on the growth and survival of cells with an APL state of differentiation but not on other cells. The distinction between initiator and promotor effects may, however, be largely artificial. We may well imagine that a genetic alteration that alone may begin the malignant process in one cell might well have a promoting effect on tumor growth if it occurred in an already malignant cell. Likewise, the distinction between genetic and epigenetic mechanisms leading to malignancy may become cloudy, in view of the apparently reversible nature of malignant transformation in at least some model systems [e.g., mouse teratocarcinomas and their normal behavior when incorporated as single cells in a blastocyst (Mintz and Illmensee, 1975)]. Evidently, changes in protein (gene) expression occurring without any alteration in DNA sequence are sufficient to produce a malignant phenotype that in turn may be reversed to a normal state in the appropriate environment.

In view of the general finding of increasingly abnormal karyotypes in cells of increasingly malignant behavior (farther down the path of clonal evolution), we may hypothesize that a crucial event in the course of such evolution may be the development of a mechanism to increase the rate at which changes in genetic expression occur (by genetic or epigenetic means). Thus, we may expect various malignancies to share at least some biochemical features in common, and these similarities may increase the more malignant the cells in question. Weber (1977) has clearly identified key rate-limiting enzymes in a number of metabolic pathways whose activities must change to permit progression down the path of clonal evolution to greater malignancy. Klein (1979) has similarly discussed the ''convergent'' evolution of karyotypic abnormalities possessing promoting effects on tumor growth. We may thus expect to find sets of proteins whose expression must be regulated in common in order to permit evolution of progressively more malignant clones of cells. Such sets need not consist of only those genes whose transcription is directly changed by a genetic alteration, but also those proteins whose expression is secondarily altered by differing regulation at any of a number of steps (e.g., RNA processing and translation).

Likewise, we may identify sets of proteins whose expression must be coordinately regulated during normal differentiation to a final functional cell. If indeed ''oncogeny is blocked ontogeny,'' as Potter stated (1978), then we may identify specific sets of proteins in which failure of coordinate regulation occurs with a resultant block in differentiation. The classification of those protein sets whose coordinate expression characterizes, on the one hand, normal growth, differentiation, and metabolism, coupled with, on the other hand, those sets of proteins characteristic of malignant progression may justify our global approach to genetic expression in human leukemias. Ultimately, we may hope to find ways of modulating these regulatory events by genetic or epigenetic means so as to reverse malignancy and achieve differentiation.

References

Bennett, J. M., Catovsky, D., Daniel, M. T., Flandrin, G., Galton, D. A. G., Gralnick, H. R., and Sultan, C. (1976). *Br. J. Haematol.* **33**, 451–458.
Bossinger, J., Miller, M. J., Vo, K.-P., Geiduschek, E. P., and Xuong, N.-H. (1979). *J. Biol. Chem.* **254**, 7986–7998.
Breitman, T. R., Selonick, S. E., and Collins, S. J. (1980). *Proc. Natl. Acad. Sci. U.S.A.* **77**, 2936–2940.
Collins, S. J., Bodner, A., Ting, R., and Gallo, R. C. (1980). *Int. J. Cancer* **25**, 213–218.
Davidson, J. B., and Case, A. L. (1982). *Science* **215**, 1398–1400.
Gallagher, R., Collins, S., Trujillo, J., McCredie, K., Ahearn, M., Tsai, S., Metzgar, R., Aulakh, G., Ting, R., Ruscetti, F., and Gallo, R. (1979). *Blood* **54**, 713–733.
Garrels, J. I. (1979). *J. Biol. Chem.* **254**, 7961–7977.
Golomb, H. M., Rowley, J., Vardiman, J., Baron, J., Locker, G., and Krasnow, G. (1976). *Arch. Intern. Med.* **136**, 825–826.
Hanash, S. M., Tubergen, D. G., Heyn, R. M., Neel, J. V., Sandy, L., Stevens, G. S., Rosenblum, B. B., and Krzesicki, R. F. (1982). *Clin. Chem. (Winston-Salem, N.C.)* **28**, 1026–1030.
Kaplan, J., Shope, T. C., and Peterson, W. D. (1974). *J. Exp. Med.* **139**, 1070–1076.
Klein, G. (1979). *Proc. Natl. Acad. Sci. U.S.A.* **76**, 2442–2446.
Klose, J., Zeindl, E., and Sperling, K. (1982). *Clin. Chem. (Winston-Salem, N.C.)* **28**, 987–992.
Lemkin, P. F., and Lipkin, L. E. (1981a). *Comput. Biomed. Res.* **14**, 272–297.
Lemkin, P. F., and Lipkin, L. E. (1981b). *Comput. Biomed. Res.* **14**, 355–380.
Lemkin, P. F., and Lipkin, L. E. (1981c). *Comput. Biomed. Res.* **14**, 407–446.
Lemkin, P. F., and Lipkin, L. E. (1983). *Electrophoresis* **4**, 71–81.
Lemkin, P. F., Lipkin, L. E., and Lester, E. P. (1982). *Clin. Chem. (Winston-Salem, N.C.)* **28**, 840–849.
Lester, E. P., Lemkin, P., Lipkin, L., and Cooper, H. L. (1980). *Clin. Chem. (Winston-Salem, N.C.)* **26**, 1392–1402.
Lester, E. P., Lemkin, P., Lipkin, L., and Cooper, H. L. (1981). *J. Immunol.* **126**, 1428–1434.
Lester, E. P., Lemkin, P., and Lipkin, L. (1982). *Clin. Chem. (Winston-Salem, N.C.)* **28**, 828–839.
Lester, E. P., Lemkin, P. F., Lowery, J. F., and Lipkin, L. E. (1983). *Electrophoresis* **3**, 364–375.
Lipkin, L. E., and Lemkin, P. F. (1980). *Clin. Chem. (Winston-Salem, N.C.)* **26**, 1403–1412.
Lotem, J., and Sachs, L. (1979). *Proc. Natl. Acad. Sci. U.S.A.* **76**, 5158–5162.
Miller, M. J., Vo, P. K., Nielsen, C., Geiduschek, E. P., and Xuong, N. H. (1982). *Clin. Chem. (Winston-Salem, N.C.)* **28**, 867–875.
Mintz, B., and Illmensee, K. (1975). *Proc. Natl. Acad. Sci. U.S.A.* **72**, 3585–3589.
O'Farrell, P. H. (1975). *J. Biol. Chem.* **250**, 4007–4021.
O'Farrell, P. Z., Goodman, H. M., and O'Farrell, P. H. (1977). *Cell* **12**, 1133–1142.
Potter, V. R. (1978). *Br. J. Cancer* **38**, 1–23.
Rovera, G., O'Brien, T. G., and Diamond, L. (1979). *Science* **204**, 868–870.
Skolnick, M. M., Sternberg, S. R., and Neal, J. V. (1982). *Clin. Chem. (Winston-Salem, N.C.)* **28**, 969–978.
Taub, R., Kirsch, I., Morton, C., Lenoir, G., Swan, D., Tronick, S., Aaronson, S., and Leder, P. (1982). *Proc. Natl. Acad. Sci. U.S.A.* **79**, 7837–7841.
Taylor, J., Anderson, N. L., Scandora, A. E., Willard, K. E., and Anderson, N. G. (1982). *Clin. Chem. (Winston-Salem, N.C.)* **28**, 861–866.
Weber, G. (1977). *N. Engl. J. Med.* **296**, 486–493, 541–551.
Willard, K. E., Giometti, C. S., Anderson, N. L., O'Connor, T. E., and Anderson, N. G. (1979). *Anal. Biochem.* **100**, 289–298.

14

Localization of Viral-Specific DNA in the Mammalian Chromosome Complement by Cytological Hybridization

ANN S. HENDERSON*

Department of Human Genetics and Development
Columbia University Health Sciences
New York, New York

I. Introduction

Some of the earliest experiments using cytological hybridization were designed to detect viral DNA in whole cells. RNA transcripts of Epstein-Barr virus (EBV) DNA were hybridized to EBV-positive cells (Nonoyama and Pagano, 1972; zur Hausen and Schulte-Holthausen, 1972). Homology to EBV DNA was found in nuclei of cells in interphase and associated with chromosomes at meta-

*Present address: Department of Biological Sciences, Hunter College, New York, New York 10021.

247

phase. Viral-synthesizing cells could be distinguished in a mixed population, but the procedures did not permit identification of individual chromosome sites. Subsequent experiments have yielded informative data using hybridization probes from various types of viral nucleic acids. Chromosome regions of viral integration have been identified in some cases. A summary of some of the research that has used cytological hybridization to detect the presence of viral-related DNA intracellularly or associated to chromosome regions is given in Table I.

The interaction of the EBV genome with human cellular DNA is of particular interest. EBV is capable of growth transformation *in vitro* of B lymphocytes of human and some nonhuman primates. The virus is maintained in a latent state in lymphocytes and is associated with at least two forms of human cancer, African Burkitt's lymphoma and anaplastic nasopharyngeal carcinoma (reviewed by Epstein and Achong, 1979). Multiple copies of the viral genome are present in infected B lymphocytes (zur Hausen *et al.*, 1972). The majority of cellular EBV DNA sequences probably exist as episomal circles formed by covalent joining of direct repeated DNA sequences at each terminus of the DNA, although there is some prior experimental evidence that at least a portion of the EBV DNA could be linked to host cell DNA (Adams and Lindahl, 1975).

Cytological and somatic cell hybridization have been used to seek a possible

TABLE I

Studies on the Association of Viral DNA with Mammalian and Avian Cells Using Cytological Hybridization

Topic	Reference
A. Adenoviruses—the cellular and chromosomal distribution of various adenoviruses has been determined in	
1. Transformed cells as compared with non-transformed cells	McDougall *et al.*, 1972; Loni and Green, 1973
2. Permissive compared with nonpermissive cells	Moar and Jones, 1975
3. Transformed and tumor cells	Dunn *et al.*, 1973
4. Chromosomes of CELO (avian adenovirus)-induced rat tumor cells	Yasue and Ishibashi, 1982
B. Epstein-Barr virus	
1. Intracellular localization	Moar and Klein, 1978; zur Hausen *et al.*, 1972, 1974
2. Chromosomal localization	Henderson *et al.*, 1983a
3. An internal repeat, IR3 DNA, has homology to many chromosome sites	Heller *et al.*, 1982b

TABLE I (*Continued*)

Topic	Reference
C. Simian virus 40 (SV40)	
1. Association with the nucleolus	Geuskens and May, 1974
2. A sequence in defective SV40 is homologous to multiple repetitive chromosome regions in monkey cells	Segal *et al.*, 1976
3. Detection of carcinogen-mediated SV40 DNA in cells	Lavi *et al.*, 1982
D. Polyoma virus	
1. Viral DNA localized in PML brain tissue	Dorries *et al.*, 1979
2. Viral DNA localized in inducible lines of polyoma-transformed cells	Neer *et al.*, 1977
E. Herpes simplex virus (HSV)	
1. Detection of HSV RNA in human tissues	McDougall *et al.*, 1979
2. Detection of HSV RNA in human sensory ganglia	Galloway *et al.*, 1979
3. HSV I DNA localized in murine chromosomes	Henderson *et al.*, 1981
4. HSV II-specific RNA localized in tumors of human uterine cervix	McDougall *et al.*, 1982
F. Murine sarcoma virus	
1. Localized to centromeric heterochromatin and other chromosome regions	Loni and Green, 1974
G. Visna virus	
1. Localized intracellularly in sheep	Brahic and Haase, 1978; Brahic *et al.*, 1981
H. Simian sarcoma leukemia virus	
1. Localized in virus-infected cells	Kaufman *et al.*, 1974
I. Murine leukemia virus	
1. Localized in mouse AKR cells	Godard and Jones, 1979
2. Localization in cells of Balb/Mo mice	Simon *et al.*, 1982
J. Measles virus	
1. Localized in cells of patients with multiple sclerosis and subacute sclerosing panencephalitis	Haase *et al.*, 1981
K. Other homologies between viral and cellular DNA	
1. Endogenous *src* genes located to a chicken microchromosome	Tereba *et al.*, 1979
2. A clustering of five defined endogenous retrovirus loci on chicken chromosome 1	Tereba and Astrin, 1982
3. Localization of *c-onc* genes to a large microchromosome in chickens	Tereba and Lai, 1982
4. Localization of *c-mos* and *c-myc* in human chromosomes	Neel *et al.*, 1982
5. Localization of *c-myb* in human chromosomes	Harper *et al.*, 1983

correlation between the presence of EBV DNA and chromosomal changes seen in transformed or infected cells (zur Hausen *et al.*, 1972; Nonoyama *et al.*, 1973; Spira *et al.*, 1977; Glasser *et al.*, 1978; Yamamoto *et al.*, 1978). Yamamoto *et al.* (1978) demonstrated an association of EBV DNA and viral antigens with human chromosome 14 by means of somatic cell hybridization between mouse fibroblasts and a human lymphoblastoid line. This association lent support to the hypothesis that the translocation, t(8;14), often observed in Burkitt tumor cells (Manolov and Manolova, 1972; Zech *et al.*, 1976), could result from the presence of viral DNA. Direct DNA homology was not localized to a specific chromosome, however, and it was assumed that EBV DNA was either not integrated or dispersed among several chromosomes (Spira *et al.*, 1977; Glasser *et al.*, 1978; Steplewski *et al.*, 1978).

Using cytological hybridization, we have demonstrated that EBV DNA is integrated into human chromosomes of EBV-positive human cell lines (Heller *et al.*, 1982b; Henderson *et al.*, 1983a). DNA with homology to one copy of the EBV genome is present at a single chromosome region in individual cell lines. The homologous region is different among independently derived cells. Chromosomal DNA with homology to EBV DNA has not been found in association with the translocation, t(8;14), or with any other chromosome regions involved in aberrations in Burkitt tumors. A small internal repeat DNA sequence in the EBV genome, IR3, is also homologous to human chromosomal DNA; the homologous DNA sequences are a distinct subset of repetitive DNA in human chromosomes (Heller *et al.*, 1982b).

Chromosome integration of EBV DNA is compared here to integration of exogenous DNA of nonviral origin (Robins *et al.*, 1981a,b; Henderson and Robins, 1982; Henderson *et al.*, 1983b). Consistent features include the following: (i) the site of integration is on a single chromosome homolog characterized by a constricted and/or achromatic region and (ii) the chromosome region of integration is different in independent integration events.

II. General Discussion of Cytological Hybridization Technique

The physical mapping of any discrete DNA sequence should theoretically be simply accomplished by direct hybridization to chromosomal DNA. On a practical level, the localization of chromosomal DNA sequences of low multiplicity is complicated by experimental factors, whereas reiterated DNA sequences can be localized under suboptimal conditions. An early problem, based on theoretical considerations related to filter hybridizations, was whether single-copy DNA sequences or DNA sequences of low multiplicity could be detected under the experimental conditions used for hybridization for chromosomes. It was subsequently demonstrated that hybridization of unique DNA sequences occurs in filter hybridizations, but the detection of such sequences is hampered by the restrictive conditions involved in annealing DNA to filters (Shoyab et al., 1974; Sambrook et al., 1975). While many kinetic factors between filter and cytological hybridizations are expected to be similar, the problems involved, as well as the means of detection and analysis, are dissimilar. Relatively small chromosomal regions can be recognized using cytological hybrids if an adequate number of metaphase plates is analyzed and the appropriate experimental conditions are maintained. For example, chromosomal regions with homology to mRNA have been reported from cytological hybridization studies (Henderson et al., 1978; Gerhard et al., 1981; Harper and Saunders, 1981; Harper et al., 1981).

The most serious problem with respect to the use of the cytological hybridization technique has developed as the result of the use of improper and suboptimal experimental conditions. Critical analyses of experimental data obtained using suboptimal conditions have hopefully resulted in the use of guidelines for determining the feasibility of chromosome assignments with cytological hybridization (Bishop and Jones, 1972; Prensky and Holmquist, 1973; Atwood et al., 1976; Henderson et al., 1978; Henderson, 1982). Guidelines are of particular importance considering the complexity of the system and opportunity for error. One is annealing a probe to an extremely complex and diverse DNA in the presence of vast amounts of protein. False localizations can occur.

Conditions and methods for the cytological hybridization reaction have been reviewed (Pardue and Gall, 1972, 1975; Hennig, 1973; Henderson, 1982). Various aspects of the hybridization reaction have been tested (Alonso et al., 1972; Szabo et al., 1975, 1977; Singh et al., 1977; Barbera et al., 1979), and some of the kinetic factors are known (Szabo et al., 1975, 1977; Henderson, 1982). The time course of the reaction, concentration dependence of the probe, and saturation levels under various experimental conditions have been determined. On an experimental level, the most critical points to be considered are the size of the chromosomal DNA to be localized, the purity and specific activity of the probe, and the efficiency of the emulsion and hybridization. The relative homogeneity of the probe is of particular importance. Nonhomologous DNA or RNA species in the probe mixture can confound the appropriate assignment by hybridization to unforeseen reiterated regions. Theoretically, the concentration of any fraction or partial fraction of the probe hybridized could be established from the time course of the reaction, but determination of the reaction time course is time-consuming and seldom done. The availability of cloned probes should solve the problem of purity of the probe, but cloned DNA, particularly as derived directly from a genomic library, may contain highly repetitive DNA sequences.

Under defined conditions, preferential chromosome labeling will occur. The criteria established in our laboratory for preferential labeling have been given previously (Henderson, 1982), but are reiterated here. These are (i) the number of DNA sequences labeled should not exceed the number inferred from reassociation kinetics or from filter-bound DNA; (ii) the time course of the reaction should be consistent with the probe concentration present in the hybridizing solution; and (iii) the efficiency of grain formation calculated from the specific activity of the probe, exposure time, and site-specific grains should not exceed the sensitivity of the emulsion. It is assumed, but not proved, that the use of cloned DNA for hybridization could result in augmentation of the hybridization signal by "tailing" or by the formation of concatenates. If this turns out to be the case, then less stringent criteria could be used.

The efficiency, E_t, is defined as the ratio of observed grains to expected disintegrations over a specific chromosome site. This assumes that all possible DNA sites are saturated and that grain counts are made at a time when the concentration of grains over the homologous chromosomal region approaches saturation. E_t is the product of the efficiency of the emulsion (E_e) and the hybridization efficiency (E_h). The efficiency of the emulsion is about 10% for [3]H (Rogers, 1973) and about 20% for [125]I (Ada et al., 1966; Prensky et al., 1973). E_h can be determined indirectly from the mean grain density by comparison with known hybridization levels obtained in independent studies using reassociation kinetics or filter hybridizations. Estimates of E_h vary. There are many experimental parameters that affect the grain density resulting from cytological hybridization. These include the method of slide preparation (see reviews above); the denaturation of chromosomal DNA (which is probably incomplete and may be variable depending on the regions involved) (Comings et al., 1973; Singh et al., 1977; Barbera et al., 1979); and the actual annealing conditions. Loss of DNA occurs under denaturation and annealing conditions (Comings et al., 1973; Barbera et al., 1979), and the presence of nucleoprotein can result in steric hindrance to hybridization.

The relationship between the various parameters of the hybridization can be expressed as (Atwood et al., 1976)

$$E_t = C(SWD)^{-1}$$

Note that E_t has defined limits and thus can serve as a measure of feasibility of the chromosome assignment. Here C is a constant (4.18 × 10[14] or Avagadro's number divided by minutes/day × 10[6]), S is the specific activity of the probe in dpm/μg, W is the molecular weight of the site(s), and D is reciprocal grains per day. An experiment is feasible if $E_t \leq E_e$. A nomogram illustrating these relationships is given in Fig. 1.

The minimum number of contiguous bases in chromosomal DNA that can be localized with cytological hybridization is not known. Chromosomal assignments have been made to presumably single sites of transcription using DNA probes of 500 to 800 bp within plasmid vectors. The use of vectors could theoretically amplify the signal by "tailing" or concatenation (Gerhard et al.,

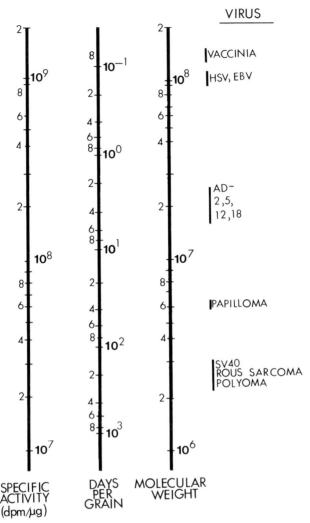

Fig. 1. Nomogram illustrating the relationships between the experimental parameters in cytological hybridization experiments. The days required to produce one grain intersects a line between the molecular weight of the site to be identified and the specific activity. The overall efficiency was assumed to be 3%, although efficiency estimates between 1 and 4% have been calculated from our laboratory data using various cloned DNA probes. Selected viruses are listed next to the approximate molecular weight. (Adapted from Henderson, 1982.)

1981; Harper and Saunders, 1981). There is a defined limit to detection by hybridization and autoradiography in a reasonable time period, since the maximum specific activity that can be obtained by nick translation of DNA with ^{125}I-labeled dCTP is in the range of 2×10^9 dpm/μg and the emulsion efficiency is fixed.

Direct grain counts can be used to determine the relative quantity of a given DNA sequence in the genome, since the number of grains present at saturation is directly proportional to the length of chromosomal DNA hybridized (Wolgemuth-Jarashow *et al.*, 1976; Szabo *et al.*, 1977; Henderson, 1982). The relative number of contiguous DNA sequences in chromosomal DNA is determined on the basis of a mean value of E_t obtained in experiments where E_h can be calculated. The copy number is calculated as

$$N = C(WE_tDS)^{-1}$$

where W is the molecular weight of an individual DNA sequence.

III. Chromosomal Integration of Epstein-Barr Virus

Chromosomal DNA with homology to EBV DNA has been shown to be present in an EBV growth transformed cell line and in cells from Burkitt tumors (Henderson *et al.*, 1983a). The physical map position of EBV DNA was determined by cytological hybridization of cloned EBV DNA fragments to human chromosomes previously identified by G banding. The EBV genome consists of about 175 kb of DNA organized into both unique and repeated sequences (Fig. 2) (reviewed by Dambaugh *et al.*, 1980a,b). Five regions of largely unique DNA sequences are formed as the result of interspersion of four classes of internal repeats (IR). Each terminus is flanked by a terminal repeat (TR). The DNA probes used for cytological hybridization were the *Eco*R1 fragments from the termini (D-IJ het) (Fig. 2) (Heller *et al.*, 1982b). Together, these fragments comprise about 85% of the EBV genome.

Specifically, chromosomal DNA with homology to EBV DNA is present on a homolog of chromosome 4 in a human cell line, IB4, derived from EBV growth transformation *in vitro* of human neonatal lymphocytes with virus from B-95 cells (King *et al.*, 1980) and in chromosome cells from the Burkitt tumor cell line, Namalwa. Chromosomal integration of EBV DNA in IB4 cells is detected on chromosome 4 at about 4q25 and is accompanied by a distinct constricted achromatic region in the chromosome. The results of hybridization, and the constricted region are illustrated in Fig. 3. The site of EBV DNA homology is stable in chromosomes of IB4 cells. Subcloned IB4 cells retain the homologous site at 4q25. The cell line, Namalwa, is latently infected with EBV. A site of EBV DNA integration is detected at a subterminal position on the short arm of

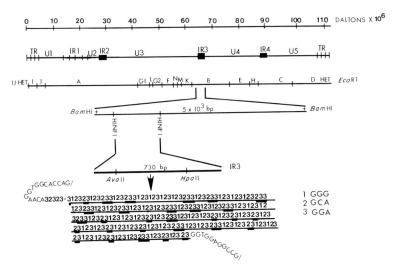

Fig. 2. Physical map of EBV DNA. The derivation of the ~730 bp IR3 *Ava*II/*Hpa*II fragment is illustrated (Heller *et al.,* 1982b). The nucleotide sequence is composed of the triplets GGG (1), GCA (2), GGA (3). Repeat units *233* and *23* are interspersed among the copies of the repeat *123*.

chromosome 1, at about 1p35, and is also accompanied by an achromatic region (Fig. 4). The relative grain distribution over the integration sites in IB4 and Namalwa chromosomes following independent hybridizations with individual cloned EBV DNA probes is given in Table II. The grain density over phytohemagglutinen (PHA)-stimulated T lymphocytes following cytological hybridization with any of the cloned EBV DNA fragments was random and of low density. No chromosome had a consistently significant grain count above background.

More tentative assignments for sites of EBV homology have been made in chromosomes of other cell lines derived from Burkitt tumors. Our earlier experiments used ^{3}H-labeled cRNA transcribed from total EBV DNA isolated from virions as a probe. An integration site was assigned in the Burkitt-derived cell line Raji to the long arm of chromosome 7 at about 7q22. The site of integration is characterized by an "expanded" achromatic area within the light G band at this region. Cloned EBV DNA fragments B and D-IJ het were hybridized to another independently cloned Raji cell line to determine if the same integration site was retained with time, laboratory manipulation, and subcloning. The integration site was retained, but as part of a translocation, t(6;7)(p21;q22), formed at a breakpoint that coincides with the site of integration. It is possible that the translocation resulted from a fragile breakpoint influenced by integration.

Each of the Raji sublines, as well as Namalwa cells, have a typical transloca-

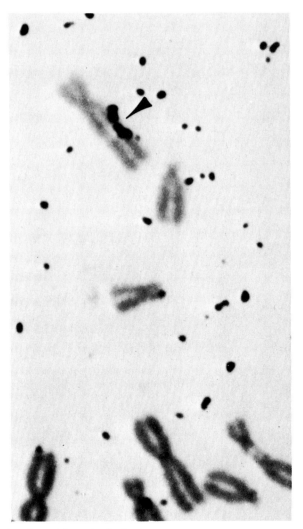

Fig. 3. Autoradiographic grain distribution over chromosome 4q25 in the cell line IB4 following cytological hybridization with nick-translated ^{125}I-labeled EBV DNA. The hybridization probe was *Eco*RI B with a specific activity of about 9×10^8 dpm/μg. The autoradiographic exposure time was 5 days. General conditions for cytological hybridization have been given previously (Henderson, 1982). The hybridization was accomplished in $3 \times$ SSC: 50% formamide at 42°C for 18 hours. The partial metaphase plate shown was chosen to illustrate both the grain density and the presence of the constricted achromatic region at 4q25. Longer exposure would result in labeling of both chromatids. The figure shows chromosomes from an unbanded preparation; chromosome 4 was identified by morphology and the presence of the achromatic region. For grain count analysis, photographs of G-banded chromosomes made prior to hybridization were compared to those of the same plate following hybridization. The chromosome complement was divided into 90 segments on the basis of G bands and other morphological features and grain counts were recorded over each individual region. The specific region of hybridization is indicated by the arrow.

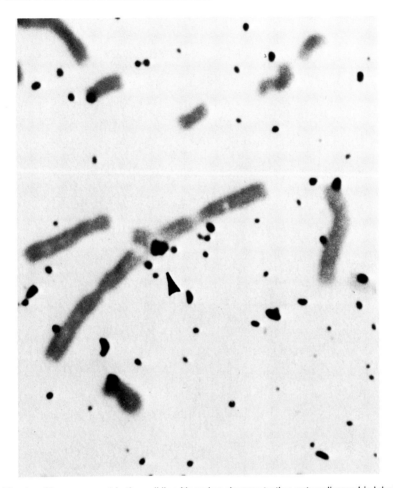

Fig. 4.   Chromosome 1 in the cell line Namalwa demonstrating autoradiographic labeling at 1p35. Specific labeling at 1p35 is indicated by an arrow. The probe used was a mixture of the cloned EBV fragments EcoR1 A, B, C + F, and D-IJ het, nick-translated with ^{125}I-labeled dCTP to a specific activity of about 1×10^9 dpm/μg. The autoradiographic exposure time was 12 days. Other conditions are given in Fig. 3.

tion between the terminal regions of chromosomes 8 and 14. A strong effort has been made to determine if chromosomal DNA sequences with homology to EBV DNA are associated with this translocation. To date, we have no evidence that homologous DNA sequences are associated with chromosomes 8 or 14 or any other chromosome involved in translocations in Burkitt tumors.

At least one copy of the complete EBV genome is integrated, since approximately equal hybridization is observed with each of the cloned DNA probes.

TABLE II

Analysis of Site-Specific Grains following Cytological Hybridization with Cloned EBV DNA

Chromosome	Probe	Specific activity (dpm/μg)	Exposure (days)	Metaphase plates analyzed	% Total grains at site	Grains/ day/ chromatid
IB4 chromosome 4q25	A	8×10^8	9	21	10	0.6
	B+K	9×10^8	6	46	12	0.7
	C+F	1.7×10^9	13	22	23	0.4
	Terminal	1.1×10^9	5	66	16	0.6
Namalwa chromosome 1p35	A	8×10^8	10	15	10	0.7
	B+K	9×10^8	7	15	11	0.6
	C+F	1.7×10^9	10	25	10	0.3
	Terminal	1.1×10^9	7	16	8	0.4

Grain count data indicates that a single integrated copy of EBV DNA is present in each cell line we have studied. In IB4, the mean of the grains from each experiment over the chromosome region in question was 2.3 grains per day per chromatid. Assuming that E_t is approximately 1% and hybridization occurred to 85% of the genome, then the number of copies of EBV DNA in IB4 DNA is 1.2. A similar calculation using data from grain counts over the region of integration in Namalwa also results in an estimate of one copy. This is consistent with data from independent experiments using reassociation kinetics and comparative autoradiographic density following Southern blotting. These methods detect one copy of EBV DNA per cell in Namalwa cells (Heller *et al.*, 1982a).

A. Chromosome Morphology

The chromosomes of IB4, Namalwa, and Raji cells have been karyotyped on the basis of G-banding patterns. The translocation, t(8;14), is found in each cell line except IB4. In Namalwa cells, there is a variant of this translocation in that a portion of chromosome 3q has been translocated to the expected breakpoint on chromosome 8 to form the translocation, [t(3;8)(q13;q24)]; the 14q+ chromosome has the expected morphology. The karyotype of IB4 cells is essentially normal with the exception of a Robertsonian translocation involving chromosome 21 and an unidentifiable small fragment. In addition to the variant in the t(8;14) translocation, Namalwa cells have several karyotypic changes including Robertsonian-like translocations (Henderson *et al.*, 1983a). The Raji cell line we are currently using has a 4q+ and an 8p+ chromosome, as well as a 7q− chromosome which results from the translocation, t(6;7). It is also trisomic for chromosome 7.

The only consistent morphological deviation seen as the result of the integration event is a constricted and/or achromatic region. There are several possible explanations for the presence of a constricted region at the integration site. A constriction could form as the result of deletion of cellular DNA. It is known that integration of SV40 DNA results in deletion of cellular DNA at the point of integration (Stringer, 1982). Integration resulting from introduction of exogenous DNA from a nonviral source can also result in deletion of cellular DNA (Henderson and Robins, 1982 and Section IV). Alternatively, the normal structural folding of chromosomal DNA could be disturbed by the presence of inserted EBV DNA. Similar chromosome changes have been seen as the result of the presence of adenoviruses. For example, adenovirus 12 (Ad-12) induces an ''uncoiling'' near the chromosome locus for thymidine kinase on human chromosome 17 (McDougall *et al.*, 1974; Ruddle and Creagon, 1975). Other ''gaps'' resulting from the presence of adenoviruses have also been associated with several regions on chromosome 1 (McDougall, 1971; McDougall *et al.*, 1979).

B. IR3 DNA

IR3 DNA is an internal repeat in the EBV genome that comprises about 2.5% of the *Eco*R1 generated fragment B (see Fig. 2). IR3 DNA codes for a portion of a polyadenylated viral RNA found in latently infected or growth transformed cell lines (van Santen *et al.*, 1981). IR3 DNA transcription does not occur in unin- fected cells. The IR3 DNA sequences in EBV DNA are variable and composed of a simple sequence repeat of three triplet elements, GGG, GCA and GGA, arranged in several major repeat units (Heller *et al.*, 1982b) (Fig. 2).

Cytological hybridization was used to follow the distribution of IR3 DNA in human chromosomes from PHA-stimulated lymphocytes, as well as some of the EBV-positive lines discussed here. The probe used was a AvaII/HpaII fragment (Heller *et al.*, 1982b and Fig. 2). The distribution of chromosomal DNA with homology to IR3 DNA in chromosomes of PHA-stimulated lymphocytes is given in Figs. 5 and 6. The distribution is multichromosomal and nonrandom; the pattern of homology is distinctly different from that described for other repeated sequences in the human genome. Consistent sites of IR3 DNA homology are seen at centromeric, subtelomeric, and telomeric regions, as well as some mid- arm regions among all autosomes and the X chromosomes. There is no detect- able homology to IR3 DNA on the Y chromosome. The distributive pattern most closely corresponds to tandem repeats located at some distance from each other along the length of the chromosome. The minimal estimate of hybridized DNA based on grain counts is between 10^8 and 10^9 daltons.

Cellular DNA(s) with homology to IR3 DNA is a new group of interrelated repetitive DNA sequences. Only a small number of sequence matches to IR3 DNA (9 to 12 bp) have been found in the Nucleic Acid Data Base (Dayhoff *et al.*, 1981). It is possible that the IR3 DNA of the EBV genome originated from a cellular source. If the origin of EBV IR3 DNA was from cellular DNA, then the association with viral DNA arose early in the evolution of EBV DNA, since all EBV isolates, as well as the related HV Papio DNA, contain IR3 DNA (Heller *et al.*, 1982a).

Chromosomal regions with homology to complete EBV DNA contain IR3 DNA repeats. One possible function of IR3 DNA in human chromosomes could be to mediate recombination between cellular and EBV DNA. A cellular–viral DNA transcription unit is possible since IR3 DNA is transcribed, (Heller *et al.*, 1982a). The hypothesis that IR3 DNA mediates viral integration has been tested in part (Henderson *et al.*, 1983a). If viral DNA recombined in a conventional fashion with cellular DNA, then the unique sequences that normally flank the EBV IR3 DNA sequences would be removed to positions at some distance from each other by the recombination event. A *Bam*Hl region in EBV DNA (Fig. 2) contains IR3 DNA and some portion of the adjacent sequences U3 and U4. When the EBV *Bam*Hl region is hybridized to cellular DNA (Namalwa) digested with

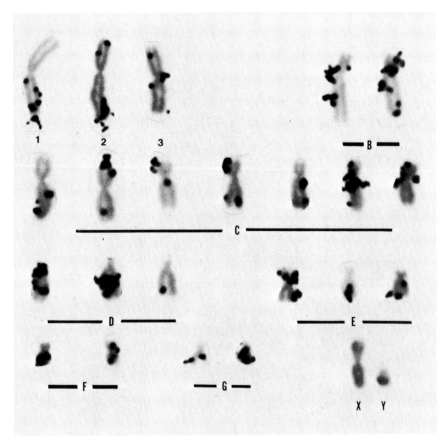

Fig. 5. Grain density over human chromosomes from PHA-stimulated lymphocytes following cytological hybridization with IR3 DNA (see Fig. 2). Chromosomes are arranged by approximate size order and morphological characteristics into chromosome groups A to G, X and Y. IR3 DNA was nick-translated to a specific activity of about 8×10^8 dpm/μg. The autoradiographic exposure was 8 days. Experimental conditions are given in Fig. 3.

*Bam*Hl, hybridization occurs at a fragment that is similar in size to the original EBV *Bam*Hl fragment. DNA containing either U3 or U4 DNA also hybridizes to this fragment, i.e., U3 and U4 have maintained the expected positions within the linear EBV genome. Conventional recombination did not occur between a circularized viral intermediate and interstitial cellular IR3 DNA, since the integrated DNA is an ordered linear representation of this portion of the EBV genome. The alternative, that IR3 DNA directs integration by linear intercalation, has no historical precedent, but is being tested directly by monitoring cloned DNA which flanks the integrated EBV DNA.

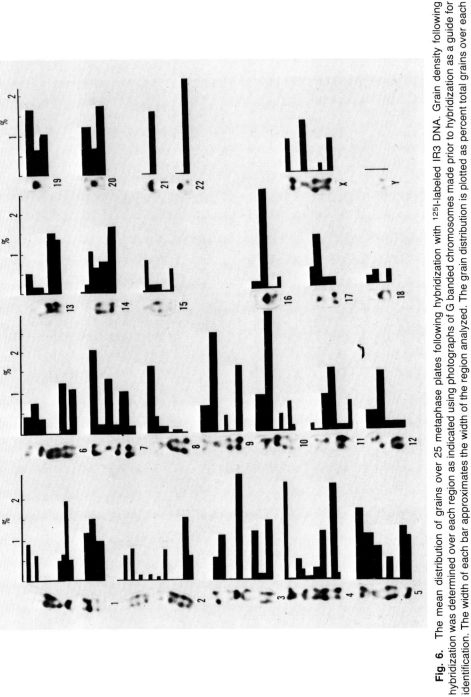

Fig. 6. The mean distribution of grains over 25 metaphase plates following hybridization with ^{125}I-labeled IR3 DNA. Grain density following hybridization was determined over each region as indicated using photographs of G banded chromosomes made prior to hybridization as a guide for identification. The width of each bar approximates the width of the region analyzed. The grain distribution is plotted as percent total grains over each version given in Fig. 5. (Reprinted from Heller et al., 1982b.)

IR3—RELATED DNA IN HUMAN CHROMOSOMES

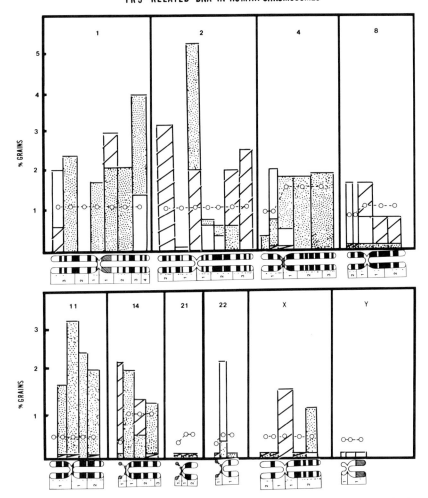

Fig. 7. Comparison of grain distribution over selected chromosomes of PHA-stimulated lymphocytes (clear bars), IB4 cells (striped bars), and Namalwa cells (stippled bars), following hybridization with ^{125}I-labeled IR3 DNA. The dashed line (- -○- - -○- -) represents the expected grain distribution based on relative chromosome length. For simplification, values that were in the expected range have been omitted; the bars represent deviations from the expected percent of total grains based on chromosome length for each region analyzed. Other experimental conditions are given in Fig. 5.

The distribution of IR3 DNA homology in chromosomes of PHA-stimulated lymphocytes from several individuals and in the cell lines, IB4 and Namalwa, has been compared. The mean grain density over specific chromosome regions is different among individuals, as well as between cell lines. The distribution of IR3-related DNA in selected chromosomes of PHA-stimulated lymphocytes, Namalwa, and IB4 cells is compared in Fig. 7. Some chromosomes show large deviations from the expected number of grains based on a random distribution. For example, chromosome 21 has a low grain density in most of the cells studied, as does the X chromosome. There are probably no or very few regions of IR3 DNA homology on the Y chromosome. Chromosome 19 is notable in that virtually every region of the chromosome has a high grain density.

The chromosomal locations of IR3 DNA homology have also been determined in the human cell line Loukes and in murine cells. Loukes was established from an American Burkitt lymphoma, and lacks detectable EBV DNA sequences. The distribution in Loukes cells was similar to that observed in chromosomes of PHA-stimulated lymphocytes, but the hybridization was more intense. IR3-related DNA sequences are present in mouse chromosomes in regions distal to the centromere and in midarm and telomeric locations. Our results show that there are fewer sites in the mouse, but these regions show more intense hybridization as measured by grain density. This correlates with the greater hybridization of IR3 to mouse DNA relative to human DNA in Southern blot hybridizations (Heller *et al.*, 1982b).

The origin region of SV40 (SV40 ori) also has homology to cellular DNA (McCutchan *et al.*, 1981; Queen *et al.*, 1981; Conrad and Botchan, 1982), although human cellular DNA homology to the SV40 ori region may be derived from a family of sequences that is not highly conserved (Conrad and Botchan, 1982). Since the SV40-related cellular DNA is GC-rich, it is possible that the homologous sequences are not extensively homologous, but share common sequences. SV40 DNA hybridizing sequences are different from IR3 DNA. Cloned SV40 and IR3 DNAs do not cross-hybridize, although both have GC-rich sequences (Heller *et al.*, 1982a). Cellular DNA with homology to SV40 ori DNA that has been sequenced is distinctly different from the DNA sequence of IR3 DNA. The relative homology of SV40 DNA hybridizing fragments to cellular DNA is much lower than that of IR3-related DNA; cellular sequences with homology to IR3 DNA can be detected under stringent hybridization conditions, suggesting extensive homology.

The role of cellular DNA sequences with homology to small portions of DNA-containing viruses remains to be defined. These DNAs could direct cellular integration or augment cellular transformation by, as yet, undefined means. The least exciting alternative, that short sequences of viral–cellular homology are a passive product of viral–cellular interactions seems unlikely. IR3 DNA is transcribed. Conrad and Botchan (1982) have suggested that the control regions of

SV40 DNA could be homologous to cellular sequences with a similar function. One of the hybridizing cellular SV40 DNA fragments has been shown to be analogous to a 72 bp repeat in the origin region of SV40, which is required for efficient early gene transcription *in vivo*. It is possible that a similar functional role for IR3 DNA will be found.

IV. Chromosomal Integration of Exogenous DNA of Nonviral Origin

Studies on the chromosome integration of exogenous DNA of nonviral origin provide a model to corroborate morphological features of viral integration. We have shown that chromosome integration occurs with the introduction of exogenous DNA into mammalian cells (Robins *et al.*, 1981a,b; Henderson and Robins, 1982; Huberman *et al.*, 1982). Human growth hormone (hGH) DNA, as well as herpes simplex tk$^+$ DNA, are present in coordinate linkage in rat chromosomes following cotransformation of these DNAs using the calcium phosphate method (Robins *et al.*, 1981a). Four independent DNA cotransformants, containing 5 to 100 hGH genes, as well as five revertants (tk$^-$) selected from each cotransformed cell line, have been studied in detail. As with viral insertion, the integration of nonviral exogenous DNA occurs on a single homolog in cloned cells from each independent DNA-mediated gene transfer event. The chromosome region carrying the inserted DNA is different for each event. These experiments demonstrate that foreign DNA is stably integrated into mammalian chromosomes. About one-half of the tk-revertants delete all transforming DNA; in 15 cases, significant deletion occurred, although some portion of the integrated sequences were retained in the expected chromosomal location.

Several types of chromosome rearrangements and morphological changes can be associated with the region of integration (Robins *et al.*, 1981b; Henderson *et al.*, 1983b). These include ''expanded'' regions, constrictions, and distortion in the normal G-banding pattern (Fig. 8). Elongated chromosomes that resulted from internal chromosomal duplication were found in three of the four DNA cotransformed cell lines. In two cell lines, integration occurred at the point of chromosomal duplication. The duplication is a repetition of the chromosome in reverse order initiating at the normal terminus of the chromosome. Thus, if the normal sequence of the chromosome were abcde, the elongated chromosome would read abcdedc. The elongated chromosomes where integration occurred are illustrated in Figs. 9 and 10. In the first case, integration has taken place at the point of internal replication on rat chromosome 4 (Figs. 9 and 10A). A visible portion of the chromosome has been deleted, and a constricted region is apparent at the juncture between the normal terminus of chromosome 4 and the repeated region. In a second cell line, integration occurred on an elongated chromosome 5

266

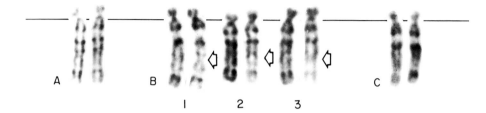

A   B   C

1   2   3

Fig. 8. Morphological changes resulting from integration of exogenous DNA into rat chromosomes. Human Growth hormone (hGH) and herpes simplex tk+ DNA were introduced into rat cells using the calcium phosphate method (Robins *et al.*, 1981a). In one DNA-mediated tranformation, approximately 50 copies of HGH DNA integrated on the long arm of chromosome 1. (A) Normal homologs of chromosome 1 in the Buffalo rat cell line. (B) Comparison of homologs of chromosome 1 where one of the homologues carries integrated DNA. The variations seen were (1) large constricted regions; (2) small constricted regions, and (3) a distortion in the banding pattern as the result of integration. This is illustrated in the homolog to the right. The region of integration is denoted by an arrow. (C) Comparison of homologs of rat chromosome 1 following reversion to the tk⁻ phenotype and deletion of all integrated sequences. The homolog to the right is noticeably shortened as the result of the deletion event.

(Fig. 10B). In this case, an extended achromatic region is seen at the integration site. Tk-revertants usually delete the inserted DNA by simply deleting the repeated portion of the chromosome. One exception is given in Fig. 10A(2). A direct excision has occurred, presumably involving dual breaks at each juncture of integrated and cellular DNA, followed by repair at the excision sites. In the example given, all integrated DNA has been deleted, but a constricted region was retained at the site where integration occurred.

We have direct evidence that integration of exogenous DNA sequences can result in deletion of endogenous cellular DNA. In one of the DNA cotransformants about 200 copies of hGH DNA have integrated at or near a region containing rDNA on a single homolog of chromosome 11 (Henderson and Robins, 1982). The direct result of the integration is deletion of over 70% of endogenous rDNA at this locus. The deletion is morphologically distinguished by the loss of satellites on the short arm of chromosome 11. It can be demonstrated that either the rDNA at the site of integration is inactivated or that the copy number is too low to detect rDNA activity. There is no NOR-specific silver stain associated with this chromosome and no participation in satellite association.

The integration of hGH DNA sequences in rat chromosomes is not a special case of the behavior of foreign DNA in mammalian cells. Human β-globin genes have been located in chromosomes of murine L cells following DNA transfer by microinjection (Huberman *et al.*, 1983). The human genes were linked to herpes

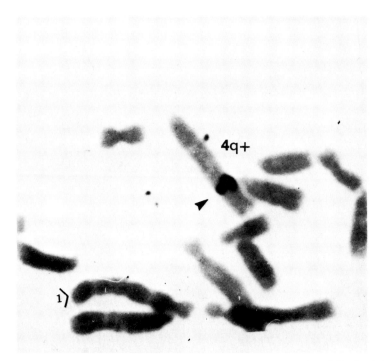

Fig. 9. Autoradiographic labeling over elongated rat chromosome 4q+ following hybridization with nick translated ^{125}I-labeled human growth hormone (hGH) DNA. DNA-mediated transfer resulted in the integration of approximately 75 copies of hGH DNA at the juncture between the normal terminus of chromosome 4 and the extended region as indicated by the arrows (Robins *et al.*, 1981a). Identification of the chromosome 4q+ was made on the basis of length; this is the longest chromosome on the metaphase plate (see chromosome 1). The specific activity of the ^{125}I-labeled hGH DNA was about 1×10^9 dpm/μg; autoradiographic exposure was for 2 days.

simplex tk+ DNA cointroduced by microinjection. Two independent DNA transfer experiments have been studied. In the first, the chromosome region carrying integrated sequences was near the terminal region of a single homolog of mouse chromosome 4. This chromosome forms part of a translocation chromosome t(4;4). A comparison of the grain density over chromosomes carrying integrated sequences in early and late passage cells revealed that a twofold amplification had occurred upon passage of the cells for an additional 30–40 generations. This observation has been confirmed by independent filter hybridizations. In a second DNA transfer experiment, integrated sequences are present at the terminal region of a homolog of chromosome 14 which is also involved in a Robertsonian translocation, t(8;14).

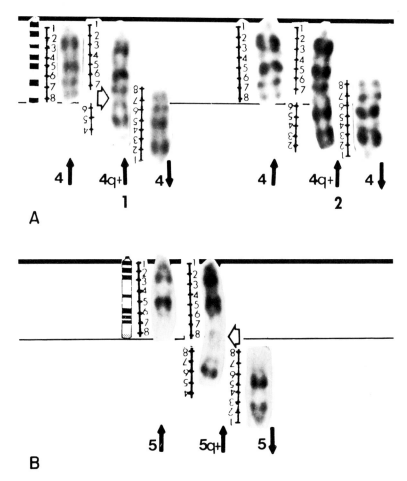

Fig. 10. Analysis of elongated chromosomes in rat cells following DNA-mediated transfer of HGH DNA. (A) 1, Normal rat chromosome 4 is compared with elongated chromosome 4q+. Experimental conditions are given in Fig. 9 and in Robins *et al.* (1981a). The normal chromosomes are arranged in the usual and inverted positions (indicated by black arrows) in order to compare the banding pattern to that of the elongated chromosome produced as the result of the inverted terminal repeat. A small constricted region and deletion of cellular chromosomal DNA is seen at the site of integration (white arrow). 2, Comparison of normal rat chromosome 4 and the elongated chromosome 4q+ following deletion of all integrated DNA sequences in a tk⁻ revertant. A constricted region is still apparent at the region where integration occurred. (B) The normal rat chromosome 5 is compared with an elongated 5q+ chromosome. DNA-mediated transfer resulted in the integration of 5 copies of hGH DNA in the elongated chromosome at the position of the normal terminus of chromosome 5 (Robins *et al.*, 1981a). The site of integration (white arrow) is morphologically distinguished by an achromatic region located between the usual terminus of chromosome 5 and the beginning of the inverted repeat region.

V. Discussion

We have shown that exogenous DNA of viral or nonviral origin can be directly incorporated into chromosomal DNA. Some general aspects of the integration process have been determined. The integration of foreign DNA occurs at a single site on one chromosome homolog that is invariant within a cell line. Stability of the integration site is maintained throughout strong selection pressures used in selecting DNA cotransformants and revertants and in long-term culture. Integration of exogenous DNA is not limited to a unique chromosome region, since independent DNA transfer experiments or viral insertions can result in different regions of chromosome integration. No gross chromosome rearrangements directly resulting from integration have been detected in our experiments. The only consistent morphological feature associated with integration is the presence of an achromatic and/or a constricted region.

The majority of questions concerning the integration process remain to be answered. It is not known how or why a given chromosome region should be selected for integration. Short or long sequence homologies are known to direct homologous recombination in specific cases. Sequence homology directs integration in yeast where yeast genes recombine with their genetic counterpart (Hinnen et al., 1978). There is no evidence, to date, that exogenous DNA is incorporated into mammalian DNA in a similar manner. For example. newly introduced SV40 genomes do not integrate into preexisting SV40 insertional sites following superinfection (Botchan et al., 1979). Exogenous DNA could also take advantage of related or unrelated breakage–reunion to integrate stably. If this were true, however, an obvious association would be found between EBV DNA and chromosomes known to participate in translocations in Burkitt tumor cells. We have been unable to make this association. Perhaps the most important information we have obtained concerns the plasticity of the chromosome. The chromosome survives the integration event in virtually an intact state.

A simple repeat array in the EBV genome, IR3, is homologous to multiple sites in human, and mouse, chromosomal DNA. This homology differs from relatedness seen in other viral–cellular DNA homologies. Sequences homologous to the SV40 ori region are present in primate DNA, but in much lower amounts, and perhaps with less complete homology (Conrad and Botchan, 1982). The IR3 DNA–cellular DNA homology also differs strongly from the relationship between retrovirus and cell transforming genes, since these are protein-encoding genes composed largely of unique sequence DNA (reviewed by Cooper, 1982).

The presence of any subset of repetitive DNAs within the mammalian genome is of interest to chromosome structure. IR3-related DNA is located throughout the genome, but the homologous sequences are not confined to any known morphologically defined region. The pattern of homology is not a simple distribution. It differs significantly from the distributive pattern of unrelated repetitive DNAs, such as those of the Alu I family. The distribution of IR3 DNA-related chromosome DNA most closely corresponds to that of large blocks of homologous sequences located at some distance from each other along the chromosome length. A similar distribution is seen when component alpha from the African green monkey (isolated from a defective SV40 virion) is hybridized to monkey chromosomes (Segal *et al.*, 1976; Rosenberg *et al.*, 1978; Singer, 1982).

The localization of virion-specific DNA in chromosomes, even in the absence of specific details of viral–cellular interactions, sets the stage for more comprehensive studies at the DNA level. A coordination of techniques from cytogenetics and molecular biology will be valuable in determining the complexities of viral–cellular interactions. The location of chromosomal DNA with homology to viral nucleic acid has bearing on questions that will determine the relationship of integration to the disease state, whether integration occurs at specific chromosome region(s), and whether associated changes in the chromosome can be used as an index of integration and/or the disease state. The most direct approach to the assignment of viral integration sites in chromosomes is cytological hybridization.

References

Ada, G. L., Humphrey, J. H., Askonas, B. A., McDevitt, H. O., and Nossal, G. J. V. (1966). *Exp. Cell Res.* **41**, 557–572.

Adams, A., and Lindahl, T. (1975). *Proc. Natl. Acad. Sci. U.S.A.* **72**, 1477–1481.

Alonso, C., Helmsing, P. J., and Berendes, H. D. (1974). *Exp. Cell Res.* **85**, 383–390.

Atwood, K. C., Yu, M. T., Eicher, E., and Henderson, A. S. (1976). *Cytogenet. Cell Genet.* **16**, 372–375.

Barbera, E., Caliani, J. J., Pages, M., and Alonso, C. (1979). *Exp. Cell Res.* **119**, 151–162.

Bishop, J. O., and Jones, K. W. (1972). *Nature (London)* **240**, 149–150.

Botchan, M., Topp, W., and Sambrook, J. (1979). *Cold Spring Harbor Symp. Quant. Biol.* **43**, 709–719.

Brahic, M., and Haase, A. T. (1978). *Proc. Natl. Acad. Sci. U.S.A.* **75**, 6125–6129.

Brahic, M., Stowring, L., Ventura, P., and Hasse, A. T. (1981). *Nature (London)* **292**, 240–242.

Comings, D. E., Avelino, E., Okado, T. A., and Wyandt, H. E. (1973). *Exp. Cell Res.* **77**, 469–493.

Conrad, S. E., and Botchan, M. R. (1982). *Mol. Cell. Biol.* **2**, 949–965.

Cooper, G. M. (1982). *Science* **218**, 801–806.

Dambaugh, T., Beisel, C., Hummel, M., King, W., Fennewald, S., Cheung, A., Heller, M., Raab-Traub, N., and Kieff, E. (1980a). *Proc. Natl. Acad. Sci. U.S.A.* **77**, 2999–3003.

Dambaugh, T., Raab-Traub, N., Heller, M., Beisel, C., Hummel, M., Cheung, A., Fennewald, S., King, W., and Kieff, E. (1980b). *Ann. N.Y. Acad. Sci.* **602**, 711–179.

Dayhoff, M. O., Chen, H. R., Hunt, L. T., Barker, W. C., Yeh, L.-S., George, D. G., and Orcutt, B. C. (1981). National Biomedical Research Foundation, Georgetown University Medical Center, Washington, D.C.

Dorries, K., Johnson, R., and ter Meulen, U. (1979). *J. Gen. Virol.* **42**, 49–57.

Dunn, A. R., Gallimore, P. H., Jones, K. W., and McDougall, J. K. (1973). *Int. J. Cancer* **11**, 628–636.

Epstein, M., Achong, B. (1979). *In* "The Epstein-Barr Virus" (M. Epstein and B. Achong, eds.), pp. 1–22. Springer-Verlag, Berlin and New York.

Galloway, D. A., Fenoglio, C., Sheuchuk, M., and McDougall, J. (1979). *Virology* **95**, 265–268.

Gerhard, D. S., Kawasaki, E. S., Bancroft, F. C., and Szabo, P. (1981). *Proc. Natl. Acad. Sci. U.S.A.* **78**, 3755–3759.

Geuskens, M., and May, E. (1974). *Exp. Cell Res.* **87**, 175–185.

Glasser, R., Nonoyama, M., Hampar, B., and Croce, C. M. (1978). *J. Cell Physiol.* **96**, 319–326.

Godard, C., and Jones, K. W. (1979). *Nucleic Acids Res.* **6**, 2849–2861.

Haase, A., Ventura, P., Gibbs, C., and Tourtellotte, W. (1981). *Science* **212**, 672–674.

Harper, M. E, and Saunders, G. (1981). *Chromosoma* **83**, 431–439.

Harper, M. E., Ulrich, A., and Saunders, G. F. (1981). *Proc. Natl. Acad. Sci. U.S.A.* **78**, 4458–4460.

Harper, M. E., Simon, M., Franchini, G., Gallo, R., and Wong-Staal, F. (1983). *Proc. Natl. Acad. Sci. U.S.A.* (in press).

Heller, M., van Santen, V., and Kieff, E. (1982a). *J. Virol.* **44**, 311–320.

Heller, M., Henderson, A., and Kieff, E. (1982b). *Proc. Natl. Acad. Sci. U.S.A.* **79**, 5916–5920.

Henderson, A. (1982). *Int. Rev. Cytol.* **76**, 1–46.

Henderson, A., and Robins, D. (1982). *Cytogenet. Cell Genet.* **34**, 310–314.

Henderson, A., Yu, M. T., and Atwood, K. C. (1978). *Cytogenet. Cell Genet.* **21**, 231–240.

Henderson, A., Yu, M. T., and Silverstein, S. (1981). *Cytogenet. Cell Genet.* **29**, 107–115.

Henderson, A., Ripley, S., Heller, M., and Kieff, E. (1983a). *Proc. Natl. Acad. Sci. U.S.A.* **80**, 1987–1991.

Henderson, A., Ripley, S., and Robins, D. (1983b). Manuscript in preparation.

Hennig, W. (1973). *Int. Rev. Cytol.* **36**, 1–44.

Hinnen, A., Hicks, J., and Fink, G. R. (1978). *Proc. Natl. Acad. Sci. U.S.A.* **75**, 1929–1933.

Huberman, M., Berg, P., Curcio, J., DePietro, J., Henderson, A., and Anderson, F. (1983). *Nucleic Acids Res.* (in press).

Kaufman, S., Gallo, R., and Miller, N. (1974). *J. Virol.* **30**, 637–641.

King, W., Powell, A. L. T., Raub-Traub, N., Hawke, M., and Kieff, E. (1980). *J. Virol.* **36**, 506–518.

Lavi, S. (1982). *J. Cell. Biochem.* **18**, 149–156.

Loni, M. C., and Green, M. (1973). *J. Virol.* **12**, 1288–1292.

Loni, M. C., and Green, M. (1974). *Proc. Natl. Acad. Sci. U.S.A.* **71**, 3418–3422.

McCutchan, T. F., and Singer, M. F. (1981). *Proc. Natl. Acad. Sci. U.S.A.* **78**, 95–99.

McDougall, J. (1971). *J. Gen. Virol.* **12**, 43–51.

McDougall, J. K., Dunn, A. R., and Jones, K. W. (1972). *Nature (London)* **236**, 346–348.

McDougall, J. K., Dunn, A. R., and Gallimore, P. H. (1974). *Cold Spring Harbor Symp. Quant. Biol.* **39**, 591–600.

McDougall, J., Galloway, D., and Fenoglio, C. (1979). *In* "Antiviral Mechanisms and the Control of Neoplasia" (P. Chandra, ed.), pp. 233–240. Plenum, New York.

McDougall, J., Crum, C., Fenoglio, C. M., Goldstein, L., and Galloway, D. (1982). *Proc. Natl. Acad. Sci. U.S.A.* **79**, 3853–3857.

Manolov, G., and Manolova, Y. (1972). *Nature (London)* **237**, 33–34.

Moar, M. H., and Jones, K. W. (1975). *Int. J. Cancer* **16**, 998–1007.

Moar, M. H., and Klein, G. (1978). *Biochim. Biophys. Acta* **519**, 49–64.

Neel, B., Jhanwar, S., Chaganti, R., and Hayward, W. (1982). *Proc. Natl. Acad. Sci. U.S.A.* **79**, 7842–7846.

Neer, A., Bara, N., and Manor, H. (1977). *Cell* **11**, 65–71.

Nonoyama, M., and Pagano, J. (1972). *Nature (London)* **238**, 169–171.
Nonoyama, M., Huang, C. H., Pagano, J. S., Klein, G., and Singh, S. (1973). *Proc. Natl. Acad. Sci. U.S.A.* **70**, 3265–3268.
Pardue, M. L., and Gall, J. G. (1972). In "Molecular Genetics and Developmental Biology" (M. Sussman, ed.), pp. 341–349. Prentice-Hall, Englewood Cliffs, New Jersey.
Pardue, M. L., and Gall, J. G. (1975). In "Methods in Cell Biology" (D. M. Prescott, ed.), Vol. 10, pp. 1–16. Academic Press, New York.
Prensky, W., and Holmquist, G. (1973). *Nature (London)* **241**, 44–45.
Prensky, W., Steffensen, D., and Hughes, W. (1973). *Proc. Natl. Acad. Sci. U.S.A.,* **70**, 1860–1864.
Queen, C., Lord, S. T., McCutchan, T. F., and Singer, M. F. (1981). *Mol. Cell. Biol.* **1**, 1061–1068.
Robins, D., Ripley, S., Henderson, A., and Axel, R. (1981a). *Cell* **23**, 29–39.
Robins, D., Axel, R., and Henderson, A. (1981b). *J. Mol. Appl. Genet.* **1**, 191–204.
Rogers, A. W. (1973). "Techniques in Autoradiography." Elsevier, London.
Rosenberg, H., Singer, M., and Rosenberg, M. (1978). *Science* **200**, 394–402.
Ruddle, F. H., and Creagan, R. P. (1975). *Annu. Rev. Genet.* **9**, 407–486.
Sambrook, J., Botchan, M., Gallimore, P., Ozanne, B., Petersson, U., Williams, J., and Sharp, P. A. (1975). *Cold Spring Harbor Symp. Quant. Biol.* **39**, 615–632.
Segal, S., Garner, M., Singer, M., and Rosenberg, M. (1976). *Cell* **9**, 247–257.
Shoyab, M., Markham, P. D., and Baluda, M. A. (1974). *J. Virol.* **14**, 225–230.
Simon, I., Lohler, J., and Jaenisch, R. (1982). *Virol.* **120**, 106–121.
Singer, M. (1982). *Int. Rev. Cytol.* **76**, 67–112.
Singh, L., Purdom, I. F., and Jones, K. W. (1977). *Chromosoma* **60**, 337–389.
Spira, J., Povey, S., Weiner, F., Klein, G., and Andersson-Anvret, G. (1977). *Int. J. Cancer* **20**, 849–853.
Steplewski, Z., Koprowski, H., Andersson-Anvret, M., and Klein, G. (1978). *J. Cell Physiol.* **97**, 1–8.
Stringer, J. R. (1982). *Nature (London)* **296**, 363–365.
Szabo, P., Elder, R., and Uhlenbeck, O. (1975). *Nucleic Acids Res.* **5**, 647–653.
Szabo, P., Elder, R., Steffensen, D. M., and Uhlenbeck, O. C. (1977). *J. Mol. Biol.* **115**, 539–563.
Tereba, A., and Astrin, S. (1982). *J. Virol.* **43**, 737–740.
Tereba, A., and Lai, M. (1982). *Virology* **116**, 654–657.
Tereba, A., Lai, M., and Murti, K. (1979). *Proc. Natl. Acad. Sci. U.S.A.* **76**, 6486–6490.
van Santen, V., Cheung, A., and Kieff, E. (1981). *Proc. Natl. Acad. Sci. U.S.A.* **78**, 1930–1934.
Wolgemuth-Jarashow, D. J., Jagiello, G. M., Atwood, K. C., and Henderson, A. S. (1976). *Cytogenet. Cell Genet.* **17**, 137–143.
Yamamoto, K., Mizuno, F., Matsuo, T., Tanaka, A., Nonoyama, M., and Osato, T. (1978). *Proc. Natl. Acad. Sci. U.S.A.* **75**, 5155–5159.
Yasue, H., and Ishibashi, M. (1982). *Virology* **116**, 99–115.
Zech, L., Haglund, V., Nilsson, K., and Klein, G. (1976). *Int. J. Cancer* **17**, 47–56.
zur Hausen, H., and Schulte-Holthausen, H. (1972). In "Oncogenesis and Herpes Viruses" (P. M. Biggs, G. de-The, and L. N. Payne, eds.), pp. 321–325. IARC, Lyon.
zur Hausen, H., Diehl, V., Wolf, J., Shulte-Holthausen, H., and Schneider, V. (1972). *Nature (London), New Biol.* **237**, 189–190.
zur Hausen, H., Schulte-Holthausen, H., Wolf, H., Dorries, K., and Egger, H. (1974). *Int. J. Cancer* **13**, 657–664.

15

A Sensitive Colorimetric Method for Visualizing Biotin-Labeled Probes Hybridized to DNA or RNA on Nitrocellulose Filters

JEFFRY J. LEARY,* DAVID J. BRIGATI,[†,‡] AND DAVID C. WARD[*,§]

Yale University School of Medicine
New Haven, Connecticut

*Department of Human Genetics.
†Department of Laboratory Medicine.
‡Present address: Department of Pathology, The Milton S. Hershey Medical Center, Pennsylvania State University, Hershey, Pennsylvania 17033.
§Department of Molecular Biophysics–Biochemistry.

I. Introduction*

Our understanding of the human genome, in both normal and malignant cells, has expanded dramatically over the past decade with the development of recombinant DNA techniques and sensitive methods for analyzing the organization, sequence complexity, and chromosomal location of specific genes or their transcripts. Each of these procedures (e.g., molecular cloning, Southern blotting, Northern blotting, and *in situ* hybridization) exploit the exquisite specificity and sensitivity that can be obtained by nucleic acid hybridization and, without exception, routinely employ polynucleotide probes of high specific radioactivity coupled with autoradiographic detection methods. In spite of the tremendous power of these analytic tools, there are serious limitations and disadvantages associated with the use of radioactively labeled hybridization probes, especially for routine application in clinical or diagnostic medicine. The short functional half-life of many radioisotopes, the expense, the personnel safety, and the isotope disposal problems, make it desirable to have alternative, but equally sensitive, methods for detecting, quantitating, or localizing specific nucleic acid sequences.

Previous reports from this laboratory have described the synthesis of biotin-labeled analogs of TTP and UTP that can be enzymatically incorporated into DNA and RNA, respectively (Langer *et al.*, 1981; Brigati *et al.*, 1983). The resulting biotin-labeled polynucleotides exhibit reassociation kinetics similar to those of biotin-free polymers, and they function effectively as hybridization probes *in situ*. Hybridization signals can be visualized by indirect immunofluorescence, immunoperoxidase or immuno-colloidal gold techniques, following incubation with a primary anti-biotin antibody, and by cytochemical methods that employ complexes of avidin and biotinylated peroxidase to detect the biotin-labeled probe. Such procedures have been applied successfully to the localization of specific polynucleotide sequences in *Drosophila* polytene chromosomes (Langer and Ward, 1981; Langer-Safer *et al.*, 1982), mammalian metaphase chromosomes (Hutchison *et al.*, 1982; Manuelidis *et al.*, 1982), cultured cell populations (Singer and Ward, 1982; Brigati *et al.*, 1983) and formalin-fixed tissue sections (Brigati *et al.*, 1983). However, none of the visualization methods used in these studies were able to detect polynucleotide se-

---

*Abbreviations: Bio-4-dUTP, Bio-11-dUTP and Bio-16-dUTP; analogs of TTP that contain a biotin molecule linked to the C-5 position of the pyrimidine ring through linker arms that are 4, 11, and 16 atoms long, respectively. Bio-4-DNA, Bio-11-DNA and Bio-16-DNA; DNA probes prepared with Bio-4, Bio-11-or Bio-16-dUTP analogs, respectively. NBT, nitro blue tetrazolium, BCIP, 5-bromo-4-chloro-3-indolyl phosphate. DAB, 3,3'-diaminobenzidine. EAC, ethyl aminocarbazole; ABAP, complexes of avidin and biotinylated alkaline phosphatase, poly ABAP, complexes of avidin and biotinylated alkaline phosphatase polymers. NaCl/Cit, standard saline citrate (0.15 M CaCl/0.015 M sodium citrate, pH 7.0).

quences present at the level of one copy per mammalian cell. It was apparent, therefore, that the routine application of biotin-labeled probes in genetic analysis would require the development of more sensitive biotin-detection systems. Here we report the synthesis of biotinylated polymers of intestinal alkaline phosphatase, and the construction of avidin (or streptavidin) enzyme polymer complexes that are 20- to 50-fold more sensitive than immuno- or affinity reagents used previously. We also describe a rapid and sensitive procedure for visualizing biotin-labeled DNA probes after hybridization to target sequences immobilized on nitrocellulose filters.

II. Materials and Methods

Affinity purified rabbit anti-biotin IgG was prepared as described (Langer-Safer *et al.*, 1982). An ammonium sulfate fraction of goat anti-biotin IgG was generously provided by Enzo Biochem Inc., New York. Biotinylated rabbit anti-goat IgG, biotinylated goat anti-rabbit IgG, and avidin DH-biotinylated horseradish peroxidase complex (Vectastain ABC kit) were purchased, or provided as gifts, from Vector Laboratories, Inc., Burlingame, California. Streptavidin (Hoffman *et al.*, 1980) was obtained from either Bethesda Research Laboratories, Inc., Gaithersberg, Maryland or Enzo Biochem Inc. Calf intestinal alkaline phosphatase (Catalog No. 567-752) and pancreatic DNAse type I were purchased from Boehringer Mannheim, Indianapolis, Indiana. Biotinyl-ε-amino caproic acid *N*-hydroxysuccinimide ester was synthesized according to Costello *et al.* (1979) or was a gift from Dr. Stanley Kline, Enzo Biochem. Inc. Disuccinimidyl suberate was a product of Pierce Chemical Co., Rockford, Illinois. Restriction endonucleases and *E. coli* DNA polymerase I were obtained from New England Biolabs, Inc., Beverly, Massachusetts. Agarose (type II), bovine serum albumin (BSA, fraction V), 5-bromo-4-chloro-3-indolyl phosphate *p*-toluidine salt, cadaverine-free base, 3,3'-diaminobenzidine tetrahydrochloride, Ficoll (type 400), ethyl aminocarbazole, herring sperm DNA (type VII), nitro blue tetrazolium (grade III), and polyvinylpyrrolidone (PVP-40) were from Sigma Chemical Co., St. Louis, Missouri. Plasmids containing human globin gene sequences were provided by Dr. Sherman Weissman, Yale University. JW101 is a 0.4×10^3 bp cDNA α-globin clone (Wilson *et al.*, 1978) and pHβC6 is a 5.2×10^3 bp genomic fragment containing the β-globin gene in pBR322 (Fukamaki *et al.*, 1982). Plasmid pMM984 (Merchlinsky *et al.*, 1983) contains the complete 5.1 kb genome of the parvovirus, minute virus of mice (MVM), cloned into pBR322. This plasmid contains a single *Xho*I site within the MVM sequence insert. Human placental DNA was a gift from Scot Van Arsdell, Yale University.

A. Polymerization and Biotinylation of Intestinal Alkaline Phosphatase

Calf intestinal alkaline phosphatase was polymerized by cross-linking with disuccinimidyl suberate (DSS). The enzyme, supplied as a 10 mg/ml solution by the manufacturer, was diluted to 1 mg/ml in ice cold NMZT buffer (3 M NaCl, 1 mM MgCl$_2$, 0.1 mM ZnCl$_2$, 30 mM triethylanolamine, pH 7.6) in a silanized glass reaction vessel or a silanized Eppendorf tube. All subsequent reactions were done at 4°C. A 5 mg/ml solution of DSS in dimethylformamide was added (10 μl/ml of enyzme solution) in two equal aliquots (~30–60 seconds apart) with gentle stirring. This solution, containing a 19-fold molar excess of DSS over enzyme, was stirred over 20 minutes during which time a cloudy precipitate appeared. Aliquots of 10 μl of cadaverine-free base (0.1 mg/ml in NMZT buffer) were added to the reaction mixture four times at 10 minute intervals. The DSS-cadaverine ratio was then made equimolar by adding another 30 μl of cadaverine solution for each milliter of reaction mixture. After stirring an additional 10 minutes, 2 μl of undiluted cadaverine-free base stock was added and the mixture stirred a further 30 minutes. The resultant clear solution was then dialyzed extensively against NMZT buffer. (The polymerization and cadaverine treatments were often repeated a second time, however these additional steps did not appear to increase the polymer size significantly since both 1× and 2× polymerized enzyme complexes detect target sequences with about equal sensitivity.)

Monomeric or polymeric forms of alkaline phosphatase were reacted with a 60-fold molar excess of biotinyl-ε-aminocaproic acid N-hydroxysuccinimide ester (BACSE) by adding 10 μl of a 20 mg/ml solution of BACSE (in dimethylformamide) for each milligram of enzyme present in the dialysis bag. After stirring the bag on a rotary shaker at 4°C for 2 hours, the reaction mixture was again extensively dialyzed against NMZT buffer. Sodium azide was added to a final concentration of 0.02% (w/v), and the biotinylated enzymes were stored at 4°C until use.

B. Preparation of Avidin-Biotinylated Alkaline Phosphatase Polymer Complexes (Poly ABAP Complexes)

The biotinylated enzyme polymer must be mixed with a slight excess of avidin to produce complexes capable of direct interaction with biotinylated probes hybridized on filters. The protein mixture that gave an optimal signal-to-noise ratio was determined empirically by analyzing the ability of various protein mixtures to discriminate between avidin-DH and biotinylated goat IgG spotted on nitrocellulose. Protein ratios were adjusted to give a strong reaction with biotinylated IgG but little, if any, signal from the avidin-DH spot. The component composition of the poly ABAP complex was further optimized for high sensitivity and specificity against Bio-16-DNA samples spotted on nitrocellulose using a constant avidin-DH concentration and varying amounts of biotinylated enzyme polymer. The optimum protein ratios should be established for each new lot of enzyme polymer to ensure maximum specificity and sensitivity. Enzyme complexes were made using avidin-DH or streptavidin, and complexes made with either biotin-binding protein gave similar results.

The poly ABAP complex used in the experiments reported here was constructed as follows: Avidin-DH (1.8 mg/ml) was diluted to a concentration of 7.2 μg/ml into AP 7.5 buffer [0.1 M Tris-HCl, pH 7.5, 0.1 M NaCl, 2 mM MgCl$_2$, 0.05% (v/v) Triton X-100]. The protein was added to a clean borosilicate glass tube prerinsed with a solution of bovine serum albumin (3%, w/v) in AP 7.5 buffer. Biotinylated alkaline phosphatase polymer (0.92 mg/ml in NMZT buffer) was then added to a final concentration of 1.8 μg/ml and complex formation allowed to proceed for at least 10 minutes prior to use. The physical and enzymatic characteristics of this poly ABAP complex will be reported elsewhere.

C. Preparation of Dot Blots

Plasmid pMM984 DNA, either linearized by *Xho*I digestion or nick-translated with Bio-11 or Bio-16-dUTP substrate (see below) was serially diluted in 50 mM Tris-Cl, pH 7.5, containing 0.3 N NaOH and 1.5 mg/ml of sheared herring sperm DNA. Appropriate dilutions were neutralized on ice with ice cold 3 N HCl, and 5 μl aliquots were spotted directly on BA-85 nitrocellulose filter sheets (Schleicher and Schuell, Keene, New Hampshire) on top of Saran wrap. Filters were air dried, baked for 4 hours at 80°C, and cut into strips containing a dilution series ranging from 0 to 128 pg of plasmid DNA per spot.

D. Preparation of Southern Blots

Agarose gels approximately 6 mm thick were prepared on a horizontal electrophoresis apparatus, and DNA samples were electrophoresed as described by Alwine *et al.* (1980). DNA was transferred to nitrocellulose sheets (BA-85 or Sartorius 11336) presaturated with 20× NaCl/Cit as described by Southern (1975) and modified by Thomas (1980), after performing the acid depurination step of Wahl *et al.* (1979). Complete transfer was ensured by using a 3-cm thick foam sponge saturated with 20× NaCl/Cit as a fluid reservoir beneath the gel. DNA filters were air dried, baked at 80°C for 2–4 hours and stored at 4°C over CaSO$_4$ until hybridized.

E. Hybridization Probes

Probes were prepared by nick translation essentially as described by Rigby *et al.* (1977). Reaction mixtures (20–200 μl) contained 40 μg/ml DNA; 200 units/ml DNA pol I; 0.005 μg/ml DNAse; 50 mM Tris-Cl, pH 7.5; 5 mM MgCl$_2$; 50 μg/ml BSA; 50 μM each dCTP, dGTP, dATP, and TTP (P-L Biochemicals, Inc., Milwaukee, Wisconsin) or Bio-dUTP analogs. Bio-4-dUTP, Bio-11-dUTP, and Bio-16-dUTP were synthesized as previously described (Langer *et al.*, 1981; Brigati *et al.*, 1983). Samples of Bio-11-dUTP and Bio-16-dUTP were also generously provided by Dr. Stanley Kline, Enzo Biochem Inc. Nick-translation reactions containing Bio-dUTP analogs were incubated for 2 hours at 14°C, while reactions with TTP were incubated for 1 hour at 14°C. Some of the Bio-dUTP reactions also contained 200 μCi/ml of [α-^{32}P]dCTP (Amersham, 410 Ci/mmole). High specific radioactivity probes were prepared as above with TTP and [α-^{32}P]dATP at 5 μM and 1000 Ci/mmole (Amersham). Nick-translated DNAs were purified and characterized as previously described (Brigati *et al.*, 1983).

F. Prehybridization and Hybridization Conditions

The general protocol outlined below was found (see Section III) to be optimal when using biotin-labeled hybridization probes. Filters were prehybridized for 2–4 hours at 42°C in 5× NaCl/Cit as per Wahl *et al.* (1979) in a sealed plastic bag using a mixture containing 45% (v/v) deionized formamide (conductivity < 10 μmho, pH 6.5 or less), 5× Denhardt's solution (Denhardt, 1966), 25 mM NaPO$_4$ buffer, pH 6.5, and sonicated herring sperm DNA (250–500 μg/ml). The hybridization buffer contained 5× NaCl/Cit, 45% (v/v) formamide, 1× Denhardt's solution, 25 mM NaPO$_4$ buffer, pH 6.5, 10% dextran sulfate [added as 20% of the final volume from a 50% (w/v) stock], 250–500 μg/ml sonicated herring sperm DNA, and 200–500 ng/ml of a DNA probe that had been nick translated with Bio-16-dUTP. The carrier and probe DNAs were heat denatured just prior to addition. Ten milliliters of hybridization mixture was used per 100 cm^2 of filter and the hybridization reaction incubated at 42°C (in a sealed bag) for 30–180 minutes. For analysis of single-copy mammalian gene sequences, hybridization was generally done to a *Cot* of 0.8 × 10^{-2} (e.g., for a probe concentration of 350 ng/ml the hybridization time was 120 minutes). Following the hybridization, filters were washed four times at room temperature, 2–3 minutes for each wash, twice with 2× NaCl/Cit–0.1% sodium dodecyl sulfate (SDS) and twice with 0.2× NaCl/Cit–0.1% SDS. Two stringent washes (15 minutes each) were done with 0.16× NaCl/Cit–0.1% SDS at 50°C. Filters were then rinsed briefly in 2× NaCl/Cit–0.1% SDS at room temperature, air dried, and mounted for autoradiography with XAR X-ray film (Kodak, Rochester, New York) or assayed for biotin as described below.

G. Colorimetric Detection of Bio-DNA Probes

Dry nitrocellulose filter blots were incubated at 42°C for 15 minutes in a 3% (w/v) solution of BSA in AP 7.5 buffer, air dried, baked at 80°C for 20–60 minutes, and then rehydrated in the BSA–AP 7.5 buffer at 42°C for 20–30 minutes. Small filter strips were treated in 13 × 100 mm glass tubes, while larger sheets were treated in polyethylene trays or heat-sealed polypropylene bags. Filters were exposed to enzyme complexes for 5 minutes at room temperature; 2–5 ml of complex were used for each 100 cm² of filter. Filters were rapidly washed three times in 250 ml of AP 7.5 and twice in AP 9.5 (0.1 M Tris-HCl, pH 9.5, 0.1 M NaCl, 5 mM MgCl$_2$). When avidin-peroxidase (ABC) complexes were used 2× NaCl/Cit was substituted for AP 7.5 and AP 9.5 buffers.

For development with ABAP or poly ABAP complexes, filters were incubated at room temperature for 0.5 to 24 hours in AP 9.5 buffer containing 0.33 mg/ml of NBT and 0.17 mg/ml of BCIP (McGadey, 1970). The phosphatase substrate solution was prepared as follows: for each 15 ml of reagent, 5 mg of NBT was suspended in 1.5 ml of AP 9.5 in a microcentrifuge tube and vortexed vigorously for 1–2 minutes, centrifuged briefly in a microfuge, and the supernatant decanted into 10 ml of AP 9.5 warmed to 35°C in a polypropylene tube. The residual NBT pellet was extracted twice more with 1.5 ml of AP 9.5 buffer, and the supernatants were pooled with the original solution. The tube was rinsed with a final 0.5 ml of AP 9.5 that was also decanted into the 15 ml NBT stock solution. BCIP (2.5 mg) was dissolved in 50 µl of N,N-dimethylformamide and added dropwise with gentle mixing into the NBT solution. Do not vortex or vigorously shake the reagent mixture, as extensive aeration can lead to the formation of undesirable precipitates. Although this reagent was generally prepared fresh, it was stable at room temperature for at least 24 hours in the dark.

Filters were incubated with the substrate solution in sealed polypropylene bags, using 10–15 ml of solution/100 cm² of filter. To reduce nonspecific background, color development should proceed in the dark or subdued light. Single-copy mammalian gene sequences generally become visible within 30 minutes, although highly colored hybridization signals require incubation times of several hours. Color development was terminated by washing filters in 10 mM Tris-HCl, 1 mM EDTA, pH 7.5. Developed blots were stored dry or in heat-sealed bags containing a small amount of 20 mM Tris-HCl, 5 mM EDTA, pH 9.5. Although the color intensity fades when the nitrocellulose sheet is dried, rewetting with buffer will restore color intensity as long as the filter has been stored without prolonged exposure to strong light.

III. Results

The general utility of biotin-labeled polynucleotides as hybridization probes depends, in large part, upon the sensitivity and speed of the probe detection method. We therefore first examined the relative efficiencies of standard immunological and affinity procedures for visualizing biotin-labeled DNA. Serial twofold dilutions of target (pMM984 plasmid) DNA, labeled with Bio-4-dUTP, Bio-11-dUTP, or Bio-16-dUTP, were mixed with a constant amount of carrier herring sperm DNA (7.5 μg) and spotted directly onto nitrocellulose strips. These strips were then incubated with various detector reagents and the sensitivity of each method determined. Results of such experiments are summarized in Table I. Indirect immunofluorescence, using a hand-held UV-light source for visualization, was a relatively insensitive procedure with detection limits near 1 ng of target DNA (lines 1 and 2 in Table I). Indirect immunoperoxidase methods, using either DAB or EAC as a substrate, were better (lines 3 and 4 in Table I), but still only 150–200 pg were seen with a Bio-11-DNA target. The peroxidase–antiperoxidase assay method of Sternberger et al. (1970) improved the sensitivity approximately twofold over that seen with the indirect immunoperoxidase technique (data not shown), but it was also not sensitive enough for the analysis of single-copy mammalian DNA sequences. With each of these immunological methods, increasing the length of the biotin "linker arm" from 4 to 11 atoms enhanced the detectability of the target by approximately fourfold. In contrast, Bio-4-DNA was not detected at all by complexes of avidin and biotinylated horseradish peroxidase [the ABC complexes of Hsu et al. (1981)]. Howev-

TABLE I

Relative Sensitivity of Biotin-Specific Reagents in Detecting Biotin-Labeled Polynucleotides Bound to Nitrocellulose Filters

Bio-DNA target	Detector reagents	Substrates	Detection limits (pg target sequence)
1. Bio-4	Anti-biotin IgG + FITC-2° Ab	—	2000–4000
2. Bio-11	Anti-biotin IgG + FITC-2° Ab	—	500–1000
3. Bio-4	Anti-biotin IgG + HRP-2° Ab	DAB/EAC	500–1000
4. Bio-11	Anti-biotin IgG + HRP-2° Ab	DAB/EAC	150–200
5. Bio-4	ABC (avidin DH - Bio HRP)	DAB/EAC	None detected
6. Bio-11	ABC	DAB/EAC	75–150
7. Bio-16	ABC	DAB/EAC	75–150
8. Bio-16	Anti-biotin IgG + Bio-2° Ab + ABC	DAB/EAC	≥100–200
9. Bio-16	ABC + Bio-DNA + ABC	DAB/EAC	≥100–200
10. Bio-16	ABAP (avidin-Bio Alk. Phos.)	NBT + BCIP	20–30
11. Bio-16	poly ABAP (avidin-poly Bio Alk. Phos.)	NBT + BCIP	1–2

er, ABC complexes revealed Bio-11-DNA and Bio-16-DNA with equal efficiency and with a sensitivity limit of less than 100 pg in a simple one-step reaction (lines 6 and 7 in Table I). Complexes made with avidin-DH and biotinylated intestinal alkaline phosphatase (ABAP complexes) were even more sensitive than ABC complexes made with peroxidase (line 10 in Table I), with detection limits between 20 and 30 pg of target DNA. Surprisingly, all attempts to increase the signal strength using multiple "sandwiching" techniques resulted in either no enhancement or a sharp decrease in signal. This was observed using either anti-biotin IgG or an ABC type complex as the primary detector (lines 8 and 9 in Table I). These observations suggested that such procedures were preferentially removing the primary detector from the filter, rather than building upon it, possibly reflecting differential affinities between the target–primary detector protein complex and the primary–secondary detector reagents. We reasoned that the simplest way to circumvent this problem was to construct covalently linked enzyme polymers that, after biotinylation, could be used in conjunction with avidin (or streptavidin) for direct probe detection. Polymers of intestinal alkaline phosphatase that retained high levels of enzymatic activity were prepared as described in Section II. As shown in Table I, line 11, this complex, termed poly ABAP, when used in conjunction with a substrate mixture of nitro blue tetrazolium and 5-bromo-4-chloro-3-indolyl phosphate, would detect 1–2 pg of target DNA with enzyme incubations of 3–4 hours. Assuming 6–10 pg of DNA per diploid mammalian cell and average "gene" size of 5×10^3 bp, 12 pg sensitivity would be required for analyzing unique sequences in a 7.5 μg sample of DNA. The poly ABAP complex thus appeared to have this capacity.

Figure 1 shows typical assay results obtained using ABC, ABAP, and poly ABAP enzyme detector complexes. Peroxidase (ABC) reactions (lane 1 in Fig. 1) generally gave higher nonspecific background on the nitrocellulose filters than ABAP or poly ABAP complexes (lanes 2 and 3 in Fig. 1, respectively), particularly if incubations with peroxidase substrates were longer than 30–60 minutes. However, using the poly ABAP detector, 1 pg of target DNA was visible without significant background noise with enzyme incubations of 3–4 hours. Since the NBT/BCIP substrate mixture did not exhibit appreciable end-product inhibition of the phosphatase activity, the intensity of the signal could be increased further by prolonging the substrate incubation period for up to 24 hours.

Having developed an enzyme complex with the capacity to detect picogram quantities of biotin-labeled DNA, the optimum conditions for using Bio-11-DNA or Bio-16-DNA as hybridization probes were investigaged. Previous *in situ* hybridization experiments (Langer-Safer *et al.,* 1982; Brigati *et al.,* 1983) indicated that biotin-labeled polynucleotides exhibited less nonspecific binding to tissues and chromosomes than comparable radiolabeled probes. These observations suggested that high Bio-DNA probe concentrations could also be used to drive hybridization reactions to target sequences on nitrocellulose. The validity

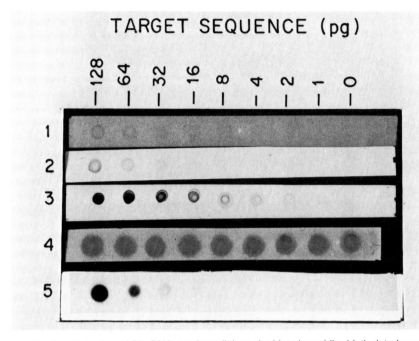

Fig. 1. Detection of Bio-DNA on nitrocellulose dot blots by avidin–biotinylated enzyme complexes. Each spot contained the indicated amount of pMM984 plasmid DNA (target sequence), labeled with Bio-16-dUTP and $[\alpha\text{-}^{32}P]$dCTP (3×10^5 cpm/μg) by nick translation, and 7.5 μg of carrier DNA. Detection systems were: (lane 1) ABC (peroxidase) complex, 1-hour reaction with DAB, (lane 2) ABAP complex, 3.75-hour reaction with NBT/BCIP, (lane 3) poly ABAP complex, 3.75-hour reaction with NBT/BCIP. Blot 4 was stained for total DNA with 0.02% Toluidene blue, while 5 is an autoradiograph of a duplicate strip exposed to film for 24 hr with screen.

of this suggestion was tested by hybridizing pMM984 DNA probes, labeled with ^{32}P alone or with both ^{32}P- and biotin-nucleotides, to replica dot-blot strips. The two probes, of identical specific radioactivity, were hybridized at various probe concentrations ranging from 5 to 1000 ng/ml (Fig. 2). The autoradiograph of the strips hybridized with ^{32}P-labeled DNA showed significant nonspecific background at all probe concentrations above 25 ng/ml (Fig. 2C). In contrast, the ^{32}P-labeled Bio-16-DNA probe gave virtually no nonspecific background noise at probe concentrations up to 750 ng/ml (Fig. 2B). This result demonstrated that a good signal-to-noise ratio could be obtained using very high concentrations of a Bio-DNA probe, thus making it possible to markedly reduce the hybridization times required to achieve any desired *Cot* value.

The autoradiographic signal from the ^{32}P-labeled Bio-16-DNA probe (Fig. 2B) was appreciably lower than that observed with the biotin-free ^{32}P-labeled

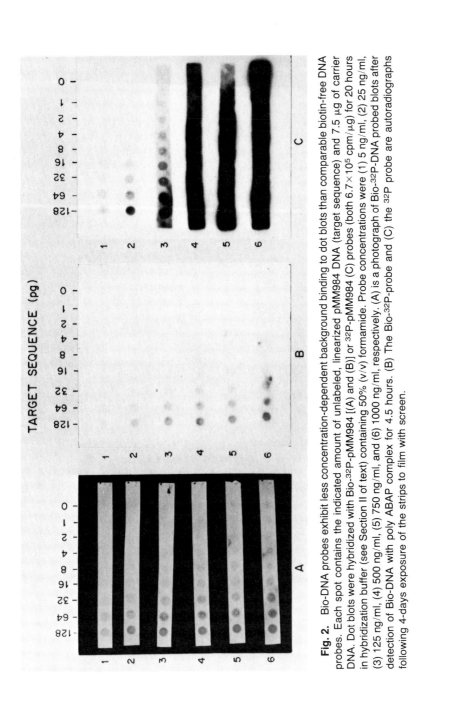

Fig. 2. Bio-DNA probes exhibit less concentration-dependent background binding to dot blots than comparable biotin-free DNA probes. Each spot contains the indicated amount of unlabeled, linearized pMM984 DNA (target sequence) and 7.5 μg of carrier DNA. Dot blots were hybridized with Bio-^{32}P-pMM984 [(A) and (B)] or ^{32}P-pMM984 (C) probes (both 6.7×10^5 cpm/μg) for 20 hours in hybridization buffer (see Section II of text) containing 50% (v/v) formamide. Probe concentrations were (1) 5 ng/ml, (2) 25 ng/ml, (3) 125 ng/ml, (4) 500 ng/ml, (5) 750 ng/ml, and (6) 1000 ng/ml, respectively. (A) is a photograph of Bio-^{32}P-DNA probed blots after detection of Bio-DNA with poly ABAP complex for 4.5 hours. (B) The Bio-^{32}P-probe and (C) the ^{32}P probe are autoradiographs following 4-days exposure of the strips to film with screen.

probe of equivalent specific radioactivity (Fig. 2C). This observation, coupled with the previous report (Langer *et al.*, 1981) that the melting temperature of biotin-labeled DNA duplexes is slightly lower than that of biotin-free DNAs, indicated that maximum specific hybridization of the Bio-16-DNA probe was not achieved under the conditions used (50% formamide buffer, 42°C). To establish a more optimal condition for probe delivery, duplicate sets of filters were hybridized (and washed) at different stringencies. This study indicated that hybridization buffers containing 45% formamide, when combined with stringent washes in 0.16 × NaCl/Cit at 50°C, gave the best signal-to-noise ratios (Fig. 3). Although decreasing the stringency further resulted in nonspecific hybridization to the carrier DNA (spot 0), there was still little nonspecific binding to the filter at a probe concentration of 500 ng/ml.

The ability of the poly ABAP detection system to visualize sequences in a Southern blot format was first analyzed in a reconstruction experiment. Various amounts of linearized pAT153 plasmid DNA were added to 10 µg samples of sheared carrier DNA and the mixtures electrophoresed on a 1.4% agarose gel. The region of the gel containing the 3.6 kb plasmid bands was transferred to nitrocellulose and the filter hybridized with a Bio-16-labeled plasmid probe. As a critical test of the potential of the system, the hybridization was done at a high stringency (in 50% formamide) to a high *Cot,* conditions which are known to give less than maximal results. Nevertheless, after a 2-hour incubation in the NBT/BCIP substrate solution the poly ABAB complex clearly detected bands containing as little as 3.1 pg of plasmid DNA (Fig. 4B). The intensity of the signal was also proportional to the amount of target sequence.

Further testing of the utility of this detector system was done by digesting human placental DNA with *Eco*RI or *Hin*dIII and transferring the resulting fragments to nitrocellulose after electrophoresis in a 1% agarose gel. The DNA was then hybridized for 2 hours with Bio-16-labeled α-globin or Bio-16-labeled β-globin probes. The α-globin probe (clone JW101) is a cDNA clone that contains only 400 nucleotides of the α-globin gene sequence; the β-globin probe (pHβC6) is a 5.2 kb genomic clone. After the hybridized probes were visualized by the poly ABAP reagent and several hours of enzyme incubation (Fig. 5), restriction fragments were observed that had sizes in good agreement with the published literature (Orkin, 1978; Van der Ploeg *et al.,* 1980; Fritsch *et al.,* 1980). The minor 2.5 kb *Eco*R1 fragment hybridized to the β-globin probe (Fig. 5, lane 3) is most likely the *Eco*R1 fragment from the 5′ region of the δ-globin gene, which cross-hybridizes with β-globin probes (Fritsch *et al.,* 1980; Mears *et al.,* 1978). Although the three *Hin*dIII fragments that hybridized with the α-globin probe (Fig. 5, lane 2) exhibit a weaker signal than the other bands observed in lanes 1, 3, and 4, this is not surprising since each of these fragments hybridized to only a subset of the 400 nucleotides present in the probe. It is clear,

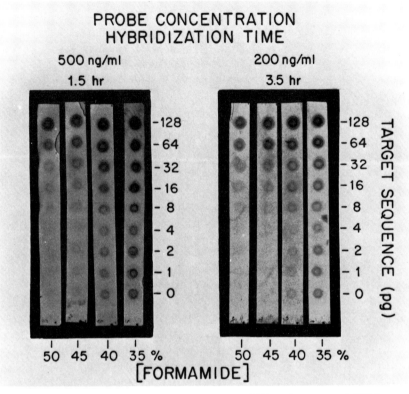

Fig. 3. Optimum specific hybridization with Bio-DNA probe occurs at 45% formamide. Dot blots contained linearized pMM984 and carrier DNA as in Fig. 2. Blots were hybridized under two Bio-16-pMM984 DNA probe and time conditions at the indicated formamide concentrations. Blots, after hybridization, were washed at 50°C in NaCl/Cit concentrations of $0.1\times$, $0.16\times$, $0.27\times$, and $0.45\times$ for hybridizations at 50, 45, 40 and 35% formamide, respectively. Bound Bio-DNA was detected with poly ABAP complex and a 1.5-hour enzyme reaction. Blots hybridized in 45% formamide have a 2- to 4-fold increase in signal over that obtained in 50% formamide without the nonspecific hybridization to carrier DNA (spot 0) detected when reactions contained 40 and 35% formamide.

however, that unique mammalian gene sequences can be visualized colorimetrically using the poly ABAP detection system. Specific RNA sequences have also been visualized on nitrocellulose by this method with similar (1–10 pg) sensitivity (data not shown). Combining Bio-DNA probes with a poly ABAP detector system thus provides a rapid and sensitive procedure for Southern, Northern, or dot blot hybridization analysis that eliminates the need for radioactive materials and autoradiography.

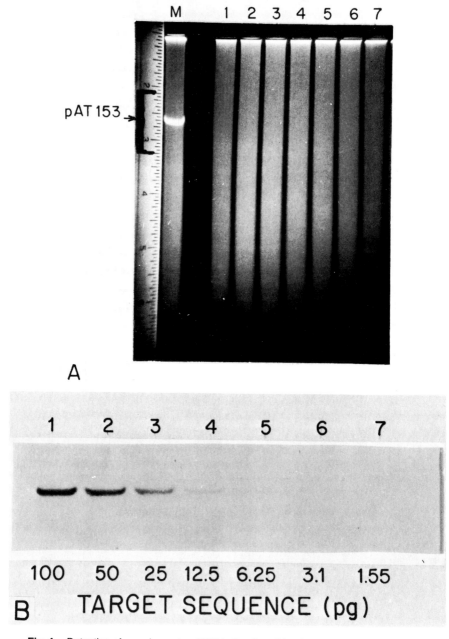

Fig. 4. Detection of complementary DNA in Southern blots by Bio-DNA hybridization and colorimetric localization is sensitive, and proportional to the amount of complementary DNA. (A) 1.4% gel was loaded with linearized plasmid (pAT153) DNA (target sequence) in 10 μg of sheared herring sperm for each lane. Lane M contained 0.6 μg of plasmid DNA to mark the location of plasmid bands after electrophoresis and ethidium bromide staining (upper panel). (B) The appropriate region of lanes 1−7 was transferred to nitrocellulose, and hybridized with Bio-16-pMM984 probe (which contains all pAT153 sequences) at 0.25 μg/ml for 18 hours in 50% formamide. Bound Bio-DNA probe was detected with poly ABAP complex in a 2-hour reaction with NBT/BCIP.

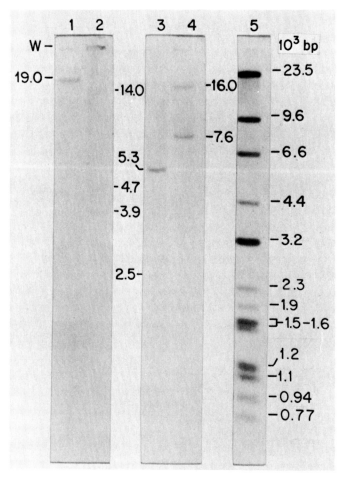

Fig. 5. Detection of α- and β-globin genes in human DNA by Southern blotting using Bio-DNA probes and poly ABAP colorimetric visualization. *Eco*R1 (lanes 1 and 3) and *Hin*dIII (lanes 2 and 4) digests of human placental DNA (15 μg/lane) were electrophoresed in a 1% agarose gel and transferred to nitrocellulose. Lanes 1 and 2 were hybridized with an α-globin probe (JW101) containing a 0.4×10^3 bp cDNA clone at 0.35 μg/ml for 2 hours in 45% formamide. Lanes 3 and 4 were hybridized with a β-globin probe (pHβC6) containing a 5.2×10^3 bp genomic clone under the same conditions. Lane 5 contained 750 pg each of λ phage *Hin*dIII and pMM984 *Pst*1 digests in 10 μg of sheared carrier DNA and was hybridized with λ and pMM984 probes. All probes were labeled with Bio-16-dUTP by nick translation. Hybridized probes were detected with poly ABAP complexes in NBT/BCIP reactions of 1 hour (lane 5), 4 hours (lanes 3 and 4), or 9 hours (lanes 1 and 2).

IV. Discussion

The hybridization and enzymatic detection protocol reported here offers several advantages over conventional procedures that use radioactive probes and autoradiographic detection. Because of their chemical stability, biotinylated DNA probes can be used over long periods of time (at least 1–2 years) and still yield highly reproducible hybridization results. Incorporation of the biotin-nucleotides into DNA alters the physical properties of the polymer such that it exhibits lower nonspecific binding to filter supports as well as to cellular or chromosomal material. By using Bio-DNA probes at high concentration, the hybridization times required for the analysis of low abundance or unique eukaryotic gene sequences can be reduced to 1 or 2 hours. This feature applies to studies using either colorimetric or autoradiographic detection methods. However, colorimetric visualization provides superior resolution, since only the intensity of the color signal increases while the size of the spot generating the signal remains constant (see Fig. 1, lanes 2 and 5). The poly ABAP enzyme complex, when used in combination with the NBT/BCIP substrate mixture, is sufficiently sensitive to visualize 1–2 pg of standard nick-translated probe after a few hours of enzyme incubation. Under these conditions the complex is detecting ~0.5 fmoles (0.5×10^{-15} moles) of biotinylated nucleotide. The sensitivity of detection can be increased four- to fivefold simply by making the nitrocellulose filter transparent (wet with toluene), and several other procedures for signal enhancement are also available. DNA probes can be labeled with two or more biotinylated nucleotides and/or 3'-end-labeled with biotinylated nucleotides using terminal transferase. Alternatively, the hybridization efficiency can be increased by using single-strand probes generated from sequences cloned in M13. Finally, the size of the enzyme polymer used to construct the poly ABAP complex can be increased by additional chemical polymerization reactions. Such studies are currently in progress. It is our expectation that a combination of these approaches will lead to colorimetric methods of polynucleotide visualization with femtogram sensitivity.

One limitation of the method at present is that the colored precipitate generated by the NBT/BCIP substrate mixture is extremely insoluble in all organic solvents tested. Therefore, it is very difficult to remove it from the nitrocellulose filter. Alternative substrates for alkaline phosphatase that generate colored precipitates that are fully soluble in organic solvents are available (Burstone, 1960); however these substrates exhibit significant end-product inhibition and are not as sensitive as the NBT/BCIP mixture for probe detection. With the development of better enzyme polymers or hybridization protocols, these alternative substrates could be used if one wishes to reprobe the same blot.

Enzyme–polymer complexes made with avidin or streptavidin could also prove quite useful for antigen detection using a biotinylated antibody intermediate, for sequence analysis by the dideoxynucleotide method (Sanger *et al.*, 1977), and for visualizing clones of interest after colony (Grunstein and Hogness, 1975) or plaque (Benton and Davis, 1977) hybridization. Such applications are currently being evaluated.

Acknowledgments

JJL was the recipient of an NIH postdoctoral Fellowship, No. AI06195. Salary support for DJB was provided by Enzo Biochem Inc. The research work was supported by Grants from the National Institutes of Health (GM-20124 and CA016038). The technical assistance of Paula Northrup is acknowledged.

References

Alwine, J. C., Kemp, D. J., Parker, B. A., Reiser, J., Renart, J., Stark, G. R., and Wahl, G. M. (1980). *Methods Enzymol.* **68**, 220–242.
Benton, W. D., and Davis, R. W. (1977). *Science* **196**, 180–182.
Brigati, D. J., Myerson, D., Leary, J. J., Spalholz, B., Travis, S. Z., Fong, C. K. Y., Hsiung, G. D., and Ward, D. C. (1983). *Virology* **126**, 32–50.
Burstone, M. S. (1960). *J. Natl. Cancer Inst.* **24**, 1199–1207.
Costello, S. M., Felix, R. T., and Giese, R. W. (1979). *Clin. Chem.* **25**, 1572–1580.
Denhardt, D. T. (1966). *Biochem. Biophys. Res. Comm.* **23**, 641–646.
Fritsch, E. F., Lawn, R. M., and Maniatis, T. (1980). *Cell* **19**, 959–972.
Fukumaki, Y., Ghosh, P. K., Benz, E. J., Jr., Reddy, V. B., Lebowitz, P., Forget, B. G., and Weissman, S. M. (1982). *Cell* **28**, 585–593.
Grunstein, M., and Hogness, D. S. (1975). *Proc. Natl. Acad. Sci. U.S.A.* **72**, 3961–3965.
Hoffman, K., Wood, S. W., Brenton, C. C., Montikeller, J. A., and Finn, F. M. (1980). *Proc. Natl. Acad. Sci. U.S.A.* **77**, 4666–4671.
Hsu, S. M., Raine, L., and Fanger, H. (1981). *J. Histochem. Cytochem.* **29**, 577–580.
Hutchison, N. J., Langer-Safer, P. R., Ward, D. C., and Hamkalo, B. A. (1982). *J. Cell Biol.* **95**, 609–618.
Langer, P. R., and Ward, D. C. (1981). *In* "Developmental Biology Using Purified Genes", *ICN-UCLA Symp. Mol. Cell. Biol.,* **23**, 647–658.
Langer, P. R., Waldrop, A. A., and Ward, D. C. (1981). *Proc. Natl. Acad. Sci. U.S.A.* **78**, 6633–6637.
Langer-Safer, P. R., Levine, M., and Ward, D. C. (1982). *Proc. Natl. Acad. Sci. U.S.A.* **79**, 4381–4385.
Manuelidis, L., Langer-Safer, P. R., and Ward, D. C. (1982). *J. Cell Biol.* **95**, 619–625.
McGadey, J. (1970). *Histochemie* **23**, 180–184.
Mears, J. G., Ramirez, F., Leibowitz, D., and Bank, A. (1978). *Cell* **15**, 15–24.
Merchlinsky, M. J., Tattersall, P. J., Leary, J. J., Cotmore, S. F., Gardiner, E. M., and Ward, D. C. (1983). *J. Virol.* **47**, 227–232.
Orkin, S. H. (1978). *Proc. Natl. Acad. Sci. U.S.A.* **75**, 5950–5954.
Rigby, P. W. J., Dieckmann, M., Rhodes, C., and Berg, P. (1977). *J. Mol. Biol.* **113**, 237–251.
Sanger, R., Nicklen, S., and Coulson, A. R. (1977). *Proc. Natl. Acad. Sci. U.S.A.* **74**, 5463–5467.
Singer, R. H., and Ward, D. C. (1982). *Proc. Natl. Acad. Sci. U.S.A.* **79**, 7331–7335.

Southern, E. M. (1975). *J. Mol. Biol.* **98,** 503–517.

Sternberger, L. A., Hardy, P. H., Jr., Cuculis, J. J., and Meyer, H. G. (1970). *J. Histochem Cytochem.* **18,** 315–333.

Thomas, P. S. (1980). *Proc. Natl. Acad. Sci. U.S.A.* **77,** 5201–5205.

Van der Ploeg, L. H. T., and Flavell, R. (1980). *Cell* **19,** 947–958.

Wahl, G. M., Stern, M., and Stark, G. R. (1979). *Proc. Natl. Acad. Sci. U.S.A.* **76,** 3683–3687.

Wilson, J. T., Wilson, L. B., deRiel, J. K., Villa-Komaroff, L., Efstratiadis, A., Forget, B. G., and Weissman, S. M. (1978). *Nucleic Acids Res.* **5,** 563–581.

16

Chromatin Structure, Globin Gene Transcription, and Erythroid Cell Differentiation

MICHAEL SHEFFERY, RICHARD A. RIFKIND, AND PAUL A. MARKS

DeWitt Wallace Research Laboratory
Memorial Sloan-Kettering Cancer Center
New York, New York

I. Introduction

Murine erythroleukemia cells (MELC) represent a relatively homogeneous population of virus-transformed erythroid precursors (Marks and Rifkind, 1978). These cells have provided a useful model for examining, in detail, alterations in chromatin structure associated with the transition of genes from a state of relatively inactive transcription to active transcription that occurs during cell differentiation.

Among the properties of MELC that make them suitable for these types of

CHROMOSOMES AND CANCER
291

analyses is the fact that cells can be maintained for an essentially unlimited period of time under appropriate *in vitro* conditions (Friend *et al.*, 1971; Reuben *et al.*, 1976). MELC (inducer-sensitive strain 745A-DS19 was employed in all studies unless otherwise noted) can be induced by a variety of agents, including dimethyl sulfoxide (DMSO) (Friend *et al.*, 1971), hexamethylene bisacetamide (HMBA) (Reuben *et al.*, 1976), butyric acid (Leder and Leder, 1975), and other agents to express characteristics of erythroid cell differentiation (Marks and Rifkind, 1978). Induced differentiation of MELC is characterized by the coordinated expression of a developmental program, including commitment to terminal cell division (Gusella *et al.*, 1976; Fibach *et al.*, 1977), and increased accumulation of α- and β-globin mRNA (Ross *et al.*, 1972; Ohta *et al.*, 1976), of α-, β^{maj}-, β^{min}-globins, and hemoglobins major (Hb^{maj}) and minor (Hb^{min}) (Boyer *et al.*, 1972; Ostertag *et al.*, 1972), of heme-synthesizing enzymes (Sassa, 1976), of membrane-associated erythroid-specific proteins [such as spectrin and glycophorin (Eisen *et al.*, 1977)], and a variety of other proteins including the chromatin-associated protein, $H1^{\circ}$ (Keppel *et al.*, 1977; Chen *et al.*, 1982). Evidence available to date indicate that all agents effective as inducers of MECL cause differentiation along the erythroid pathway (Marks and Rifkind, 1978).

A number of laboratories, including our own, have provided data that suggests that the virally transformed MELC are blocked at a stage in the erythroid lineage that is relatively late in erythropoiesis, e.g., CFU-e (Fig. 1) (for references, see Marks and Rifkind, 1978). MELC are more differentiated and more restricted in potential than pluripotent hematopoietic stem cells. In view of the evidence that differentiation potential in MELC is restricted primarily to the erythroid line, it is reasonable to suggest that certain molecular events, required to determine

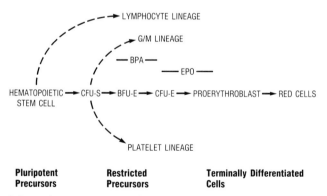

Fig. 1. Schematic representation of sequential stages of hematopoietic cell development. The pluripotent precursors, hematopoietic stem cells, produce the lymphocyte lineage and precursors (CFU-s) of granulocyte/macrophages, erythroid cells, and platelets. Erythroid precursors (BFU-e) differentiate to CFU-e: both are precursors of restricted potential and, in turn, generate proerythroblasts and terminally differentiated red cells.

erythroid-specific lineage characteristics have already occurred in MELC. On the other hand, those molecular events that are required for the transition from CFU-e to the full expression of terminal erythroid cell differentiation occur only as inducer-mediated terminal differentiation proceeds.

In the present chapter, we focus on investigations in our laboratory that have examined the effects of inducer on the expression of α- and β-globin genes during inducer-mediated MELC differentiation. Terminal erythroid cell differentiation of normal erythroid precursors requires the action of the erythropoietic hormone, erythropoietin (Marks and Rifkind, 1978). Viral transformed MELC appear to have become erythropoietin independent and do not require the hormone for growth in culture, and the hormone does not induce them to express characteristics of terminal erythroid cell differentiation. On the other hand, a broad series of chemicals will induce differentiation of MELC, including the expression of α- and β-globin genes (Table I).

In this chapter, we specifically address two aspects of inducer-mediated MELC expression of α- and β-globin genes. First, we have found that different inducers cause different patterns of expression of the α- and β-globin genes, during MELC differentiation, which appears due, in part, to the fact that inducers act at different levels of control of globin gene expression. Second, using various assays to evaluate chromatin structure, we have found that transcriptional activation of globin structural genes is associated with a complex set of changes in the configuration of globin gene chromatin (Hofer *et al.*, 1982; Sheffery *et al.*, 1982, 1983a,b). Certain patterns of chromatin structure have been established prior to the block in MELC erythropoiesis, and these changes are stably propagated. These patterns, it is suggested, represent, at a molecular level, the developmental history of this transformed erythroid precursor. Other alterations in chromatin structure occur during the course of inducer-mediated MELC differentiation and the expression of the α- and β-globin genes. These changes pre-

TABLE I

Inducers of MELC Erythroid Differentiation[a]

Polar compounds:	Dimethyl sulfoxide
	Hexamethylene bisacetamide
Fatty acids:	Butyric acid
DNA intercalators:	Actinomycin
Modified bases:	Azacytidine
Phosphodiesterase inhibitors:	Methylisoxanthine
Ion-flux agents:	Ouabain
Physical agents:	UV, X-ray
Posttranscription-acting agent:	Hemin

[a] For detailed references, see review by Marks and Rifkind (1978).

sumably reflect, in part, molecular events characteristic of the final stages of differentiation of this lineage. Taken together, these findings suggest that the transition from a relatively inactive to an actively transcribed set of genes, using the globin genes as a model, appears to involve a multi-step process which is characterized, at least in part, by a series of alterations in chromatin configuration in the domain of these genes.

II. Different Effects of Inducers on Expression of Globin Genes in MELC Differentiation

Murine erythroleukemia cells accumulate two types of hemoglobin, containing three species of globin polypeptides (α, β^{maj}, and β^{min}). Thus, inducer-mediated accumulation of hemoglobin may involve the coordinated expression of at least three different genes. All inducers of MELC (Table I) can increase the accumulation of hemoglobin. It has been found that in uninduced MELC, there is a low but detectable level of Hb^{min} reflecting a low level of α- and β^{min}-globin gene expression in uninduced MELC (Nudel et al., 1977a; Lowenhaupt and Lingrel, 1979). Polar-planar compounds, such as HMBA and DMSO, induce the accumulation of twofold or more of Hb^{maj} than Hb^{min}. Butyric and propionic acids induce approximately equal amounts of Hb^{maj} and Hb^{min}. Hemin induces the accumulation of predominately Hb^{min} (Nudel et al., 1977a; Curtis et al., 1980).

Studies of the rates of accumulation of α-, β^{maj}, and β^{min}-globin mRNA show that these reflect closely the relative rates of accumulation of Hb^{maj} and Hb^{min} in MELC induced with the different agents studied, including DMSO, HMBA, butyric acid, and hemin (Nudel et al., 1977a). We have, however, found differences in the kinetics of appearance, as well as in the relative amounts of α-, and β-globin mRNA, with different inducers (Table II) (Nudel et al., 1977a). When MELC are cultured in the presence of HMBA, DMSO, or butyric acid, accumulation of α-globin mRNA can be detected in the cytoplasm by 12 to 16 hours (Table II) (Nudel et al., 1977a,b). Cytoplasmic accumulation of β-globin mRNA sequences is not detected until about 8 hours later, in the presence of these inducers. By 48 hours there is an approximately tenfold increase in the globin mRNA content of induced MELC. Hemin, by comparison, unlike the polar compounds (such as DMSO and HMBA) or the fatty acids (such as butyric acid), rapidly (by 6 hours) and simultaneously initiates the accumulation of both α- and β-globin mMRA. Although the principal β-like mRNA induced by the polar inducers is β^{maj} mRNA, hemin initiates accumulation of β^{min} globin mRNA (Nudel et al., 1977a; Curtis et al., 1980), which is the principal β-globin found in uninduced MELC.

TABLE II

Effect of Inducers on α- and β-Globin mRNA Accumulation in MELC

Time in culture (hours)	mRNA	mRNA (μg) produced[a]			
		DMSO	HMBA	Butyric acid	Hemin
3	α	—	—	—	33
	β	—	—	—	12
6	α	—	—	—	22
	β	—	—	—	7
8	α	40	50	26	—
	β	12	10	13	—
12	α	40	23	17	14
	β	12	10	13	5
16	α	22	10	10	10
	β	12	10	13	3
24	α	9	3	1.2	4.3
	β	11	9	2.1	2.0
40	α	1.8	0.9	0.9	3.2
	β	3.0	1.6	1.1	1
72	α	0.8	0.3	0.9	—
	β	0.8	0.3	0.6	—
96	α	0.4	0.4	0.9	—
	β	0.3	0.4	0.6	—

[a] Cytoplasmic RNA prepared from MELC cultured with inducers for the indicated times were hybridized to α- and β-globin cDNA (Nudel *et al.*, 1977b). Results are expressed as micrograms of RNA required to achieve 50% protection of cDNA. The lower the amount of RNA required, the greater the amount of mRNA for α- or for β-globin accumulated in the MELC.

III. Inducer-Mediated Effects on Globin Gene Transcription

The finding of differences in patterns of hemoglobins and globin mRNA accumulation in MELC induced with different agents has led us to study the molecular level at which inducers may affect control of gene expression. We turned first to investigate transcriptional control of the α_1- and β^{maj}-globin genes. For these studies, we employed the technique of the nuclear chain elongation transcription assay (Hofer *et al.*, 1982). We have compared the effects of two inducers of MELC, namely, HMBA and hemin. Isolated nuclei, prepared from cells cultured with one or the other of these agents, were incubated with [^{32}P]UTP for 5 minutes. RNA polymerase II-generated RNA molecules, already associated with DNA templates, will be elongated with [^{32}P]UTP under these conditions, and the level of radioactivity associated with the gene-specific nascent RNA may be taken as a measure of gene-specific transcriptional activity (Hofer *et al.*, 1982). RNA was isolated from the nuclei and hybridized to a series of double-stranded subclones prepared from the β^{maj}-globin gene (Fig. 2) and from the α_1 globin gene (Fig. 3) (Hofer *et al.*, 1982; Sheffery *et al.*, 1983b). For the β^{maj}-globin gene domain, restriction enzyme-generated fragments extending approximately 1.5 kb upstream (5' end) to approximately 1.4 kb downstream (3' end) from the structural gene were prepared. Of these, fragment A (upstream) and fragments E and F (downstream) did not contain sequences corresponding to the structural portions of the β^{maj}-globin gene (Fig. 2). For the α_1-globin gene domain, restriction enzyme-generated fragments extending approximately 2.3 kb upstream and 0.4 kb downstream from the structural gene were prepared. Of these, fragments Z and A (upstream) and fragment E2 (downstream) did not contain sequences corresponding to the structural sequences of the α_1-globin gene (Fig. 3). For the β^{maj}-globin gene, fragments B, C, and D and for the α_1-globin gene, fragments B, C, D and E1 contain structural sequences (Figs. 2 and 3).

In the ^{32}P-labeled nuclear chain elongation transcript RNA isolated from nuclei of MELC cultured with HMBA for 48 hours, the transcripts show a markedly increased hybridization to αB, αC, and αD fragments of the α_1-globin gene and to βB, βC, βE and βF of the β-globin gene (Fig. 4, HMBA) compared with comparable preparations from MELC cultured either without inducer (Fig. 4, control) or with hemin (Fig. 4, hemin). Individual dot hybridizations were

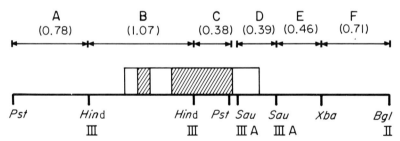

Fig. 2. β^{maj}-Globin gene subclones. The location of the β^{maj}-globin gene is schematically represented on a restriction endonuclease fragment containing the gene that has been cleaved with the different restriction endonucleases indicated (Hofer *et al.*, 1982). The cleavage sites for the different restriction endonucleases are as determined by Tilghman *et al.* (1977) and Konkel *et al.* (1978). The position of the three exons are shown by the open boxes, and of the two introns, by the hatched boxes. The cap site corresponds to the leftward (5') end of the open box and the putative poly(A) addition site to the rightward (3') end of the open box. Subclones prepared across this fragment are indicated by letter designations above the gene. Numbers in parenthesis indicate approximate lengths (in kb) of subclones. Restriction endonuclease sites used in construction of subcloned fragments are indicated by letter abbreviations across the bottom of the figure.

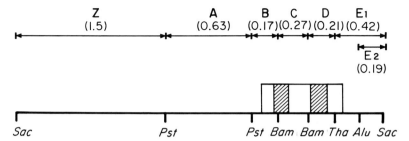

Fig. 3. α_1-Globin gene subclones. The location of the α_1-globin gene is schematically represented on a SacI restriction endonuclease fragment containing the gene. The position of three exons are shown by the open boxes and of the two introns by the hatched boxes. The gene is represented beginning at the cap site (5') end (leftward) and ending at the 3' putative poly(A) addition site (rightward). Subclones prepared across the SacI fragment are indicated by letter designations above the gene. Numbers in parenthesis indicate approximate lengths (in kb) of subclones. Restriction endonuclease sites used in construction of subcloned fragments are indicated by letter abbreviations across the bottom of the figure.

CONTROL		HMBA		HEMIN	
αA	βA	αA	βA	αA	βA
αB	βB	αB	βB	αB	βB
αC	βC	αC	βC	αC	βC
αD	βE	αD	βE	αD	βE
αE$_1$	βF	αE$_1$	βF	αE$_1$	βF
αE$_2$		αE$_2$		αE$_2$	
liv	Igα	liv	Igα	liv	Igα
pUC	pBr	pUC	pBr	pUC	pBr

Fig. 4. Dot hybridization of RNA labeled in isolated nuclei prepared from MELC cultured for 48 hours without inducer (control) or with 5mM HMBA or with 0.1mM hemin. β^{maj}- and α_1-globin gene subcloned fragments are designated according to the schema illustrated in Figs. 2 and 3, respectively. Each subclone was immobilized in the designated location as dots on nitrocellulose filters and hybridized to RNA prepared from 5 minute [32P]UTP pulse-labeled nuclei in the nuclear chain elongation transcription assay (Hofer et al., 1982). An equivalent number of counts was added to each filter, and autoradiographs of washed filters are illustrated. Other dots shown were used as controls: a cDNA clone that hybridizes to nuclear RNA transcripts prepared from uninduced (control) and induced MELC is designated "liv." The plasmid vehicle used to construct subclones of α_1 and β^{maj} fragments are designated pUC and pBr. Igα designates a cloned Igα gene employed, as control, for a gene not expressed in MELC.

quantitifed by densitometry or by assaying for radioactivity in a liquid scintillation counter (Tilghman *et al.*, 1977; Sheffery *et al.*, 1983b). Transcription of
both the α_1- and β^{maj}-globin genes increases approximately 10- to 20-fold after
48 hours of culture with HMBA. It was noted, in addition, that hybridization to
β^{maj} fragment B was also detected in uninduced MELC (Fig. 4, control, βB
fragment). Darnell and co-workers (Hofer *et al.*, 1982; Salditt-Georgieff *et al.*,
1983) have suggested that this might represent either transcription of the β^{min}-
globin gene (which has some homology in the βB region) or premature termination of some β^{maj}-globin gene transcripts in uninduced MELC; the exact reason
for this hybridization remains unclear. No similar phenomena is detected in the
α_1-globin gene (compare αB and αC with βB, control column, Fig. 4). These
findings suggest that the HMBA-mediated increase in accumulation of α- and β-
globin mRNA reflects, primarily, control of gene expression exercised at the
level of transcription. By comparison, hemin appears to effect an increase in
globin mRNA accumulation without accelerating the rate of transcription (Profous-Juchelka *et al.*, 1983). By implication, this means that hemin acts at a
posttranscriptional level, influencing the processing, transport, or stability of a
low but constitutive level of transcript. This mechanism appears consistent with
the known effect of hemin in augmenting the content of Hb^{min}, which is the
principal hemoglobin, although at very low level, of uninduced MELC (Curtis *et
al.*, 1980).

Little hybridization of nuclear chain elongation transcripts is detected to frag-
ment αA, which is 5' to the α_1-cap site, or to βA, which is 5' to the β^{maj}-cap
site, suggesting that *in vitro* transcription initiates normally, at or close to the cap
site. The hybridization observed to the βE and βF fragments, as previously noted
(Hofer *et al.*, 1982), suggests that there may be a transcription termination site
for the β^{maj}-globin gene, approximately 1.5 kb downstream from the 3' end of
this structural gene. By comparison, the absence of substantial hybridization to
the E$_2$ fragment (Fig. 3), which begins only 50 bp downstream from the putative
poly(A) addition site, suggests that the termination site for the α_1-globin gene
lies close to the 3' end of that structural gene.

IV. Alterations in Chromatin Structure in Globin Gene
Domains

From the findings summarized above, it is clear that during HMBA-induced
MELC differentiation there is a 10- to 20-fold increase in the rate of transcription
of the α_1- and β^{maj}-globin genes. Studies from a number of laboratories have
established that alterations in DNA and chromatin structure are associated with
gene expression in differentiating cell systems (for reviews, see Nudel *et al.*,
1977; Tilghman *et al.*, 1977; Alter and Goff, 1978a,b; Konkel *et al.*, 1978;
Lowenhaupt and Lingrel, 1979; Marks *et al.*, 1979; Curtis *et al.*, 1980; Elgin,

1981; Igo-Kemenes *et al.*, 1982; Weisbrod, 1982; Profous-Juchelka *et al.*, 1983; Salditt-Georgieff, 1983). These include changes in the pattern of DNA methylation (Doerfler, 1981; Felsenfeld and McGhee, 1982), in binding of high mobility group (HMG) proteins 14 and 17 (Weisbrod and Weintraub, 1979), in sensitivity of chromatin to digestion by DNase I (Garel and Axel, 1976; Weintraub and Groudine, 1976), and in the appearance of sites or regions that are hypersensitive to digestion by DNase I, usually (but not invariably) found upstream of the 5' end of active (or potentially active) genes (Elgin, 1981; Larsen and Weintraub, 1982). Sites of S_1 nuclease sensitivity have recently been demonstrated to be associated with, but not necessarily identical to, sites of DNase I hypersensitivity (Larsen and Weintraub, 1982; Sheffery *et al.*, 1983b). McGee and co-workers (1981) have demonstrated that the DNase I hypersensitive region adjacent to the active chick β-globin gene is in a configuration suggesting the absence of normal nucleosomal structures and the presence of a stretch of protein-free DNA.

In our laboratory several features of DNA and chromatin configuration have been examined in detail with respect to the changes in gene expression at the globin loci that occur during induced MELC differentiation (Sheffery *et al.*, 1982). We have evaluated alterations in chromatin structure in the domain of the α_1- and β^{maj}-globin structural genes by the following assays: (1) determination of the pattern of DNA methylation, (2) determination of the sensitivity to DNase I, and (3) determination of the pattern of chromatin sites hypersensitive to DNase I digestion. Certain patterns of chromatin and DNA are found in uninduced MELC that fail to change upon induction of terminal cell differentiation; these include the pattern of DNA methylation about both the α_1 and β^{maj} genes and the general sensitivity of these genes to DNase I. On the other hand, other changes are specifically initiated during induction of differentiation; these include the development of DNase I hypersensitive sites 5' to both the α_1 and β^{maj} genes. Thus, certain changes in chromatin structure have already occurred, presumably during the developmental history of the erythroid lineage, and are stably propagated in the virus-transformed, developmentally arrested MELC. Additional changes in chromatin structure occur only when exposure to inducers initiates terminal differentiation.

A. DNA Methylation

The pattern of DNA methylation has been cited as a heritable molecular characteristic that, at least in many instances, distinguishes expressed and unexpressed genes (Doerfler, 1981; Felsenfled and McGhee, 1982). In general, relative hypomethylation is associated with activation of transcription of a structural gene sequence; however, not all potential methylation sites within a domain need be unmethylated, and unique sites may well be critical for active transcription. For example, in the rabbit β-globin domain, demethylation of some, but not all, methylated sites correlates with gene activity (Shen and Maniatis, 1980). A small

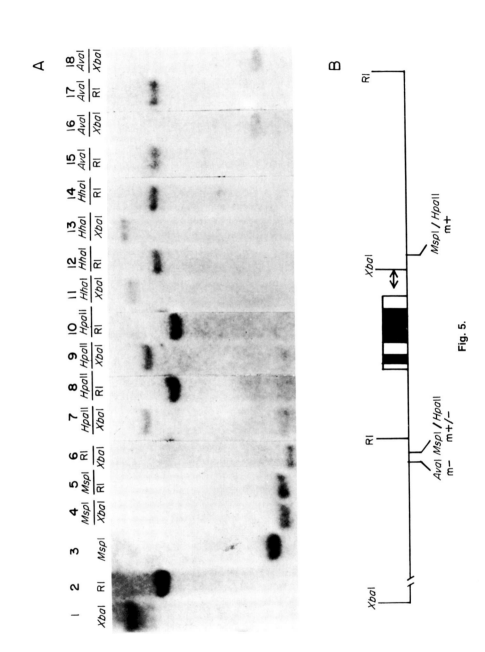

Fig. 5.

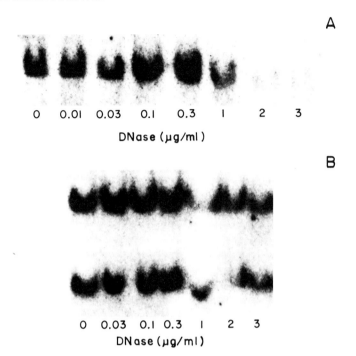

A

0   0.01   0.03   0.1   0.3   1   2   3

DNase (µg/ml)

B

0   0.03   0.1   0.3   1   2   3

DNase (µg/ml)

Fig. 6. DNase I sensitivity of chromatin containing the β^{maj}-globin gene and the Igα gene. Nuclei were prepared from MELC cultured without inducer and digested with the concentrations of DNase I indicated below each lane. Purified DNA, following this digestion, was then incubated with EcoR1 and the resultant digest analyzed for the presence of β^{maj}-globin gene (A) or the Igα gene (B). EcoR1 digestion produces two Igα gene fragments of about 2.5 and 1.8 kb. These data are from Sheffery et al. (1982).

Fig. 5. Pattern of DNA methylation near the β^{maj}-globin gene. Total genomic DNA was purified from MELC cultured without or with 4 mM HMBA for 48 hours. (A) Samples of DNA were incubated with restriction endonucleases indicated above each lane, numbered 1 through 18. DNA from cells cultured without inducer was placed in lanes 1–8, 11, 12, 15, and 16 and from HMBA cultures, lanes 9, 10, 13, 14, 17, and 18. DNA prepared from the cells was digested with the restriction endonucleases, electrophoresed, blotted onto nitrocellulose (Southern, 1975), and hybridized with radioactively labeled β^{maj}-globin gene-specific probe (see legend to Fig. 7) (Sheffery, 1982). Lanes 1–6, 7–10, 11–14, and 15–18 are from separate radioautograms, and exact comparison of fragment mobilities is not possible. (B) Schematic representation of the β^{maj}-globin gene domain indicating the restriction endonuclease sites MspI, HpaII, and AvaI. m+, fully methylated site; m+/−, partially methylated site; m−, unmethylated site. RI, EcoRI. These data are from Sheffery et al. (1982).

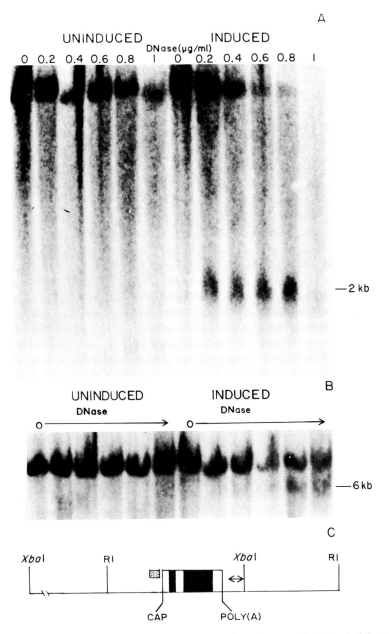

Fig. 7. Hypersensitivity to DNase I of a chromatin region near the 5′ end of the β^maj-globin gene in induced MELC. (A) Nuclei were prepared from uninduced (left) or HMBA-induced (right) MELC and digested with the concentration of DNase I (in g/ml) indicated above each lane. DNA was purified, digested with *Xba*I and analyzed by the method of Southern (1975) with a β^maj-globin gene-specific probe (indicated by the double-headed arrow). A DNase I-generated subfragment of 2 kb is indicated. (B) DNA was purified from a

decrease in overall DNA methylation has been described during induced differentiation of MELC (Christman *et al.*, 1980).

We have examined the pattern of DNA methylation in the region of the β^{maj}- and α_1-globin genes during HMBA-mediated MELC differentiation. Cytosine methylation in the nucleotide sequence, CCGG, was assayed by use of the methyl-sensitive isoschizomer-pair of restriction enzymes, *Msp*I and *Hpa*II, and other restriction enzymes (Fig. 5) (Sheffery *et al.*, 1982). Compared to the nucleotide and methylation pattern in the chick (Weintraub *et al.*, 1981), there are relatively few potentially methylated sites in the MELC globin gene domains that can be assayed by these restriction enzymes. Of the sites assayed and mapped near the β^{maj}-globin gene, one site is fully methylated, one is partially methylated, and one is unmethylated, in uninduced cells (Fig. 5). Most sites (but not all) assayed near the α_1-globin genes are unmethylated in uninduced cells. No detectable change in the pattern of DNA methylation around either the α_1- or β^{maj}-globin genes was observed during HMBA-mediated differentiation. It would appear that, within the limits of resolution of this assay, the pattern of globin gene methylation is established and stably propagated at a developmental stage in erythropoiesis prior to the stage represented by the MELC. This pattern is not required to change during subsequent transition to active globin gene expression.

B. DNase I Sensitivity

Previous studies of the accessibility of MELC chromatin digestion by DNase I, as assayed by liquid hybridization (Miller *et al.*, 1978), suggested that the globin gene-associated chromatin of uninduced MELC is in an "active" configuration relatively accessible to nuclease action, as compared to the chromatin about other genes not expressed in erythroid cells. We have examined, by the method of Southern (1975), the DNase I accessibility of α_1- and β^{maj}-globin genes, in comparison with the sensitivity of another gene locus Igα, which is not

DNase I digestion series as in (A) above and then digested with *Eco*RI, and the fragments generated by this digestion were analyzed by the method of Southern employing the β^{maj}-globin gene probe. Increasing concentrations (from zero) of DNase I are indicated by the arrows above the lanes. A DNase I-generated subfragment of about 6 kb was detected in preparations from cell nuclei of HMBA induced cells. (C) Schematic representation of a restriction endonuclease map around the β^{maj}-globin gene showing the location of adjacent *Eco*RI and *Xba*I sites. The 5' and 3' ends of β^{maj}-globin gene are indicated as cap and poly(A), respectively. The size and location of the β^{maj}-globin gene-specific probe sequence (Sheffery *et al.*, 1982) is indicated by the double-headed arrow extending from the 3' *Xba*I site. The probe is located in the 3' flanking sequence of the β^{maj}-globin gene and does not cross-react with the β^{min}-globin gene. The β^{maj}-globin gene is represented by the open (exon) and solid (intron) boxes. The DNase I-hypersensitive region (stippled box), is mapped from data presented in (A) and (C). These data are from Sheffery *et al.* (1982).

expressed in MELC. The β^{maj}- and α_1-globin genes are distinctly more sensitive to digestion by DNase I than is the Igα gene, in both uninduced and induced MELC (Fig. 6). Taken together, the observations on methylation pattern and general DNase I sensitivity suggest that the α_1- and β^{maj}-globin gene domains of MELC, before their induction to full transcriptional activity, are in a differentiation-specific configuration compatible with and perhaps essential for the induction of globin gene expression.

C. DNase I Hypersensitivity Sites

Recently, we have obtained the first evidence for alterations in chromatin structure associated with inducer-mediated activation of globin gene transcription (Sheffery *et al.*, 1982). During HMBA-induced differentiation of MELC, specific sites, displaying a six- to tenfold increase in DNase I sensitivity, appear in chromatin regions near the 5′ end of the α_1- and β^{maj}-globin genes (Fig. 7). The DNase I hypersensitive site near the β^{maj}-globin gene maps to an approximately 200 bp region in the 5′ flanking region of the gene. Although our mapping of the DNase I hypersensitive sites in the region of the α genes is somewhat less precise, the present data suggest that a DNase I hypersensitive site is generated, during activation of globin gene expression, 5′ to the α_1-globin gene (Sheffery *et al.*, 1983b). These changes in globin gene chromatin structure, which are recognized as DNase I hypersensitive regions, then represent changes at the molecular level associated with the late stages of induced terminal differentiation.

V. Summary

This chapter summarizes evidence that the transition from relatively inactive to actively expressed globin genes associated with HMBA-induced MELC differentiation involves a complex series of alterations in the chromatin structure of the genes. We suggest that these virus-transformed cells, CFU-e-like erythroid precursors, have globin gene chromatin structure, characterized at least in part, by a particular DNA methylation pattern and a general increased level of DNase I sensitivity that reflects the cells' developmental progression in the erythroid lineage to a stage of potential globin gene transcription. In this model, these features of chromatin structure of the globin genes may be associated with the restriction in developmental potential characteristic of progression in the hemopoietic lineage to a CFU-e-like stage of erythropoiesis, at which the transformed MELC appear to be blocked. These changes in chromatin structure are stably propagated in MELC and constitute, as it were, the molecular phenotype of this developmental stage.

The major increase in globin gene transcription that is associated with HMBA-mediated terminal differentiation of MELC is accompanied by further changes in chromatin structure, as indicated, in part, by the appearance of DNase I hypersensitive sites 5' to both the α_1- and β^{maj}-globin genes. Taken together these observations suggest that a multi-step alteration in chromatin structure is associated with the developmental history of erythroid cells and with the increased globin gene transcription that occurs at the final stages of differentiation.

Acknowledgments

The research studies reviewed in this chapter from the laboratories of the authors were supported, in part, by grants from the National Cancer Institute (PO1-CA-31768 and CA-08748), The American Cancer Society (CH-68), and the Bristol-Myers Cancer Grant Program.

References

Alter, B. P., and Goff, S. C. (1978a). *Blood* **50,** 867–876.
Alter, B. P., and Goff, S. C. (1978b). *Blood* **52,** 1047–1057.
Boyer, S. H., Wuu, K. D., Noyes, A. M., Young, R., Scher, W., Friend, C., Preisler, H., and Bank, A. (1972). *Blood* **40,** 823–835.
Chen, Z. X., Banks, J., Rifkind, R. A., and Marks, P. A. (1982). *Proc. Natl. Acad. Sci. U.S.A.* **79,** 471–475.
Christman, J. K., Weich, N., Schoenbrun, B., Schneiderman, N., and Acs, G. (1980). *J. Cell Biol.* **86,** 366–370.
Curtis, P., Finnigan, A. C., and Rovera, G. (1980). *J. Biol. Chem.* **255,** 8971–8974.
Doefler, W. (1981). *J. Gen. Virol.* **57,** 1–20.
Elgin, S. C. R. (1981). *Cell* **27,** 413–415.
Eisen, H., Nasi, S., Georopulos, C. P., Arndt-Jovin, D., and Ostertag, W. (1977). *Cell* **10,** 680–695.
Felsenfeld, G., and McGhee, J. (1982). *Nature (London)* **296,** 602–603.
Fibach, E., Reuben, R. C., Rifkind, R. A., and Marks, P. A. (1977). *Cancer Res.* **37,** 440–444.
Friend, C., Scher, W., Holland, J. G., and Sato, T. (1971). *Proc. Natl. Acad. Sci. U.S.A.* **68,** 378–82.
Garel, A., and Axel, R. (1976). *Proc. Natl. Acad. Sci. U.S.A.* **73,** 3966–3970.
Gusella, J., Geller, R., Clarke, B., Weeks, V., and Housman, D. (1976). *Cell* **9,** 221–229.
Hofer, E., Hofer-Warbinek, R., and Darnell, J. E. (1982). *J. Cell* **29,** 887–893.
Igo-Kemenes, T., Horz, W., and Zachau, H. G. (1982). *Annu. Rev. Biochem.* **51,** 89–121.
Keppel, F., Allet, B., and Eisen, H. (1977). *Proc. Natl. Acad. Sci. U.S.A.* **74,** 653–656.
Konkel, D. A., Tilghman, S. M., and Leder, P. (1978). *Cell* **15,** 1125–1132.
Larsen, A., and Weintraub, H. (1982). *Cell* **29,** 609–622.
Leder, A., and Leder, P. (1975). *Cell* **5,** 319–322.
Lowenhaupt, K., and Lingrel, J. B. (1979). *Proc. Natl. Acad. Sci. U.S.A.* **76,** 5173–5177.
McGhee, J. D., Wood, W. I., Dolan, M., Engel, J. D., and Felsenfeld, G. (1981). *Cell* **27,** 45–55.
Marks, P. A., and Rifkind, R. A. (1978). *Annu. Rev. Biochem.* **47,** 419–448.
Marks, P. A., Rifkind, R. A., Bank, A., Terada, M., Gambari, R., Fibach, E., Maniatis, G., and Reuben, R. (1979). *In* "Cellular and Molecular Regulation of Hemoglobin Switching" (G. Stamatoyannopoulos and A. W. Neinhuis, eds.), pp. 437–455. Grune & Stratton, New York.

Miller, D. M., Turner, P., Nienhuis, A. W., Axelrod, D. E., and Gopalakrishnan, T. V. (1978). *Cell* **14**, 511–524.

Nudel, U., Salmon, J., Fibach, E., Terada, M., Rifkind, R. A., Marks, P. A., and Bank, A. (1977a). *Cell* **12**, 463–469.

Nudel, U., Salmon, J. D., Terada, M., Bank, A., Rifkind, R. A., and Marks, P. A. (1977b). *Proc. Natl. Acad. Sci. U.S.A.* **74**, 1100–1104.

Ohta, Y., Tanaka, M., Terada, M., Miller, O. J., Bank, A., Marks, P. A., and Rifkind, R. A. (1976). *Proc. Natl. Acad. Sci. U.S.A.* **73**, 1232–1236.

Ostertag, W., Melderis, H., Steinheider, G., Kluge, N., and Dube, S. (1972). *Nature (London), New Biol.* **239**, 231–234.

Profous-Juchelka, H. R., Reuben, R. C., Marks, P. A., and Rifkind, R. A. (1983). *Mol. Cell. Biol.* **3**, 229–234.

Reuben, R. C., Wife, R. L., Breslow, R., Rifkind, R. A., and Marks, P. A. (1976). *Proc. Natl. Acad. Sci. U.S.A.* **73**, 862–866.

Ross, J., Ikawa, Y., and Leder, P. (1972). *Proc. Natl. Acad. Sci. U.S.A.* **69**, 3620–3623.

Salditt-Georgieff, M., Sheffery, M., Krauter, K., Darnell, J. E., Rifkind, R. A., and Marks, P. A. (1983). Submitted for publication.

Sassa, S. (1976). *J. Exp. Med.* **143**, 305–315.

Sheffery, M., Rifkind, R. A., and Marks, P. A. (1982). *Proc. Natl. Acad. Sci. U.S.A.* **79**, 1180–1184.

Sheffery, M., Rifkind, R. A., and Marks, P. A. (1983a). *Proc. Natl. Acad. Sci. U.S.A.* **80**, 3349–3353.

Sheffery, M., Rifkind, R. A., and Marks, P. A. (1983b). Submitted for publication.

Shen, J. C.-K., and Maniatis, T. (1980). *Proc. Natl. Acad. Sci. U.S.A.* **77**, 6634–6638.

Southern, E. M. (1975). *J. Mol. Biol.* **98**, 503–517.

Tilghman, S. M., Teimeier, D. C., Polsky, F., Edgell, M. H., Seidman, J. G., Leder, A., Enquist, L. W., Norman, B., and Leder, P. (1977). *Proc. Natl. Acad. Sci. U.S.A.* **74**, 4406–4410.

Weintraub, H., and Groudine, M. (1976). *Science* **193**, 848–856.

Weintraub, H., Larsen, A., and Groudine, M. (1981). *Cell* **24**, 333–344.

Weisbrod, S. (1982). *Nature (London)* **297**, 289–295.

Weisbrod, S., and Weintraub, H. (1979). *Proc. Natl. Acad. Sci. U.S.A.* **76**, 630–634.

PART IV

Relationship of Chromosome
Changes to Neoplastic
Transformation

Introduction

JOHN E. ULTMANN

> Section of Hematology/Oncology
> and the Cancer Research Center
> The University of Chicago
> Chicago, Illinois

The preceding chapters have presented evidence that carcinogenesis may lead to activation of transforming genes, that this damage can be localized to a precise gene locus, and that resultant changes lead not only to alteration of gene expression measurable by biochemical tests but also to consistent nonrandom karyotypic changes.

These developments now permit us to correlate gene and/or chromosome abnormalities with (1) characteristic morphologic expression, i.e., t(15q+; 17q−): acute promyelocytic leukemia; (2) characteristic clinical behavior, i.e., −5 and/or −7: preleukemic phase leading to acute leukemia in the elderly occupationally exposed patients; and (3) characteristic response to drug(s) and in some instances drug resistance: amplification of the dihydrofolate reductase (DHFR) gene leading to methotrexate resistance.

We are on the frontier of an information explosion correlating structure with gene function, gene product with disease, response of disease to drugs, and failure to respond!! What is needed to optimize these correlations are carefully planned epidemiologic studies searching out the causal factors in patients that might have been responsible for the disease and specific gene abnormalities. Appropriate controls will be essential to establish firm relationships: Exposed individuals who do not have the disease and who may or may not have the gene/chromosome defect will have to be identified. Patients with disease and specific chromosome defects who deny known chemical exposure will have to be thoroughly investigated to search for new, unsuspected causes.

Next we need careful clinical analysis to detect minor expressions of disease

CHROMOSOMES AND CANCER **309**

commonly or always associated with abnormal gene or chromosome defect or abnormal gene product. Until recently, the disease syndromes had been thoroughly described and the discovery of the gene or chromosome abnormality followed. More recently, the discovery of microgranular promyelocytic leukemia [previously an acute myelogenous leukemia (AML) with unexplained coagulopathy] followed the description of the characteristic but unexplained 15q+; 17q− defect in cases of atypical AML. Now, we are entering a phase where gene/chromosome/gene product abnormalities are in search of disease or of subsets of syndromes.

The whole system of tumor classification will have to change. In addition to the morphologic characteristic, we will have to consider receptor sites, immunologic surface markers, and gene or chromosome characteristics in nomenclature. Previously unexplained variations in presentation, course, response, etc., may be more ascribable to these characteristics than morphology.

Finally, the complexity of tumor heterogeneity as controlled by variations in gene structure, variability of chromosome abnormalities, and differences in gene products must be examined (or reexamined) to account for true drug resistance.

The clinicians have a lot of catching up to do. The papers we have heard in this Symposium are a challenge to complement the progress that has been made in the laboratory.

17

Clinical Significance of Chromosome Patterns in Malignant Diseases*

MARILYN G. PEARSON, RICHARD A. LARSON,
AND HARVEY M. GOLOMB

Section of Hematology/Oncology
The University of Chicago
Chicago, Illinois

I. Introduction

With the development of sophisticated banding techniques, cytogenetic analysis of malignant cells has become a useful diagnostic and prognostic tool in hematology and oncology. Acute and chronic leukemias have been the most

*Supported in part by PHS Grants CA-19266 and AM 07134-07 from The Department of Health and Human Services and by The Harry Greenberg Foundation. Dr. Larson is a Fellow of The Leukemia Society of America.

extensively studied diseases cytogenetically, in part because suitable tissue (blood or bone marrow) and adequate metaphase cells are readily obtainable. Specific chromosomal abnormalities correlate with well-defined clinical and morphological subsets of leukemia, and favorable and unfavorable prognostic groups have been identified.

Clonal chromosomal abnormalities have also been found in other myeloproliferative and lymphoproliferative diseases and in certain solid tumors. The clinical application of these data has not yet been established. However, it appears that a specific cytogenetic abnormality may be associated with the development of a unique malignancy. This chapter will document the clinical relevance and specificity of chromosome abnormalities in malignant diseases.

II. Acute Nonlymphocytic Leukemia (ANLL)

Several large series have documented that one or more abnormal clones may be identified at the time of diagnosis in myeloblasts from bone marrow or peripheral blood in 50% or more of patients with ANLL *de novo* (Table I). These clonal chromosome abnormalities are acquired features of the malignant cell line; that is, they are not present in uninvolved tissues such as normal fibroblasts (Rowley, 1980a).

In recent years the frequency with which these abnormal karyotypes are detected has increased. Before banding techniques were available, the overall number of chromosomes present in each cell could distinguish between hypo-

TABLE I

Frequency of Normal and Abnormal Karyotypes in Adults with ANLL

Reference	Number of patients[a]	Normal	Abnormal
Oshimura *et al.* (1976)	38	22(58)[b]	16(42)[b]
Mitelman *et al.* (1976)	30	13(43)	17(57)
Alimena *et al.* (1977)	30	14(43)	16(57)
Philip *et al.* (1978)	40	19(47)	21(53)
1st Int. Workshop Chromosomes Leukemia (1978)	279	140(50)	139(50)
Golomb *et al.* (1978)	90	44(49)	46(51)
Hossfeld *et al.* (1979)	48	22(46)	26(54)
Hagemeijer *et al.* (1981)	86	39(45)	47(55)
Yunis *et al.* (1981)	24	0	24(100)
Larson *et al.* (1983)	53	18(34)	35(66)

[a] Excluding those with inadequate metaphases.
[b] Numbers in parentheses are percent normal or abnormal.

diploid (<46) or hyperdiploid (>46) clones. Banding techniques with Giemsa staining or quinacrine fluorescence are necessary to identify pseudodiploid clones; these are cells that contain structural rearrangements or deletions but have a modal chromosome number of 46. Increasing use of 24- to 48-hour cultures of leukemic cell suspensions with or without conditioned media or cell cycle active agents such as methotrexate have allowed the identification of subtle clonal abnormalities that might have been missed using only direct bone marrow preparations (Yunis et al., 1981; Knuutila et al., 1981). Advanced culture techniques may also provide a larger number of analyzable mitoses.

Clearly, as techniques have improved, the cytogeneticist's ability to detect the presence of an abnormal clone has increased. For example, among 140 consecutive ANLL patients studied at the University of Chicago between 1970 and 1981, the identification of a cytogenetically abnormal clone increased in frequency from 49% of the first 49 patients (through 1976) to 66% of the 53 patients studied after 1978 (Larson et al., 1983). Indeed, Yunis et al. (1981) have recently reported that all patients with ANLL may have clonal chromosome abnormalities. Using methotrexate cell synchronization and Colcemid inhibition of mitotic spindle formation, these authors studied prometaphase (850-band stage) chromosomes in 26 patients. All of the patients in whom adequate material was obtained (24 of the 26) were shown to have clonal abnormalities. This contrasts with the 40–60% incidence of aneuploidy reported in earlier series (Table I).

When a patient with ANLL attains a complete remission after chemotherapy, the previously observed abnormal clone is characteristically absent from bone marrow cells. The reappearance of the same abnormal clone even at a time when the bone marrow appears morphologically normal may herald disease relapse. The appearance of additional karyotype abnormalities (clonal evolution) occurs frequently and may portend a poor prognosis (Testa et al., 1979).

The presence or absence of cytogenetically normal cells has been shown to correlate with clinical course, including response to remission induction therapy and overall survival (Table II). In 1973, Sakurai and Sandberg showed that the median survival was only one-third as long for patients whose bone marrow had only abnormal metaphase cells (AA) as for patients who had only normal metaphase cells (NN). Patients with both normal and abnormal metaphase cells (AN) had an intermediate survival. Many investigators have reported similar results. For example, Hossfeld et al. (1979) reported on 48 patients with ANLL, all of whom had been treated according to a single protocol. The complete remission (CR) rate of NN patients was 73%, that of AN patients was 60%, and that of AA patients was 36%. As might be expected, the respective median survival times paralleled the remission rates for each group.

Among 124 patients with ANLL de novo who were treated at the University of Chicago between 1970 and 1981, the 53 with an initially normal karyotype had a significantly longer median survival than did the 16 in whom no normal meta-

TABLE II

Median Survival of ANLL Patients according to Karyotype

	Median survival (months)		
Reference	NN[a]	AN[a]	AA[a]
Sakurai and Sandberg (1973)	11.5	10.3	3.2
Nilsson et al. (1977)	10.1	6.5	2.0
Alimena et al. (1977)	7.0		2.0
1st Int. Workshop Chromosomes Leuk. (1978)	8.0	5.0	3.5
Hossfeld et al. (1979)	12.5	8.5	4.0
Larson et al. (1983)	11.0	8.0	2.5

[a] NN, normal metaphases only; AN, normal and abnormal metaphases; AA, abnormal metaphases only.

phase cells were found (Larson et al., 1983). Twenty-seven NN patients (51%) attained CR and lived a median of 11 months, whereas only 4 AA patients (25%) attained CR and had a median survival of only 2½ months. Again, the 55 AN patients had an intermediate course with 21 (39%) attaining CR and a median survival of 8 months. Once our patients attained a complete remission, there was no significant difference in median survival between those patients with entirely normal karyotypes and those with initially abnormal karyotypes.

It is now possible to group patients with ANLL by well-defined morphologic criteria as defined by the FAB Cooperative Group (Bennett et al., 1976). When we compared initial karyotypes within each morphologic subset of ANLL, the value of cytogenetic studies in predicting survival was significant only for patients with acute myelogenous leukemia (AML with or without maturation, M2 and M1). When considered together as AML, our 24 NN patients had a median survival of 12 months versus 2 months for the 5 AA patients. The 28 AN patients lived a median of 9 months. Among patients with the second most common subtype of ANLL, acute myelomonocytic leukemia (AMMoL, M4), the median survivals for 23 NN (9½ months), 15 AN (10 months), and 7 AA patients (8 months) were not statistically different. These results are consistent with our earlier studies (Golomb et al., 1976, 1978) and with data from the First International Workshop on Chromosomes in Leukemia (1978). In that multi-institutional study, the 137 AML (M1 and M2) patients had median survivals of 8 months for NN, 5 months for AN, and 3½ months for AA patients. Among the 67 M4 and M5 [acute monocytic leukemia (AMoL)] patients there were no observable differences, with a median survival of 6 months for NN, 5 months for AN, and 7 months for AA patients.

As the medical management of patients with acute leukemia has improved during the past decade, the prognostic importance of initial karyotype grouping based merely on the presence or absence of any abnormal clone has decreased. Within our own institution, we found no significant differences in the remission rate or median survival times when our most recent 68 ANLL patients were compared according to their initial cytogenetic subgroup.

The real significance of karyotype analysis at the time of diagnosis probably resides in the presence of specific clonal chromosome abnormalities, some of which have now been identified (Rowley, 1981). Among the most common abnormalities in ANLL is the loss of an entire chromosome 7. Patients with monosomy 7 have been noted to have more infections and more days with fever above 39°C than patients with normal karyotypes (Borgstrom et al., 1980). This may be related to the fact that neutrophils lacking one chromosome 7 have been found to be defective in several granulocyte functions, including chemotaxis (Ruutu et al., 1977). Monosomy 7 in ANLL thus may predict a poor prognosis if few of these patients survive induction therapy due to infectious complications. In our own experience, however, 4 of 9 treated patients with monosomy 7 achieved a complete remission, and the median survival of the entire group of 11 patients was 6½ months, not different from that for our total group of 148 patients.

About 10% of patients with M2 leukemia have a translocation involving the long arms of chromosome 8 and 21: t(8;21)(q22;q22). When 48 patients with this abnormality were studied in the Second International Workshop on Chromosomes in Leukemia (1980), all 43 with adequate bone marrow specimens were classified as M2 by FAB criteria. As shown in Table III, t(8;21) occurred either as an isolated abnormality or together with other abnormalities, but in all cases it was associated with a good response to induction chemotherapy. However, the median survival was short (5½ months) in the 16 patients (33%) in whom t(8;21) was associated with loss of a sex chromosome. In contrast, the 18 patients (38%) with only t(8;21) had a median survival of 14 months. Within this group, the median survival time in AN patients (>26 months in males; >21½ months in females) was considerably longer than in AA patients (6½ months in males; 9½ months in females). Of 23 patients who were alive 1 year after diagnosis, 19 were initially AN; of 11 patients alive at 2 years, all were initially AN.

Among the best recognized structural rearrangements in ANLL karyotypes is t(15;17), identified only in leukemic patients with acute promyelocytic leukemia (APL: M3) of either the hypergranular type or the microgranular variant (Testa et al., 1978; Golomb et al., 1979). Our cytogenetics laboratory was able to identify the t(15;17) abnormality in blood or bone marrow cells from each of 25 patients with APL de novo who had adequate cytogenetic specimens. The frequency with which t(15;17) is detected in patients with APL has a curious geographic variation (Table III). Among 82 cases from around the world that were studied recently in the Fourth International Workshop on Chromosomes in Leukemia (1983), 50 (61%) had t(15;17), but 28 (34%) had no detectable cytogenetic

TABLE III

Structural Rearrangements in ANLL

Reference	No. of patients	Karyotype	CR (%)	Median survival (months)
t(8;21)—M2 leukemia				
2nd Int. Workshop Chromosomes Leuk. (1980)	48	t(8;21) only: 18 (38%)	72	14
		t(8;21)-X or -Y: 16 (33%)	62.5	6
		t(8;21) and other: 14 (29%)	85	16
Trujillo et al. (1979)	32	t(8;21) only: 14 (44%)		
		t(8;21)-X or -Y: 10 (31%)	84.4	20
		t(8;21) and other: 8 (25%)		
Berger et al. (1982b)	10	t(8;21) only: 2 (20%)		
		t(8;21)-X or -Y: 9 (90%)	100	NR[a]
		t(8;21) and other: 1 (10%)		

Reference	No. of patients	No. with t(15;17)	Karyotype	CR (%)	Median survival (months)
t(15;17)-M3 and M3 variant leukemia					
1st Int. Workshop Chromosomes Leuk. (1978)	17	9 (54%)	NR	NR	NR
Teerenhovi et al. (1978)	12	0	NR	NR	NR
2nd Int. Workshop Chromosomes Leuk. (1980)	80	33 (41%)	t(15;17): 23 (29%)	26	1
			t(15;17) and other: 10 (12%)	30	2
			Other only: 7 (9%)	29	5
			Normal: 40 (50%)	45	4
Golomb et al. (1979)	6	6 (100%)	NR	50	NR
Van Den Berghe et al. (1979)	15	11 (75%)	NR	NR	NR

[a] NR, not reported.

abnormality, and 4 had an abnormality other than t(15;17). Eight of 9 APL patients from Japan, 6 of 9 from Australia, 5 of 9 from South Africa, and all 5 from Paris had t(15;17). In contrast, all 6 APL patients from London, all 3 from Helsinki, and 7 of 11 from Rome had a normal karyotype. Reasons for this geographic variation in frequency are still unknown, but may be related to methodology.

Morphologically, APL, and especially the microgranular variant, is frequently confused with the subtype of AML in which some maturation is present in the myeloid cells (M2). Clinically, APL is most common in patients under 30 and is characterized by the occurrence of disseminated intravascular coagulation (DIC) during induction chemotherapy (Jones and Saleem, 1978; Golomb et al., 1980). Prompt therapy with low doses of heparin and with platelet transfusions has reduced the incidence of fatal hemorrhage, while anthracycline-based chemotherapy regimens have been able to produce a high percentage of complete remissions in this disease. In addition, the duration of these remissions may be longer than that seen with other forms of acute leukemia in adults. Thus, the rapid identification of the important t(15;17) marker can identify a group of young patients with acute leukemia who may benefit from prophylactic heparin therapy while undergoing induction chemotherapy. Careful attention to the expected complication of DIC can thus offer these APL patients a greater chance for successful remission induction and perhaps a long survival.

Bloomfield and Arthur (1982) have recently described another cytogenetic abnormality associated with characteristic morphologic findings. Four of their 41 patients with ANLL had as their only chromosome abnormality a partial deletion of the long arm of chromosome 16 (16q−). These patients differed in age, FAB classification (2 with M2 and 2 with M4), and initial leukocyte count. The only unifying feature was significant bone marrow eosinophilia. Two of the three treated patients had remained in continuous complete remission for longer than 10 and 19 months.

At the University of Chicago, we have identified a similar group of patients with an abnormality of chromosome 16 and bone marrow eosinophilia (Larson et al., 1982). In all 8, however, the specific abnormality was inv(16)(p13q22) and not merely a deletion of 16q. The percentage of eosinophils in the bone marrow was variable, but in all cases studied, these eosinophils were abnormal morphologically and cytochemically. All 8 of these patients had M4 leukemia. Again, 5 of the 7 treated patients achieved a complete remission. Thus, this unique chromosome abnormality may suggest a favorable prognosis.

Berger and his colleagues (1982a) have reported that a translocation or deletion of the long arm of chromosome 11 (11q−) is closely associated with acute monocytic leukemia (M5), another subset of ANLL which may be characterized by prolonged first remissions. Other investigators have identified t(9;11) in association with monocytic leukemias, suggesting that the critical determinant may reside on the long arm of chromosome 11 (Hagemeijer et al., 1982).

Abnormalities of the long arm of chromosome 3 have also been described in several patients with ANLL (Sweet *et al.*, 1979; Norrby *et al.*, 1982; Bernstein *et al.*, 1982). These have included both inversions and translocations. Many of these patients have been noted to have abnormal platelets and megakaryocytes with peripheral thrombocytosis and small, hypolobulated megakaryocytes in the bone marrow. No other unifying characteristics have been identified, but only a small number of patients have so far been described.

III. Secondary ANLL

Of increasing interest have been characteristic chromosome abnormalities found in patients who develop ANLL after prior chemotherapy and/or radiotherapy for other disorders, such as Hodgkin's disease; non-Hodgkin's lymphoma; breast, lung, colon, and ovarian cancer; multiple myeloma; hairy cell leukemia; or renal transplantation (Rowley *et al.*, 1977, 1981; Whang-Peng *et al.*, 1979). Most often, these patients have the morphologic characteristics of M1 or M2 leukemia, although erythroleukemia (M6) has also been seen. Often, all three hematopoietic cell lines are involved in a myelodysplastic disorder.

Characteristic chromosomal abnormalities are present in patients with secondary leukemia. Karyotypes are most often hypodiploid with loss of all or part of chromosome 5 and/or 7 (Table IV). In our own series of 46 patients, 39 had abnormalities of chromosome 5 and/or chromosome 7, and 4 had different abnormalities (Albain *et al.*, 1982). The median survival from the time of initial bone marrow dysfunction was 10 months for patients with abnormalities of either chromosome 5 or 7, 5 months with abnormalities of both chromosomes 5 and 7, and 12 months for the other 7 patients. Three of the last 7 patients achieved a complete remission compared to only one of the patients with abnormalities of chromosome 5 and/or 7.

TABLE IV

Clonal Chromosome Abnormalities in Secondary ANLL

References	Number of patients	Number abnormal	Number with −5/5q− or −7/7q−
Preisler and Lyman (1977)	10	10 (100%)	2 (20%)
Whang-Peng *et al.* (1979)	8	8 (100%)	5/5 (100%)
Albain *et al.* (1982)[a]	46	43 (94%)	39 (91%)
Pedersen-Bjergaard and Larson (1982)	17	15 (88%)	12 (80%)

[a] Includes patients previously published (Rowley *et al.*, 1977, 1981).

Many patients with secondary leukemia die during prolonged periods of marrow hypoplasia after conventional remission induction chemotherapy. Since a paucity of normal hematopoietic stem cells may underlie secondary leukemia, it has been suggested that therapy with high-dose cytosine arabinosine alone (an S phase active drug) may spare the remaining stem cells from significant toxicity and result in a more rapid marrow recovery (Preisler *et al.*, 1983). This remains to be proved.

Recently, a subgroup of patients who appear to have ANLL *de novo* have been identified who also have abnormalities of chromosome 5 and/or 7. Although by definition, none of these patients have received prior cytotoxic therapy, several epidemiological studies have shown that a significant fraction have had occupational or avocational exposure to possible carcinogens, such as chemical solvents, insecticides, or petroleum products (Mitelman *et al.*, 1978; Rowley *et al.*, 1982; Golomb *et al.*, 1982). Of interest, neither −5/5q− nor −7/7q− are commonly seen in childhood ANLL (Benedict *et al.*, 1979). The mechanism by which environmental agents are mutagenic in these patients is unknown, but may be similar to the effects of alkylating agents or ionizing radiation in patients who develop treatment-induced ANLL. In the future, as effective remission induction regimens are developed for patients with treatment-induced leukemia (such as high-dose cytosine arabinoside) it may be reasonable to use the same protocols for patients with ANLL *de novo* who have −5/5q− or −7/7q− and occupational exposure to potential mutagens.

IV. Chronic Myelogenous Leukemia (CML) and Other Ph[1]-Positive Leukemias

The first consistent chromosome abnormality associated with human malignancy was described in 1960 by Nowell and Hungerford in two patients with chronic myelogenous leukemia (CML). Now universally known as the Philadelphia (Ph[1]) chromosome in honor of its city of origin, it was initially characterized by its discoverers as an abnormally small G group chromosome.

In 1973, Rowley reported ten Ph[1]-positive patients with CML in whom additional material was found at the end of the long arm of chromosome 9 (9q+) using Giemsa and quinacrine banding. The staining characteristics were similar to those of the missing long arm of chromosome 22, suggesting a balanced translocation t(9;22)(q34;q11). Measurements of DNA content confirmed that the amount of DNA missing from chromosome 22 equaled that added to chromosome 9 (Mayall *et al.*, 1977). The Ph[1] is found in 90–95% of patients with CML, and the absence of this specific marker should suggest the possibility that the patient actually has a myeloproliferative disease other than CML.

Since the initial recognition of the Ph[1] chromosome, it has been shown that the translocation, which invariably involves chromosome 22, may not always have chromosome 9 as the other involved chromosome. In a literature review by Rowley (1980b), 29 CML patients had a simple translocation involving chromosome 22 and some chromosome other than 9. Of these, the most commonly involved chromosomes included 12 (p arm) and 17. More complex translocations in 31 patients almost invariably involved chromosomes 9 and 22 as well as one or more other chromosomes. Again, chromosome 17 was most frequently involved in these complex translocations. The presence of a variant Ph[1] translocation does not appear to influence survival, as these patients have a clinical course that parallels that of patients with the more typical 9;22 translocation.

The clinical course and survival of patients with Ph[1]-positive CML are significantly better than those of patients with Ph[1]-negative disease (40 versus 15 months median survival) (Whang-Peng et al., 1968). Of note is that when the Ph[1] chromosome in chronic phase CML is associated with loss of a Y chromosome (approximately 8–10% of male patients), survival is improved over patients with the Ph[1] alone (6 years versus 3½ years) (Sandberg, 1980). The explanation for this survival advantage is unclear.

When patients with CML are treated and a remission is achieved, the bone marrow morphology and leukocyte alkaline phosphatase (LAP) score may return to normal. However, when such a "remission" bone marrow is analyzed cytogenetically, the Ph[1] clone persists, and the percentage of Ph[1]-positive cells in the bone marrow remains unchanged. Attempts have been made to eradicate the Ph[1]-positive clone with aggressive cytotoxic therapy, but only rarely can this be achieved. Enzyme studies using glucose-6-phosphate dehydrogenase (G-6-PD) isoenzyme techniques as well as cytogenetic studies have shown that all three hematopoietic cell lines are involved in the malignant clone (Fialkow and Jacobson, 1977; Fitzgerald et al., 1971). This suggests that the cell of origin of CML is a multipotent stem cell, and this cell may be very resistant to current chemotherapy. Aggressive chemotherapy with subsequent bone marrow transplantation has been successful in eradicating the Ph[1]-positive cell line and restoring normal hematopoiesis.

As CML accelerates, the appearance of new abnormalities within the original Ph[1]-positive clone may be of clinical use in diagnosing the blast phase (Whang-Peng et al., 1968; Rowley, 1980b; Fleischman et al., 1981). In roughly one-third of patients, no clonal evolution is found, while in two-thirds new aneuploid clones are seen. About 90% of these cases are hyperdiploid. The most frequent additional abnormalities include a second Ph[1] chromosome (about 30–50% of cases), +8 (about 40%), iso-17q (about 25%), +19 (about 15%), and +21 (about 10%) (Sandberg, 1980). If blast crisis is successfully treated, these additional abnormalities frequently disappear, leaving behind the initial Ph[1] marker.

Recently, the Ph[1] marker has been described in diseases other than CML, including both ALL and ANLL (Table V). The relationship between these disorders is not yet clear, but the presence of the Ph[1] here generally predicts a poor prognosis.

TABLE V

Ph¹ (+) Diseases Other Than CML

Disease	Number of patients	Associated abnormalities
ALL	64	Ph¹, −7, −8, −15, −17, −20, −X, +5, +8, i(17q), t(1;14), t(2;7)
CML presenting as ALL	12	NR[a]
ANLL	15	Ph¹, +17, t(7;10), t(8;21)

[a] NR, not reported.

V. Acute Lymphoblastic Leukemia (ALL)

The Third International Workshop on Chromosomes in Leukemia, held in Lund, Sweden, in 1981, was devoted to ALL. Although nonrandom chromosome abnormalities had been recognized in a large percentage of patients with ALL (66% of 330 cases evaluated by the Workshop), clinical correlations with specific karyotype abnormalities had not been as well detailed as those in ANLL.

Among patients with abnormal karyotypes, 53% demonstrated pseudodiploidy, and 37% were hyperdiploid, while only 10% were hypodiploid. Of the 218 aneuploid patients, the most common structural rearrangements were translocations (46%) (Table VI). These included t(9;22)—the Ph¹ chromosome—in 21%, t(4;11) in 9%, t(8;14) in 8%, other 14q+ in 7%, and 6q− in 6%. The Ph¹ chromosome was more commonly seen in adults, while 6q− was seen predominantly in children. The t(8;14) abnormality was seen most often in patients with L3 leukemia, which may be a leukemic form of Burkitt's lymphoma. All 15 cases of B-ALL and 70% of the non-B, non-T ALL cases had clonal abnormalities, while only 39% of patients with T-ALL did so. As in ANLL, the presence of aneuploid clones was a significant negative prognostic factor independent of such known prognostic factors as age, WBC count, and FAB morphology. An additional 60 patients with ALL studied at the University of Minnesota have been reported by Bloomfield et al. (1981). Thirty-seven were adults, and 23 were children (1–15 years of age); 60% were classified morphologically as L1, 34% were L2, and 2 cases were L3. Cell surface markers revealed 47 cases of non-B, non-T ALL (78%), nine cases of T-ALL (15%), and 4 cases of B-ALL (7%). Clonal chromosome abnormalities were detected in 51 of the 60 patients (85%). All patients with B-ALL and 91% of patients with non-B, non-T ALL had clonal abnormalities, in contrast to only 44% of patients with T-ALL. Again, the common structural abnormalities seen were t(9;22) in 5 patients and t(4;11) in 4 patients. In addition, 4 patients had t(1;3) and 3 patients had t(11;14).

Translocation (4;11) in ALL has been associated with a short survival. Arthur et al. (1982) have reported five ALL patients who had t(4;11) as the only

TABLE VI

Frequency of Structural Abnormalities in ALL

References	No. of patients	Aneuploid patients	Abnormality	No. of patients	Percentage of total	Percentage of aneuploid
3rd Int. Workshop Chromosomes in Leukemia (1981)	330	218 (66%)	Ph[1]	45	14	21
			t(4;11)	19	6	7
			t(8;14)	17	5	8
			6q−	16	5	7
			Other 14q+	15	5	7
Bloomfield *et al.* 1981	60	51 (85%)	Ph[1]	5	8	10
			t(4;11)	4	7	8
			t(11;14)	3	5	6
			t(1;3)	4	7	8
			Other 14q+	5	8	10

karyotype abnormality at diagnosis. All had initial leukocyte counts of $>150 \times 10^9$/liter and non-B, non-T ALL. Four of five achieved initial complete remission; however, median remission duration and survival were very short ($2\frac{1}{2}$ and 8 months, respectively). ALL patients with t(8;14) and t(9;22) have also been reported to have a poor prognosis. Because the response to standard therapy has been poor in these high-risk patients, early bone marrow transplantation during first remission may be beneficial for patients with t(4;11), t(9;22), or t(8;14).

Another subgroup of ALL which has been identified cytogenetically consists of patients with near-haploid karyotypes. Only 17 patients with near-haploid ($N = 26$–28) ALL have been reported (Brodeur et al., 1981a; Sandberg et al., 1982). Despite high initial complete remission rates, survival was poor (10 months median in Brodeur's series). Commonly, in these patients, a hyperdiploid clone was found whose modal number was exactly double that of the near-haploid clone. In at least one patient, the near-haploid clone was detected initially by flow cytometry and only retrospectively by cytogenetic review of a bone marrow sample. The authors suggest that a near-haploid clone imparts a poor prognosis, but until other patients with hyperdiploid karyotypes are examined by flow cytometry to detect the presence of an unsuspected near-haploid cell line, the exact meaning of a near-haploid clone remains unknown.

Much of the data on adult T cell leukemia comes from Japan; reported abnormalities have included trisomy 7/7q+ (Ueshima et al., 1981) and 14q+ (Miyoshi et al., 1981), previously associated almost exclusively with B cell neoplasms. T-ALL is uncommon elsewhere in the world, and consistent chromosome abnormalities have not been well defined in other populations.

VI. Other Hematologic Diseases

Bone marrow and lymphoid tissue from patients with other hematologic diseases have been studied cytogenetically, and clonal chromosome abnormalities have been found in both lymphoproliferative and myeloproliferative disorders (Table VII).

In chronic lymphocytic leukemia (CLL) and multiple myeloma, the majority of patients studied have had normal karyotypes (Autio et al., 1979; Gahrton et al., 1980; Liang et al., 1979). This has been attributed in both instances to the low mitotic rates of these malignant cell populations, leading to cytogenetic analysis of spontaneously dividing normal cells that coexist in the tissues studied (lymph node and/or bone marrow). However, in both CLL and myeloma, a 14q+ marker chromosome has been identified, and in myeloma, an abnormality of 1q has been associated with the 14q+ marker.

Neoplastic lymphocytes in CLL may be stimulated to divide with polyclonal B cell mitogens. A recent review of 134 CLL patients by Gahrton and Robert

TABLE VII

Chromosome Abnormalities in Other Hematologic Diseases

Disease	Rearrangement	Frequency (%)
Non-Hodgkin's lymphoma		
Burkitt's	t(8;14)	80–90
Poorly differentiated lymphocytic	14q+	86
Diffuse histiocytic	14q+	54
Follicular center cell (small, large, and mixed cell)	t(14;18)	85
Angioimmunoblastic lymphadenopathy	+3	60
Chronic lymphocytic leukemia	+12	30

(1982) identified 34 patients with clonal abnormalities, 16 of whom (47%) had trisomy 12. Patients with trisomy 12 appeared to have a shorter interval between diagnosis and the need for treatment. No clear association was found between the immunoglobulin chain expressed by CLL cells and their karyotype.

Among the non-Hodgkin's lymphomas, complex chromosome abnormalities are a common finding (Sandberg, 1980; Rowley and Fukuhara, 1980). Burkitt's lymphoma cells, both African and non-African types, commonly contain a 14q+ chromosome, most frequently as a balanced translocation t(8;14)(q24;q32) (Zech et al., 1976; Zhang et al., 1982). Other variant translocations include t(2;8) (p12;q24) and t(8;22)(q24;q11). Of interest is the observation that patients with t(2;8) express κ light chains on their cell surface, while those with t(8;22) express only λ light chains, consistent with the observation that the κ gene is on chromosome 2 and the λ gene is on chromosome 22. Other malignant lymphomas have also been shown to have chromosome abnormalities, again most commonly a 14q+. Common donor chromosomes include 8, 11, 18, or the other 14. These diseases are usually of B cell origin, suggesting a specific role for chromosome 14 in the regulation of B lymphocyte proliferation.

Cytogenetic data in Hodgkin's disease is less available. In a review of the published literature on karyotypes in Hodgkin's disease, Sandberg (1980) was able to find only 118 cases. No consistent chromosome abnormalities were noted. Thirty-two patients had normal karyotypes, 55 had anomalies in the triploid range, 25 in the tetraploid range, and 23 in the diploid range. A 14q+ was occasionally reported, but much less frequently than in the non-Hodgkin's lymphomas. With the lack of widespread agreement on the cell of origin of Hodgkin's disease and only a small number of patients studied, the significance of the cytogenetic abnormalities which have been reported to date is unknown.

Recently, clonal chromosome abnormalities have been reported in angioimmunoblastic lymphadenopathy (AILD) (Kaneko et al., 1982). When lymph nodes from five patients were studied at the University of Chicago, clonal chromosome abnormalities were found in four. All were hyperdiploid. An extra chromosome 3, seen in cells from four patients, was clonal in two and nonclonal in two others. The lymph nodes in all five patients still contained at least 50% normal cells. The presence of unrelated abnormal karyotypes suggested that AILD might not be monoclonal in its early stages, but that as the disease evolves one clone may be selected and predominate in the late stage. Despite its original description as a benign proliferative process, the presence of clonal chromosome abnormalities implies malignancy, and patients with this disease may benefit from aggressive chemotherapy.

In myeloproliferative diseases, such as myelofibrosis with myeloid metaplasia (MMM), essential thrombocythemia (ET), and polycythemia vera (PV), clonal chromosome abnormalities have also been described. Because of the overlap among these entities and their tendency to evolve into acute leukemia, specific chromosome abnormalities for each myeloproliferative syndrome are difficult to define. The most commonly described abnormalities in MMM include trisomy 8 and 9, and either partial or complete monosomy 7. A further change in karyotype may signal evolution to acute leukemia (Sandberg, 1980).

One hundred seventy cases of ET were analyzed during the Third International Workshop on Chromosomes in Leukemia (1981) and only 5% of patients had a definite abnormality that was accepted by all the Workshop participants. Previously it had been reported that 21q− was a specific abnormality in ET; however, of 13 patients with 21q− studied at the Workshop, 11 were from a single institution, and the absence of band 21q22 in these karyotypes was not uniformly accepted by the Workshop participants. Data currently available do not reveal consistent karyotype abnormalities in ET.

Polycythemia vera is the most extensively studied of the myeloproliferative disorders after CML. Here again, evidence of specific and/or consistent chromosome abnormalities is lacking. The largest reported series consists of 149 patients collected by a cooperative group (Wurster-Hill et al., 1976). They report a 32% incidence of aneuploidy, but no single abnormality was seen in more than four cases. Of note is that 20q−, previously thought to be common in PV, was not seen in any of these patients. The relationship between karyotype, treatment, and development of acute leukemia has also not been established.

VII. Solid Tumors

Technical problems have hindered cytogenetic analyses of solid tumors (Table VIII). Sufficient numbers of tumor cells for analysis can be obtained only with difficulty, and this often requires multiple surgical biopsies. In only a few reports have consistent abnormalities been demonstrated either in similar tumors from different patients or from different sites of involvement within the same patient.

TABLE VIII

Clonal Chromosome Abnormalities in Solid Tumors

Disease	Specific clonal abnormalities noted	References
Colon cancer	+8, −17, others	Reichmann et al. (1981)
Neuroblastoma	1p−	Brodeur et al. (1981b)
		Gilbert et al. (1982)
Retinoblastoma	13q−	Balaban-Malenbaum et al. (1981)
		Balaban (1982)
Wilm's tumor	11p−	Riccardi et al. (1978, 1980)
		Kaneko et al. (1981)
		Slater and deKraker (1982)
Small cell lung cancer	del 3(p14;p23)	Whang-Peng et al. (1982a,b)
Renal cell carcinoma	t(3;11)(p23 or 24;p15)	Pathak et al. (1982)
Testis cancer	1p−	Wang et al. (1980)
Ovarian cancer	t(6;14) or 6q−/14q+	Wake et al. (1980)
		Atkin and Baker (1981)

In addition, some interesting preliminary data are available from cytogenetic analysis of continuous tumor cell lines growing in culture.

Reichmann et al. (1981) reported banding studies on 31 large bowel tumors, 28 primary, and 3 metastatic. It appeared that certain aberrations, especially gain of chromosome 8 and loss of chromosome 17, were nonrandom. However, modal chromosome numbers ranged from 44 to 91, and in many cases only an approximate karyotype could be obtained based on certain consistency seen in most of the analyzed cells.

Twelve patients with ovarian cancer have been reported by Wake et al., (1980), all of whom had either a 6q− or 14q+ or both [t(6;14)(q21;q24)]. These data have been confirmed by Atkin and Baker (1981). This abnormality has been correlated with papillary serous adenocarcinoma histology, but further clinical correlation is lacking.

In human neuroblastoma, both primary tumors and perpetual cell lines, a significant number of patients have been found to have an abnormality of the short arm of chromosome 1, most frequently loss of part of the short arm (1p−) but also translocations (Brodeur et al., 1981b; Gilbert et al., 1982). No information is currently available concerning prognostic or therapeutic significance of this chromosome abnormality.

Childhood Wilm's tumor has been associated with aniridia. A consistent deletion of the short arm of chromosome 11 has been found in unaffected cells of these individuals, suggesting a constitutional abnormality (Riccardi et al., 1978, 1980). Kaneko et al. (1981) have recently reported a patient without aniridia whose peripheral blood cells were karyotypically normal, but whose tumor cells in culture all contained the 11p−. These results have been confirmed by Slater and deKraker (1982). Similarly, childhood retinoblastoma has been associated with both a constitutional and tumor-isolated abnormality of the long arm of chromosome 13 (13q−) (Balaban-Malenbaum et al., 1981; Balaban et al., 1982). Again, the clinical significance of these abnormalities is not yet clear.

Specific chromosome abnormalities have also been reported in cell lines from small cell carcinoma of the lung [16 of 16 cell lines had a del 3(p14;p23)] (Whang-Peng et al., 1982a,b), familial renal cell carcinoma [t(3;11)(p23 or 24;p15)] (Pathak et al., 1982), and testicular tumors (1q−) (Wang et al., 1980). Again, no clinical applications are as yet possible.

Kristoffersson et al. (1981) recently described a new technique of fine needle aspiration to obtain tissue suitable for cytogenetic analysis. Their experience has been predominantly with malignant lymphoma, but if this procedure can be expanded to include solid tumors, a noninvasive method of studying the karyotype of solid tumors may lead to increasing data concerning consistent chromosome abnormalities in these diseases.

Another area of current investigation is the use of cytogenetic preparations to evaluate malignant effusions (DeWald et al., 1982). This appears to be a useful adjunct to standard cytologic techniques and can increase the diagnostic yield to greater than 80% (as constrasted to 50% with cytology alone). This technique is not yet widely available.

Other solid tumors have been studied in small series of patients, but consistent cytogenetic abnormalities have not been detected.

VIII. Summary

In human leukemias, the role of cytogenetic analysis as a predictor of clinical outcome has been well established. Specific chromosome translocations are associated with unique morphological subtypes. In CML, the first human malignancy associated with a specific chromosome marker, the presence of the Ph[1] has been shown to predict an improved survival. Lymphomas of B cell origin frequently have a 14q+ abnormality suggesting that chromosome 14 may play a role in B cell proliferation.

Other hematologic malignancies and solid tumors have been variably associated with clonal chromosome abnormalities. Advanced banding techniques and the use of DNA probes and restriction enzymes for gene mapping may soon provide more information to define the precise contribution of specific chromosome abnormalities to oncogenesis and tumor growth. This in turn may lead to more effective therapies.

Acknowledgments

Supported in part by PHS Grants CA-19266 and AM 07134-07 from The Department of Health and Human Services and by The Harry Greenberg Foundation. Dr. Larson is a Fellow of The Leukemia Society of America.

References

Albain, K. S., LeBeau, M. M., Rowley, J. D., Golomb, H. M., and Vardiman, J. W.(1982). *Blood* **60**, Suppl. 1, 119a.

Alimena, G., Annimol, L., Balestrazzi, P., Montuoro, A., and Dallapiccola, B. (1977). *Acta Hematol.* **58**, 234–239.

Arthur, D. C., Bloomfield, C. D., Lindquist, L. L., and Newbit, M. E., Jr. (1982). *Blood* **59**, 96–99.

Atkin, N. B., and Baker, M. C. (1981). *Cancer Genet. Cytogenet.* **3**, 275–276.

Autio, K., Turunen, O., Penttila, O., Eramaa, E., dela Chapelle, A., and Schroder, J. (1979). *Cancer Genet. Cytogenet.* **1**, 147–155.

Balaban, G., Gilbert, F., Nichols, W., Meadows, A. T., and Shields, J. (1982). *Cancer Genet. Cytogenet.* **6**, 213–221.

Balaban-Malenbaum, G., Gilbert, F., Nichols, W. W., Hill, R., Shields, J., and Meadows, A. T. (1981). *Cancer Genet. Cytogenet.* **3**, 243–250.

Benedict, W. F., Lange, M., Greene, J., Derencsenyl, A., and Alfi, O. (1979). *Blood* **54**, 818–823.

Bennett, J. M., Catovsky, D., Daniel, M. T., Flandrin, G., Galton, D. A. G., Gralnick, H. R., and Sultan, C. (1976). *Br. J. Haematol.* **33**, 451–458.

Berger, R., Bernheim, A., Siquax, F., Daniel, M.-T., Valensi, F., and Flandrin, G. (1982a). *Leuk. Res.* **6**, 17–26.

Berger, R., Bernheim, A., Daniel, M.-T., Valensi, F., Siquax, F., and Flandrin, G. (1982b). *Blood* **59**, 171–178.

Bernstein, R., Pinto, M. R., Behr, A., and Mendelow, B. (1982). *Blood* **60**, 613–617.

Bloomfield, C. D., and Arthur, D. C. (1982). *Proc. ASCO* **1**, 191.

Bloomfield, C. D., Linquist, L. L., Arthur, D., McKenna, R. W., Lebein, T. W., Peterson, B. A., and Nesbit, M. E. (1981). *Cancer Res.* **41**, 4838–4843.

Borgstrom, G. H., Teerenhovi, L., Vuopio, P., dela Chapelle, A., Van Den Berghe, H., Brandt, L., Golomb, H. M., Louwagle, A., Mitelman, F., Rowley, J. D., and Sandberg, A. A. (1980). *Cancer Genet. Cytogenet.* **2**, 115–126.

Brodeur, G. M., Williams, D. L., Look, A. T., Bowman, P., and Kalwinsky, D. K. (1981a). *Blood* **58**, 14–19.

Brodeur, G. M., Green, A. A., Hayes, F. A., Williams, K. J., Williams, D. L., and Tsiatis, A. A. (1981b). *Cancer Res.* **41**, 4678–4686.

DeWald, G. W., Hicks, G. A., Dines, D. E., and Gordon, H. (1982). *Mayo Clin. Proc.* **57**, 488–494.

Fialkow, P. J., and Jacobson, R. J. (1977). *Am. J. Med.* **63**, 125–130.

First International Workshop on Chromosomes in Leukemia (1978). *Br. J. Haematol.* **39**, 311–316.

Fitzgerald, P. H., Pickering, A. F., and Eiby, J. R. (1971). *Br. J. Haematol.* **21**, 473–480.

Fleischman, E. W., Prigogina, E. L., Volkova, M. A., Frenkel, M. A., Zakhartchenko, N. A., Konstantinova, L. N., Puchkova, G. P., and Balakirev, S. A. (1981). *Hum. Genet.* **58**, 285–293.

Fourth International Workshop on Chromosomes in Leukemia (1983). *Cancer Genet. Cytogenet.* (in press).

Gahrton, G., and Robert, K.-H. (1982). *Cancer Genet. Cytogenet.* **6**, 171–181.

Gahrton, G., Robert, K.-H., Friberg, K., Zech, L., and Bird, A. G. (1980). *Lancet* **i**, 146–147.

Gilbert, F., Balaban, G., Moorhead, P., Bianchi, S., and Schlesinger, H. (1982). *Cancer Genet. Cytogenet.* **7**, 33–42.

Golomb, H. M., Vardiman, J., and Rowley, J. D. (1976). *Blood* **48**, 9–21.

Golomb, H. M., Vardiman, J., Rowley, J. D., Testa, J. R., and Mintz, U. (1978). *N. Engl. J. Med.* **299**, 613–619.

Golomb, H. M., Testa, J. R., Vardiman, J. W., Butler, A. E., and Rowley, J. D. (1979). *Cancer Genet. Cytogenet.* **1**, 69–78.

Golomb, H. M., Rowley, J. D., Vardiman, J. W., Testa, J. R., and Butler, A. (1980). *Blood* **55**, 253–259.

Golomb, H. M., Alimena, G., Rowley, J. D., Vardiman, J. W., Testa, J. R., and Sovik, C. (1982). *Blood* **60**, 404–411.

Hagemeijer, A., Hahlen, K., and Abels, J. (1981). *Cancer Genet. Cytogenet.* **3**, 109–124.

Hagemeijer, A., Hahlen, K., Sizoo, W., and Abels, J. (1982). *Cancer Genet. Cytogenet.* **5**, 95–105.

Hossfeld, D. K., Faltermeier, M., and Wendehorst, E. (1979). *Blut* **38**, 377–382.

Jones, M. E., and Saleem, A. (1978). *Am. J. Med.* **65**, 673–677.

Kaneko, Y., Eques, C., and Rowley, J. D. (1981). *Cancer Res.* **41**, 4577–4578.

Kaneko, Y., Larson, R. A., Variakojis, D., Haren, J. M., and Rowley, J. D. (1982). *Blood* **60**, 877–887.

Knuutila, S., Vuopio, P., Elonen, E., Siimes, M., Kovanen, R., Borgstrom, G. H., and dela Chapelle, A. (1981). *Blood* **518**, 369–375.

Kristoffersson, U., Olsson, H., Mark-Vendel, E., and Mitelman, F. (1981). *Cancer Genet. Cytogenet.* **4**, 53–60.

Larson, R. A., LeBeau, M. M., Bitter, M. A., Vardiman, J. V., Golomb, H. M., and Rowley, J. D. (1982). *Blood* **60**, Suppl. 1, 131a.

Larson, R. A., LeBeau, M. M., Vardiman, J. W., Testa, J. R., Golomb, H. M., and Rowley, J. D. (1983). *Cancer Genet. Cytogenet.* (in press).

Liang, W., Hopper, J. E., and Rowley, J. D. (1979). *Cancer (Philadelphia)* **44**, 630–644.

Mayall, B. H., Carrano, A. V., Moore, D. H., II, and Rowley, J. D. (1977). *Cancer Res.* **37**, 3590–3593.

Mitelman, F., Nilsson, P. G., Levan, G., and Brandt, L. (1976). *Int. J. Cancer* **18**, 31–38.

Mitelman, F., Brandt, L., and Nilsson, P. G. (1978). *Blood* **52**, 1229–1237.

Miyoshi, I., Miyamoto, K., Sumida, M., Nishihara, R., Lai, M., Yoshimoto, S., Sato, J., and Kimura, I. (1981). *Cancer Genet. Cytogenet.* **3**, 251–259.

Nilsson, P. G., Brandt, L., and Mitelman, F. (1977). *Leuk. Res.* **1**, 31–34.

Norrby, A., Ridell, B., Swolin, B., and Westin, J. (1982). *Cancer Genet. Cytogenet.* **5**, 257–263.

Nowell, P. C., and Hungerford, D. A. (1960). *Science* **132**, 1197.

Oshimura, M., Hayata, I., Kakati, S., and Sandberg, A. A. (1976). *Cancer (Philadelphia)* **38**, 748–761.

Pathak, S., Strong, L. C., Ferrell, R. E., and Trindade, A. (1982). *Science* **217**, 939–941.

Pedersen-Bjergaard, J., and Larsen, S. O. (1982). *N. Engl. J. Med.* **307**, 965–971.

Philip, P., Kroghjensen, M., Killman, S. A., Drivsholm, A., and Hansen, N. E. (1978). *Leuk. Res.* **2**, 201–212.

Preisler, H. D., and Lyman, G. H. (1977). *Am. J. Hematol.* **3**, 209–218.

Preisler, H. D., Early, A. P., Raza, A., Vlahides, G., Browman, G., and Marinello, M. J. (1983). *N. Engl. J. Med.* **308**, 21–23.

Reichmann, A., Martin, P., and Levin, B. (1981). *Int. J. Cancer.* **28**, 431–440.

Riccardi, V. M., Sujansky, E., Smith, A. C., and Francke, U. (1978). *Pediatrics* **61**, 604–610.

Riccardi, V. M., Hittner, H. M., Francke, U., Yunis, J. J., Ledbetter, D., and Borges, W. (1980). *Cancer Genet. Cytogenet.* **2**, 131–137.

Rowley, J. D. (1973). *Nature (London)* **243**, 290–293.

Rowley, J. D. (1980a). *Annu. Rev. Genet.* **14**, 17–39.

Rowley, J. D. (1980b). *Clin. Haematol.* **9**, 55–86.

Rowley, J. D. (1981). *In* "Genes, Chromosomes, and Neoplasia" (F. E. Arrighi, P. N. Rao, and E. Stubblefield, eds.), pp. 273–296. Raven, New York.

Rowley, J. D., and Fukuhara, S. (1980). *Semin. Oncol.* **7**, 255–266.

Rowley, J. D., Golomb, H. M., and Vardiman, J. W. (1977). *Blood* **50**, 759–770.

Rowley, J. D., Golomb, H. M., and Vardiman, J. W. (1981). *Blood* **58**, 759–767.

Rowley, J. D., Alimena, G., Garson, O. M., Hagemeijer, A., Mitelman, F., and Prigogina, E. L. (1982). *Blood* **59**, 1013–1022.

Ruutu, P., Ruutu, T., Vuopio, P., Kosunen, T. U., and dela Chapelle, A. (1977). *Nature (London)* **265**, 146–147.

Sakurai, M., and Sandberg, A. A. (1973). *Blood* **41**, 93–104.

Sandberg, A. A. (1980). "The Chromosomes in Human Cancer and Leukemia." Elsevier, New York.

Sandberg, A. A., Wake, N., and Kohno, S. (1982). *Cancer Genet. Cytogenet.* **5**, 293–307.

Second International Workshop on Chromosomes in Leukemia (1980). *Cancer Genet. Cytogenet.* **2**, 89–113.

Slater, R. M., and deKraker, J. (1982). *Cancer Genet. Cytogenet.* **5**, 237–245.

Sweet, D. L., Golomb, H. M., Rowley, J. D., and Vardiman, J. W. (1979). *Cancer Genet. Cytogenet.* **1**, 33–37.

Teerenhovi, L., Borgstrom, G. H., Mitelman, F., Brandt, L., Vuopio, P., Timonen, T., Almquist, A., and dela Chapelle, A. (1978). *Lancet.* **ii**, 797.

Testa, J. R., Golomb, H. M., Rowley, J. D., Vardiman, J. W., and Sweet, D. L.,, Jr. (1978). *Blood* **52**, 272–280.

Testa, J. R., Mintz, U., Rowley, J. D., Vardiman, J. W., and Golomb, H. M. (1979). *Cancer Res.* **39**, 3619–3627.

Third International Workshop on Chromosomes in Leukemia (1981). *Cancer Genet. Cytogenet.* **4**, 95–142.

Trujillo, J. M., Cork, A., Ahearn, M. J., Youness, E. L., and McCredi, K.B. (1979). *Blood* **53**, 695–706.

Ueshima, Y., Fukuhara, S., Hattori, T., Uchiyama, T., Takatsuki, K., and Uchino, H. (1981). *Blood* **58**, 420–425.

Van Den Berghe, H., Louwagi, A., Broeckart-Van Orshoven, A., David, G., Verwilghen, R., Michaux, J. L., Ferrant, A., and Sokal, G. (1979). *Cancer (Philadelphia)* **43**, 558–562.

Wake, N., Hreshchyshyn, M. M., Piver, S. M., Matsui, S., and Sandberg, A. A. (1980). *Cancer Res.* **40**, 4512–4518.

Wang, N., Trend, B., Bronson, D. L., and Fraley, E. E. (1980). *Cancer Res.* **40**, 796–802.

Whang-Peng, J., Canellos, G. P., Carbone, P. P., and Tjio, J. H. (1968). *Blood* **32**, 755–766.

Whang-Peng, J., Knutsen, T., O'Connell, J. F., and Brereton, H. D. (1979). *Cancer (Philadelphia)* **44**, 1592–1600.

Whang-Peng, J., Kao-Shan, C. S., Lee, E. C., Bunn, P. A.,Carney, D. N., Gazdar, A. F., and Minna, J. D. (1982a). *Science* **215**, 181–182.

Whang-Peng, J., Bunn, P. A., Kao-Shan, C. S., Lee, E. C., Carney, D. N., Gazdar, A., and Minna, J. D. (1982b). *Cancer Genet. Cytogenet.* **6**, 119–134.

Wurster-Hill, D., Whang-Peng, J., McIntyre, O. R., Hsu, L. Y. F., Hirschhorn, K., Modan, B., Pisciotta, A. V., Pierce, R., Balderak, S. P., Weinfeld, A., and Murphy, S. (1976). *Semin. Hematol.* **13,** 13–32.
Yunis, J. J., Bloomfield, C. D., and Ensrud, K. (1981). *N. Engl. J. Med.* **305,** 135–139.
Zech, L., Haglund, U., Nilsson, K., and Klein, G. (1976). *Int. J. Cancer* **17,** 47–56.
Zhang, S., Zech, L., and Klein, G. (1982). *Int. J. Cancer* **29,** 153–157.

18

Chromosomes and Cancer: From Molecules to Man—An Overview

H. JOHN EVANS

Medical Research Council
Clinical and Population Cytogenetics Unit
Western General Hospital
Edinburgh, Scotland

The central theme of this Symposium has been to examine the relationship between chromosome structure, DNA organization, and transcription, all in the context of neoplastic change. The timing of this Symposium has been particularly appropriate because of what can only be described as the plethora of remarkable findings that have emerged in the last few years. These have culminated in recent months in the dramatic demonstrations of associations between a number of proto-oncogenes in the human genome and the chromosomes, and indeed chromosomal sites, involved in structural changes in certain malignant disorders. Although we have focused our attention at the DNA and chromosomal levels, the papers delivered at this Symposium have nevertheless covered a very wide field so that in my attempt at an overview my discussion will be somewhat uneven and will very much reflect a personal angle. I shall, of course, not attempt to review all the aspects that were so ably covered, but pick out some of the findings, principles, and questions that appear to me to be of particular significance at the present time, and raise a number of other questions and introduce a few other findings that we did not spend much time on, and which I think may be important.

I should like to look at these under a series of headings and begin with the status of our knowledge, or lack of knowledge, on chromosome structure, for alterations in chromosome structure were originally proposed to be causally associated with cancer almost 70 years ago (Boveri, 1914), and Boveri's original hypothesis has received very strong support in recent years, not least from the work carried out in the laboratories of one of our hosts—Dr. Janet Rowley.

I. Chromosome Architecture

Structure and function are intimately related, and the problem of how nature utilizes nuclear and chromosomal proteins in the packaging of the 2 meters of DNA that is distributed in a precise way over the 46 chromosomes in the human complement, in a manner that enables the accurate transcription, replication, and segregation of this DNA, is still something of a mystery. For sometime we were puzzled by the way in which histone proteins were associated with the DNA, but we now have a good understanding—at least at the architectural level—of histone–DNA structure in the nucleosome, but what of the equally abundant acidic proteins that appear to be involved more in the anatomy, as opposed to the physiology, of the chromosome?

There is good evidence that interphase chromosomes are anchored at various points to the nuclear membrane and that anchorage at the telomeres and at blocks of heterochromatin may be relatively permanent; it is equally clear that the structural continuity of the chromosome is retained, either directly or indirectly, in interphase. Dr. Laemmli and others have provided evidence for a protein scaffold ("core") in metaphase chromosomes and in interphase chromatin which plays a major role in chromosome folding, and that folding in interphase is also determined by the peripheral lamina proteins (Laemmli et al., Chapter 1). One of the two proteins attributed to the scaffold is a DNA-binding protein, but how this binding occurs and to what parts of the DNA is not known. Jeppesen and Gooderham in my laboratory have also isolated and characterized at least one scaffold protein (Gooderham and Jeppesen, 1983) and have cloned a number of short DNA fragments that bind to the protein core. These fragments have been sequenced and shown to contain repeated sequences, but we have yet to determine how these are arranged along the chromosome and how they interact with the DNA.

I should point out that the view that there is a protein scaffold to the chromosome that anchors loops of DNA of some 50–100 kb in length is not universally accepted, and there is some question concerning the methods of preparation that reveal such structures. For example, Cook and his colleagues (McCready *et al.*, 1982) provide evidence for a somewhat different structure, referred to as the nuclear cage and consisting of RNA and protein, to which the linear DNA is attached in large loops of around 220 kb in length and which are present throughout the cell cycle, including mitosis. There is some evidence that the replication and transcription machinery are attached to the cage, for sites of active transcription or replication appear to be associated with the cage proteins and RNA, whereas inactive sites are not so associated. The implication then is that DNA is only replicated or transcribed when it becomes attached to the cage and passes through the appropriate fixed machinery.

These two models of the scaffold plus peripheral lamina proteins and the nuclear cage may not be entirely incompatible, and this is an area where I would expect to see significant advances in the near future.

While discussing chromosome architecture, I should like to comment on one aspect of chromosome structure that has provided an enormously powerful tool in cytogenetics, namely, the structures that are responsible for the patterns of bands that we can see in fixed and processed chromsomes. At metaphase some 300 chromosome- and site-specific bands may be identified in a haploid human complement. As Dr. Jorge Yunis (this Symposium) has pointed out, the higher resolution of prometaphase and prophase chromosomes reveals up to a thousand or more bands (ISCN, 1981) and, perhaps not surprisingly, uncovers far more chromosome variation in human malignant cells than has been evident previously. I have no wish to comment on the underlying structures that give rise to these bands, but I should like to consider their cytological resolution under the microscope in relation to our genetic resolution at the gene cluster level.

By analogy with bacteria, and before the realization that many genes in man are present in clusters and have various intervening and flanking DNA sequences, it was considered that a metaphase band could contain sufficient DNA to code for 100 or more genes, even if only 10% of the genome contained functionally required and expressed sequences. Various estimates suggest that at most 10% of the 3×10^9 nucleotides in the human genome consist of coding and regulatory sequences (Bishop, 1974), and recent work has shown that gene clustering may be very common, as seen, for example, in the genes of the major histocompatibility complex, the immunoglobulins, and hemoglobin, to name but a few. A unit of expressed information, therefore, such as hemoglobin, may involve around 7×10^4 bp: others may involve more or less. If we take a round figure of 5×10^4 bp for a gene cluster and 10% of the total DNA content, or $3 \times$

10^8 bp as expressed or functional DNA, then this would suggest that the genome may contain of the order of 6000 gene clusters. In other words, each of the 1000 or so prophase bands that we see at the cytological level could contain from around 1–10 gene clusters so that our cytological resolution may, for practical purposes, be rather better than we once thought. However, not all genes are clustered, and I think it unlikely that we are going usefully to resolve finer detail with nonspecific staining techniques, and in this regard I am rather less optimistic than Dr. Yunis. The way ahead here is surely to utilize single copy specific probes with attached labels, and I shall refer to this later.

II. Transcription

In nature's world structure can rarely be divorced from function, and the search for structural change in relation to transcription is yielding exciting dividends. Here, however, we must remember that at most 10–20% of the DNA in a mammalian genome is ever transcribed, so that when we come to examine chromosome structure in the context of transcription, then only a minority of the DNA is ever in a form that may even predispose it to transcription, let alone be actively involved in the process. To the cytologist studying electron microscope pictures of transcribing regions of lampbrush chromosomes of amphibia, or polytene chromosomes of flies, there is little doubt that gene activation is directly preceded by the chromatin fiber changing from a closely packed rope to a more open structure, but our knowledge of how, and indeed why, this change comes about is fragmentary.

Transcription is obviously a multistep process, and as Dr. Chambon and others have shown, it does not simply involve access to a defined polymerase binding site. The picture of the TATA box as a simple eukaryotic promoter, in the prokaryotic sense, is not valid and, in addition to the cap site and TATA box regions, sequences located upstream are necessary for the efficient initiation of transcription although transcription can be initiated at a variety of sites (Hen *et al.*, Chapter 2). Before this process can begin it is necessary for the chromatin to change its state, and this has been elegantly demonstrated by Dr. Weintraub and his colleagues, particularly through the use of nonspecific nucleases.

Nuclease digestion experiments with pancreatic DNase I show that actively transcribed genes are sensitive to cutting, but I should emphasize that this is not an exclusive prerogative of active genes (Miller *et al.*, 1978). Studies with DNase II, which primarily cuts between nucleosomes, shows that the confirmation of active nucleosomes differs from the bulk of nucleosomes, and that this may be due, at least in part, to the binding of the HMG proteins 14 and 17. These two proteins are clearly involved in the transcription process, and fluorescent labeled antibodies to them reveal that they are specifically associated with transcriptionally active puffs in salivary gland polytene chromosomes (Mayfield *et al.*, 1978). Quite a lot of evidence implies that part of the transcriptional process may involve the creation of a nucleosome-free region proximal to the polymerase complex (e.g., Lamb and Daneholt, 1979), and this region may indeed include the nuclease hypersensitive site that is cut with a single-strand-specific S_1 nuclease at the 5' end of the chick globin gene. The *in vitro* studies on the transcription of the *TK* gene inserted into a plasmid which is then introduced into the *Xenopus* oocyte system show that coiled continuous circles are necessary for transcription, linear DNA being ineffective, so that the acidic DNA-binding structural proteins of the chromosome may be important in maintaining the supercoiled state. DNA-binding nonstructural proteins require recognition sites on the chromosome that may well be provided by the proposed "hairpin" structures arising as a result of intrastrand pairing of "foldback" repeated DNA sequences upstream from the TATA box region. Histone acetylation, HMG 14 and 17 phosphorylation, and particular undermethylation of the DNA are also associated with gene activity, and although each one of these features is considered necessary, not one is in itself sufficient for transcription. Moreover, as Dr. Sheffery pointed out (Sheffery *et al.*, Chapter 17), there is more than one way to induce a piece of DNA to undergo transcription, and I might add here that the tumor promoter TPA has recently been shown to induce transcription of a normally nonexpressed episomal virus in mouse embryo cells which then results in the transformation of these cells (Amtmann and Sauer, 1982).

Two further important points that emerged from Dr. Harold Weintraub's discussion (Weintraub, this Symposium) that are worth reemphasizing are (1) that a change in chromatin structure that may herald the process of transcription can occur long before the actual process is itself set in train and (2) that the alteration in structure that is associated with transcription is retained throughout the process of cell division and is passed on to descendant daughter cells. This last point is very important in the context of carcinogenesis where we are concerned with continued proliferation and, presumably, continued expression of DNA sequences that maintain the cell and its descendants in a proliferative cycle.

In recent times there has been considerable discussion of the role of methylation in inactivating gene sequences, and the correlation between methylation and inactivation (considered as being possibly due to the methyl groups preventing polymerase attachment) and demethylation and gene activation is by no means unequivocal. Recent evidence concerning the reactivation of inactive human or mouse gene loci following the incorporation of 5-azacytidine has been interpreted as being a consequence of demethylation (Mohandas *et al.*, 1981; Venolia *et al.*, 1982; but see Miller *et al.*, 1982). Methylation is also one factor that has stimulated further interest in the possibility that an altered form of DNA,

Z-DNA, may be present in inactive parts of the genome and may be involved in the transcription process. This is something which we have not discussed and which I would like to comment on.

Z-DNA is a reversible structural form that is only entered into by tracts of DNA containing regularly alternating purines and pyrimidines (Wang *et al.*, 1979). The Z conformation is stabilized under conditions of high salt or, as Felsenfeld and colleagues first showed last year (Behe and Felsenfeld, 1981), under conditions of low salt if the DNA is methylated at the C-5 position in tracts of (dC-dG) and this stabilization by methylation is something I shall return to.

Z-DNA is readily demonstrated with synthesized oligonucleotides *in vitro,* but recent evidence indicates that this form of DNA may also be present *in vivo.* Rich and his colleagues (Nordheim *et al.*, 1981) purified Z-DNA antibodies from sera from immunized rabbits and, by indirect immunofluorescence, showed that these antibodies bound specifically to the interband regions of *Drosophila* salivary gland chromosomes, even in the presence of poly(dG-dC)·poly(dG-dC) in the B conformation, but no binding occurred if the chromosome preparations were preincubated with Z-forms of poly(dG-dC) DNA. These results thus imply that Z-DNA is present and that it is more abundant, or more accessible, in the interband regions of *Drosophila* chromosomes, and it is these regions that are known to contain the structural genes in this species. This is an important finding, as indeed is the report of Singleton *et al.* (1982) that Z-DNA formation is induced by supercoiling in plasmid pRW751 under physiological conditions of ionic strength and superhelical density. Z-DNA is normally unstable in physiological salt conditions *in vitro,* but it clearly can be stabilized by supercoiling and by the presence of cationic polyamines, such as spermidine, that are normally present in nuclei.

Are Z-DNA sequences relevant to man? Hamada and Kakunaga (1982) have recently shown that a cloned human cardiac muscle actin gene has an intron with a sequence of 50 alternating dT and dG residues, and using this, and a probe specific for poly(dT-dG), they show that the human genome contains a very large number (up to 10^5) of highly dispersed potential Z-DNA-forming sequences. The relevance of Z-DNA in our context is that it is clear that demethylation of this kind of DNA renders it unstable and makes it revert to its B form. If Z-DNA exists throughout the genome, then its demethylation would allow unwinding of B-DNA at some distance removed from the Z region, or it could allow for the binding of DNA-binding proteins and, in this way, could act as a trigger for transcription. There is evidence that the junction between these Z and B forms of DNA are sensitive to S_1 nuclease and that there may be a single-stranded break at that site (Singleton *et al.*, 1982). Whether this would predispose to spontaneous or mutagen-induced chromosome structural rearrangements being preferentially involved at such sites is unknown, but Z-DNA could be very important in terms of being responsible for genetic position effects in chromosome translocations.

III. DNA Transfection, Oncogenes, and Chromosome Anomalies in Cancer

I tie these three topics together since one of the highlights of our Symposium has been the presentation and discussion of evidence linking all three.

A. DNA Transfection and Oncogenes

Let me remind you that Dr. Cooper and his colleagues (Krontiris and Cooper, 1981) and Weinberg and his colleagues (Shih *et al.*, 1981) were originally responsible for demonstrating that transformation of mouse NIH3T3 cells could result from DNA transfection using DNA from human tumor cells. Since then there has been a spate of reports on transformation by transfection using DNAs from various species ranging from birds to man, and from a wide variety of tumors, including human bladder, colon, and lung carcinoma; lymphoid and myeloid malignancies; mammary and neuroblastoma tumors; and, recently, a variety of sarcomas (Marshall *et al.*, 1982). These two groups and many others have gone on to identify the transforming sequences in some of these DNAs— which are referred to as cellular oncogenes or *c-onc* genes—and it is evident that these are essentially the cellular counterparts of the transforming viral sequences, or *v-onc* genes, of various acute transforming retroviruses. The transfection experiments show that *c-onc* genes surrounded by their normal flanking sequences cannot transform, but ligation of these genes to a viral transcription regulatory sequence makes them active in transformation in most (Blair *et al.*, 1981; Chang *et al.*, 1982), but not all (Watson *et al.*, 1982), cases. Overall, the evidence from these experiments implies that transformation following transfection results from the activation of the *c-onc* sequences due to the DNA rearrangement that occurs during donor DNA integration.

It is generally accepted that the retroviral *v-onc* genes are derived by recombination from the normal cellular sequences or *c-onc* genes. There are now some score or more different isolates of acute transforming retroviruses, and a number of these have been shown to have *v-onc* genes homologous, or closely similar, to human genomic sequences (e.g., Santos *et al.*, 1982). The human genome obviously contains a number of these oncogenes, and in our discussion the question was asked, "How many oncogenes are there in man?" The argument is put forward that these oncogenes may well be involved in differentiation, and so the answer to the question might be that there may be as many oncogenes as there are differentiation pathways. However, the genome is not usually profligate, and in many cases I would expect that different differentiation pathways may not infrequently utilize common DNA sequences, but even so we might expect that there may be as many as 50–100 sequences that might take on the role of oncogenes. What is clear is that these genes are highly conserved throughout evolution for oncogenes in chick, mouse, rat, cat, and man are closely similar if not identical.

Dr. Lane (see Cooper and Lane, Chapter 3) showed in her presentation that two different c-ras genes are involved in three different human carcinomas of bladder, lung, and colon, so that ras gene family would appear to be a multigene family that could be involved in a variety of human epithelial tumors. In the same way she has identified three different genes associated with different B cell leukemias and two other genes associated with T cell leukemias, and each of these genes present in the leukemia cells can produce transformation of mouse 3T3 cells in culture. Much of the evidence would suggest that, in contrast to the ras gene family, other c-onc genes may represent single copy sequences in cellular DNA. Moreover, and of great importance, it seems clear that different transforming c-onc genes are activated in different types of tumors, but the same gene is activated in independent tumors of the same type, whether these tumors are induced by chemicals, radiations, or viruses (Cooper, 1982).

The normal role of the c-onc sequences in the cell is unknown, but they must be involved in controlling cell growth, development, and differentiation. The likelihood would be that these genes are involved in differentiation in embryonic tissues and in differentiating pathways in adult proliferating tissues, as for instance we see in the elegant work on the oncogenes in the different kinds of pre-B, intermediate B, and mature B cell leukemias that we have referred to (see Cooper and Lane, Chapter 3). In addition, the work of Westin et al. (1982) on the human c-amv gene, the homolog of which (v-amv) causes myeloid leukemia in chickens, has shown that this gene is expressed in immature lymphoid T cells, but is turned off in mature T and B lymphocytes. I am aware of only one publication describing attempts to search for RNA transcripts of c-onc sequences in embryos, where Müller et al. (1982) report developmental stage and tissue specific expression of c-onc genes in mouse embryos and in early postnatal development. The relevant probes are available, and a clear and important aim is for us to learn more concerning the function of these c-onc sequences in normal ontogeny. In the case of the v-onc genes we already know that they are expressed at high levels in virus-transformed cells as, for example, in the case of pp60[src] phosphoprotein in chicken cells transformed by RSV, where the levels are 100 times higher than cellular pp60 in normal cells (Collett et al., 1978). The proteins produced by some of these oncogenes are in some cases known to be phosphokinases, and in the case of the Harvey and Kirsten murine sarcoma viruses the nucleotide sequences of their p21 transforming proteins have recently been determined (Dhar.et al., 1982; Tsuchida et al., 1982). The mechanism whereby these proteins act in the cell so that alterations in cell membrane or microfilament structure, etc., result in a continued proliferation of that cell is not known (e.g., see Collett et al., 1981), and this is clearly a major question that is yet to be resolved. In the case of the oncogenes in human tumors, the presumption would be that the relevant c-oncogene is being expressed either (1) at the wrong time, (2) is overexpressed, or (3) is expressed in the wrong way, i.e., is mutated. I say presumption, since there is some evidence for each of these three possibilities, but we require more information on this point, and I shall return to this when we consider *c-onc* genes in relation to chromosome anomalies.

B. Chromosome Anomalies in Cancer

The search for consistent, and hence informative, chromosome anomalies associated with specific neoplasms has proved rewarding in a number of instances and Golomb (see Pearson *et al.*, Chapter 17), Mitelman (see Chapter 4), and Rowley (see Chapter 8) gave very convincing summaries of the significant acquired chromosome abnormalities and Francke (see Chapter 6) gave a summary of the inherited constitutional changes that predispose to cancer. I am not going to spend time recapitulating details, but I should like to make three points.

1. The acquired changes involving trisomy 8, monosomy 5, and deletions of 5q, and monosomy 7 and deletions of 7q, have for some time been emerging as consistent findings in various myeloproliferative malignancies, and the findings from a number of recent surveys emphasize the significance of abnormalities involving these particular chromosomes. In the context of Dr. Rowley's findings of the possible importance of environmental mutagens in inducing such changes, I think it worth pointing out that many electrophilic mutagens may react with the centrioles, which are responsible for the orderly segregation of chromosomes at mitosis, and that a whole variety of such things as fatty acids and metals, which are important agents in oncogenesis, produce aneuploidy in mutagen test systems (Zimmerman, 1982). Chromosome structural changes then are not the only consequences of exposure to mutagens, and we should pay greater attention to induced aneuploidy, particularly in the context of induced malignancy.

2. Dr. Mitelman commented upon the paucity of our information on chromosome changes in solid tumors, and I should like to reemphasize this point. We really do need to have much more information on solid tumors since epithelial cancers—carcinomas—are a major form of cancer in man, and we must improve our techniques to enable us to look at the chromosomes in these tumor cells in the solid phase and not simply in derived cells that appear later in effusions.

3. The inherited constitutional anomalies discussed by Dr. Francke, and which predispose to specific cancers, certainly tell us that we require additional changes over and above the specific chromosome anomaly to initiate a malignant growth. The point that needs emphasizing here is that there are many other dominantly inherited cancer predispositions that are in a different class from the childhood malignancies discussed. It seems very probable that in these familial cases there may well be associated specific chromosomal changes, and I believe

that there is a very strong case for us to extend the application of high resolution banding techniques to studies on families where we have good evidence for a dominant inheritance of cancer.

During our discussions we occasionally referred to possible ways in which chromosome abnormalities may produce their oncogenic effects and I would like to summarize these briefly. Although there is quite a wide variety of different chromosomal structural changes that occur spontaneously, or can be induced by mutagens, we can essentially consider that all chromosome anomalies involve principally one of three kinds of change.

1. Deficiency follows as simple deletion or chromosome loss (monosomy). Both of these different kinds of changes can result in a loss of a suppressor and the uncovering of a suppressed gene or gene cluster. We might also note that if the deletion is intercalary then this may result in the bringing together of two originally well-spaced regions of the chromosome following rejoining of the proximal and distal broken ends and lead to a "position effect."

2. Duplication can arise following a simple rearrangement or by chromosome segregation giving trisomy or polysomy. In all cases we are essentially considering an amplification of either a chromosome segment or of a whole chromosome. The amplification in these cases is at a level somewhat less than that discussed by Biedler *et al.* (Chapter 7), but nevertheless may result in increased amounts of transcription of relevant duplicated sequences.

3. Transposition can occur either within chromosomes or as translocations between chromosomes, and here I would include the interpolation of mobile DNA inserts as discussed by J. A. Shapiro (this Symposium). Transpositions can result in four kinds of effects: (1) deletion mutation, (2) point mutation, (3) transfer of active loci resulting in their juxtaposition to inactive sites—whether these be heterochromatin, Z-DNA or turned-off genes—and leading to their suppression, or (4) transfer of inactive loci to active sites, so that the active site promoting machinery activates the transposed and originally quiescent sequence.

There is evidence that each of these three kinds of chromosomal change could be important in activating DNA sequences in the human genome that may be relevant to carcinogenesis, and this leads me to turn to consider the possible association of such chromosomal changes with the presence of *c-onc* sequences in the human genome.

C. Human *c*-oncogenes and Chromosome Anomalies

One of the major excitements in recent weeks has been the use of *c-onc* gene probes to map the locations of some of these sequences in the human genome and to examine their distribution in relation to the chromosomes involved in specific changes in certain neoplasms. In this regard most of us have been especially interested in chromosome 8, not least because of its involvement in Burkitt's lymphoma, and it may be appropriate here to mention that Denis Burkitt and Tony Epstein were the recipients of the cancer research prize donated by the organizers of this Symposium, Bristol-Myers, earlier this year for their work on the lymphoma that bears Dr. Burkitt's name.

The Burkitt's lymphoma story is an exciting one in terms of chromosome rearrangement, gene action, and carcinogenesis and, of course, began with a demonstration of a consistent association between the lymphoma and an 8q;14q translocation that resulted in morphologically distinguishable 8q− and 14q+ chromosomes (Manolov and Monolova, 1972; Zech et al., 1976). It was later shown that the gene cluster for Ig heavy chain was on chromosome 14q and then two other consistent translocations were discovered in about 5% of Burkitt's lymphoma cases, namely, 2;8 and 8;22, with the same 8q24 region involved in all translocations. Earlier this year it was shown that the κ Ig light chain was located in the proximal part of 2p, in the general area of the locus involved in the 2;8 translocation, and the λ light chain was located on the long arm of chromosome 22. In each case, therefore, the q24 region of chromosome 8 underwent exchange with a chromosome region that coded for one of the Ig clusters in a B cell that is an Ig producer (Fig. 1).

C. M. Croce and R. Taub (this Symposium) presented evidence obtained by the elegant studies of their groups that the c-myc oncogene, which is the equivalent of the v-myc of the avian retrovirus MC29 that causes B cell lymphoma in the chick, is located in, or is just distal to, the 8q24 band in man. Moreover, the c-myc gene appears to be transferred to the 14q+ from the 8q− in all the cases so far looked at. Croce showed that in a number of instances the c-myc gene recombined with the Ig C_μ human gene, and Taub also produced evidence for comigration in gels of c-myc and the C_μ switch region. However, it seems clear that the point of exchange in the Ig cluster is not a fixed one and may differ between different Burkitt lines. These dramatic demonstrations raise a number of questions, and I want to briefly address myself to two of them.

First, how does this exchange take place? The most obvious answer to this question is that the exchange event takes place during the normal processing of the Ig genes and may involve an abnormal switching between one of the Ig switches and the DNA sequence on 8q24 associated with, and on the proximal side of, the c-myc gene and which may perhaps share some homologous sequences in the Ig cluster. Evidence from mutagenesis experiments would suggest that translocations between chromosomes take place during DNA replication, and that regions that are involved in nonhomologous exchange must be close together in space and undergo replication at the same time for an exchange event to take place. It is not known, however, if the Ig DNA processing takes place during an S phase, but I would guess that it does, at least in those cases where aberrant translocations result.

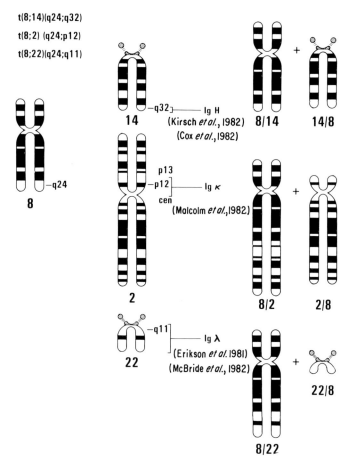

t(8;14)(q24;q32)
t(8;2) (q24;p12)
t(8;22)(q24;q11)

8

14 (Kirsch et al., 1982) 8/14 14/8
(Cox et al., 1982)

— q32⏋— Ig H

2

p13
— p12⏋— Ig κ
cen
(Malcolm et al., 1982)

8/2 2/8

22

— q11⏋— Ig λ
⏌(Erikson et al. 1981)
(McBride et al., 1982)

8/22 22/8

Fig. 1. Diagram illustrating the three different translocations involving 8q24 and the Ig loci in Burkitt's lymphoma.

Second, the DNA processing of an Ig cluster is part of the differentiation process that eventually results in the Ig cluster in the processed chromosome being expressed, whereas the Ig cluster on the homologous chromosome may be processed but not activated due to allelic exclusion. The expectation would therefore be that the 14q+ chromosome in the 8;14 translocation that retains its promotor, and much of the Ig sequences should express its Ig heavy chain and not the normal 14. Similarly, those lymphomas with 2;8 translocations should express the chromosome 2 κ light chain, and 8;22 translocations the chromosome 22 λ light chain. Insofar as the light chains are concerned, Lenoir et al. (1982) have recently shown complete concordance in a number of instances between the type of light chain expressed and the light chain coding chromosome involved in translocation with chromosome 8 (Table I). In my own laboratory we have analyzed the Ig heavy chains produced in 14 lymphoma cell lines carrying the 8;14 translocation, and in some 600 other non-Burkitt lymphoblastoid cell lines not having such translocations. All the non-Burkitt cells produce a normal heavy chain, but three of the t8;14 cell lines produce no detectable heavy chain at all, and one produces an abnormal heavy chain, having a molecular weight some 30% less than normal—a reduction that is not due to differences in glycosylation (McIntosh et al., 1983). These two sets of findings therefore are in accordance with expectation. The implication that follows is that the c-myc gene is transferred from its quiescent location at 8q24 to come under the influence of the Ig promotor on chromosome 14 (or 2 or 22) and is turned on. In discussion Croce indicated that there was some evidence that in a few instances the c-myc gene sequences were amplified, and it would be important to establish the level of c-myc transcription and demonstrate and identify the corresponding protein in these transformed cells. One puzzle that emerged was that in Croce's hybrids between the Burkitt's lymphoma line DAUDI and the nonproducing mouse myeloma cells, those hybrids containing the normal human chromosome 14 apparently produced and secreted IgM, whereas those with the 14q+ did not. This result may seem discrepant in terms of what we have learned so far about the molecular biology of the 8;14 translocations, but there are clearly many other questions that we have to answer before we have a complete picture of the events, and their consequences, that are involved in these exchanges involving an *onc* gene and Ig clusters in Burkitt's lymphoma.

In addition to the c-myc gene, the assignment of two other c-onc genes has been reported at this Symposium, viz., c-Ha-ras-l on 11p by Francke (see Chapter 6) and c-fes on 15q by Sheer et al. (see Chapter 10). A number of other groups have recently assigned other *onc* genes, and Table II lists nine human

TABLE I

Burkitt's Lymphoma: Concordance with Ig Light Chains Secreted and Ig Coded by Translocated Chromosome[a]

No. of lymphomas	Translocation	Light chain Ig coded by chromosome involved	Ig secreted
3	t(2;8)	κ	3 κ
7	t(8;22)	λ	7 λ
17	t(8;14)		9 κ
			8 λ

[a] From Lenoir et al. (1982).

c-onc genes and the eight chromosomes to which they have been assigned. This table also lists the major malignancies in which these particular chromosomes are involved, and this listing invites speculation. For example, is *c-mos* located at 8q22 (the site involved in acute myelogenous leukemia) and *c-fes* at 15q22 (the site involved in acute promyelocytic leukemia)? These are questions that will shortly be answered. The approaches here will involve the use of probes on blots of DNAs from hybrid cells carrying informative translocations or deletions of chromosomes of interest, and in this context the powerful technology of chromosome sorting, as discussed by Drs. Carrano and Young, could make an important contribution in isolating specifically rearranged chromosomes or chromosome segments (see Carrano *et al.*, Chapter 11). Already a number of laboratories have obtained specific chromosome libraries using flow sorting machines, and these are going to prove useful in detailing the sequence domains associated with *c-onc* genes (see Young *et al.*, Chapter 12). Another requirement is the improvement of the old and the development of new methods of locating relatively unique short sequences of DNA, < 2kb long, in chromosome preparations *in situ*. In this regard the novel immunological approach using biotin-labeled probes described by Leary *et al.* (see Chapter 15), and which already offers some advantages over radiolabeled probes in analyzing blots, looks very promising.

One question that we have already referred to is, can we detect RNA transcripts of *c-onc* genes listed in Table II in any of the tumors having specific abnormalities of the relevant chromosome? The answer may well be yes, but these are early days and the picture is, as yet, by no means clear. For example, the *c-myc* gene that we have seen to be associated with, and possibly amplified in, Burkitt's lymphoma is also amplified in the human acute promyelocytic leukemia (APL) cell line HL-60, as well as in original leukemic cells from the patient, but it is not amplified in other similar APL cell lines (Collins and Groudine, 1982; Dalla-Favera *et al.*, 1982a). However, *c-myc*-related RNA is present in all these cell lines so that this locus is expressed, or overexpressed, whether or not the *c-myc* sequences are amplified, perhaps in the form of double minutes as seems possible in HL-60. The specific translocation associated with APL is the t15;17, *c-fes* is on chromosome 15, but whether there are *fes*-related RNAs in these cells is not yet known. Similarly, transcripts related to *c-sis*, which is on chromosome 22, have not been detected in B cell tumors or in CML cells carrying the 9;22 translocation, but are present in sarcomas and gliomas, although whether the latter had abnormalities involving chromosome 22 was not determined (Swan *et al.*, 1982). Our knowledge concerning the expression of *c-onc* sequences associated with specific chromosome anomalies in malignant cells is therefore still somewhat fragmentary, but this is an area of active study so that it will not be long before we have a much clearer picture of the activity and importance of these *c-onc* sequences and of the role played by chromosomal anomalies in their activation.

TABLE II

Assigned Human "c-onc" Genes

Chromosome no.	Site	c-onc	Retrovirus	References	Major malignancy[a]	Translocation, monosomy, deletion, or trisomy	Site
						Major acquired or inherited chromosomal anomalies	
6	6q22–24	*myb*	Avian myeloblastosis	Dalla-Favera et al. (1982b) Harper et al. (1983)	ALL Ovarian carcinoma	del 6 6;14	6q21–25 6q21
8	8q24	*myc*	Avian myelocytomatosis	Croce[b] Taub[b] Taub et al. (1982) Sakaguchi (1983) Neel et al. (1982)	Burkitt's lymphoma ANLL Renal cell carcinoma	8;14; 2;8; 8;22 3;8	8q24
	8q22	*mos*	Moloney murine sarcoma	Rechavi et al. (1982) Prakash et al. (1982) Neel et al. (1982)	AML	8;21	8q22
9	9q34	*abl*	Abelson leukemia	Heisterkamp et al. (1982) de Klein et al. (1982)	CML	9;22	9q34

(continued)

TABLE II (*Continued*)

Chromosome no.	Site	c-onc	Retrovirus	References	Major acquired or inherited chromosomal anomalies		
					Major malignancy[a]	Translocation, monosomy, deletion, or trisomy	Site
11	11p13	ras^{H}-1	Harvey sarcoma	McBride et al. (1982b) de Martinville et al. (1983)	Wilm's tumor	del 11p	11p13
				Francke (Chapter 6)	ALL	4;11	11q23
12		ras^{K}-2	Kirsten sarcoma	Sakaguchi (1983)	B-CLL	tris. 12	tris. 12
15	15q 24–25	fes	Feline sarcoma	Dalla-Favera et al. (1982b) Heisterkamp et al. (1982) Sheer et al. (Chapter 10) Harper et al. (1983)	APL	15;17	15q22 (15q24–25?)
20		src	Rous sarcoma	Sakaguchi et al. (1983)	Mult. end. neo. 2	del 20p	20p12.2
22		sis	Simian sarcoma	Swan et al. (1982)	CML Meningioma	9;22 mon. 22	22q11 mon. 22

[a] AML, acute myelogenous leukemia; CML, chronic myelogenous leukemia; ALL, acute lymphocytic leukemia; B-ALL, B cell acute lymphocytic leukemia; APL, acute promyelocytic leukemia; Mult. end. neo. 2, Multiple endocrine neoplasia type 2.

The question was asked about the relation, in terms of chromosome assignment, of c-onc genes in man and mouse. It has been argued that these genes have been conserved throughout evolution and that they are common to a wide variety of vertebrates and so we might expect that they might be associated with similar linkage groups in man and mouse. I need hardly remind you of the elegant work of George Klein's group (Klein, 1981) on trisomy 15 in mouse T cell leukemias and the 12;15 and 6;15 translocations in the B cell plasmacytomas which were discussed by Spira (see Chapter 5). It may come as no surprise therefore to see that the c-myc gene in the mouse maps to chromosome 15, paralleling the assignment of c-myc to chromosome 8 in man. Other assigned c-onc genes in the mouse that have been assigned in man are summarized in Table III and these clearly show the expected syntenic relationships.

While referring to the mouse, I should like to draw attention to one interesting finding from Spira's work that may have an important relevance to man. This is the demonstration that the chromosomes 15 of different strains of mice appear to have different potencies with regard to their involvement in malignant transformation. Whether this offers a possible explanation for some of the geographical variation in the involvement of particular chromosome changes in certain human leukemias referred to by Mitelman might be worthy of consideration.

TABLE III

Chromosome Assignment of c-onc Genes in Man and Mouse

Onc gene and associated markers	Chromosome No.		References
	Man	Mouse	
c-src	20	2	Sakaguchi et al. (1983)
Inosine triphosphate	20	2	
Adenosine deaminase	20	2	
c-fes	15	2	
β₂-Microglobulin	15	2	Sheer et al. (Chapter 10)
Sorbitol dehydrogenase	15	2	Heisterkamp et al. (1982)
c-abl	9	2	
Adenylate kinase 1	9	2	Heisterkamp et al. (1982)
c-myc	8	15	Croce[a]
			Taub[a]
			Sakaguchi (1983)

[a] Results reported at this Symposium.

IV. Concluding Comments

Despite the obvious importance of, and the excitement associated with, the very considerable advances in our understanding of the relevance of oncogenes in carcinogenesis, I think I must emphasize that cancer is a multiple of diseases, and it would have been quite impossible for us to discuss all aspects of this problem in one symposium. I should perhaps mention that we have hardly referred to the directly transforming DNA viruses, such as those of the herpes family, which clearly cause cancer in animals and probably man; we have not discussed the importance of promoting substances, except in a brief reference to their possible effects in promoting transcription, or the suppressing effects of certain human chromosomes on the tumorigenicity of hybrid malignant cells (Klinger, 1982); and we have barely touched upon the mechanisms of action of hormones and of physical and chemical carcinogens. We must also not forget that *in vitro* cellular transformation by an oncogene is a ''dominant'' one-step process, but human carcinogenesis proceeds in many steps, so that oncogene activation can only be one of several events involved in the process of carcinogenesis.

Notwithstanding my qualifications, the demonstrations that a normal human gene can be activated at the wrong time, or in the wrong place, by transposition to sites of transcriptionally active endogenous sequences in the genome, or by linkage to a retroviral long terminal repeat segment, with the consequent acquisition by the cell of malignant properties, constitute a really remarkable, exciting, and major advance in our understanding of one very important aspect of the process of carcinogenesis. These findings of course raise numerous questions, many of which have been explored at this Symposium. One which we did not have time to consider is whether oncogene activation is relevant in interpreting the remarkable data on mice and rats showing that exposure to mutagens not only induces cancers in the parents, but increases their incidence in the offspring and later generations (Nomura, 1982). Another, which we touched upon, is whether oncogenes are involved in the development of inherited childhood cancers that are clearly associated with abnormalities in differentiation, as, for example, in the kidney in Wilms tumor, in the same way as may be the case in the acquired abnormalities of differentiation in the leukemias? It is tempting to consider that these kinds of predispositions may result from inherited genomic changes that affect the expression of potentially oncogenic differentiation genes. Now that we are beginning to define these oncogenes, their constituent DNA sequences, RNA transcripts, and the proteins they produce, we are well along the road toward an understanding of the events that occur at the genomic and cellular levels that are of significance in the development of cancers. This in turn opens up new opportunities for the development of new diagnostic and therapeutic approaches, and our expectation for the future is surely that we can translate these dramatic advances at the cellular and molecular levels into practical achievements in the clinic.

References

Amtmann, E., and Sauer, G. (1982). *Nature (London)* **296**, 675–677.
Behe, M., and Felsenfeld, G. (1981). *Proc. Natl. Acad. Sci. U.S.A.* **78**, 1619–1623.
Bishop, J. O. (1974). *Cell* **2**, 81–86.
Blair, D. G., Oskarsson, M., Wood, T. G., McClements, W. L., Fischinger, P. J., and Vande Woude, G. G. (1981). *Science* **212**, 941–943.
Boveri, T. (1914). "Zur Frage der Entstehung maligner Tumoren". Fischer, Jena.
Chang, E. H., Furth, M. E., Scolnick, E. M., and Lowy, D. R. (1982). *Nature (London)* **297**, 479–483.
Collett, M. S., Brugge, J. S., and Erikson, R. L. (1978). *Cell* **15**, 1363–1369.
Collett, M. S., Erikson, E., Purchio, A. F., and Erikson, R. L. (1981). *In* "Genes, Chromosomes, and Neoplasia" (F. E. Arrighi, P. N. Rao, and E. Stubblefield, eds.), pp. 105–122. Raven, New York.
Collins, S., and Groudine, M. (1982). *Nature (London)* **298**, 679–681.
Cooper, G. M. (1982). *Science* **218**, 801–806.
Cox, W. D., Markovic, V. D., and Teshima, I. E. (1982). *Nature (London)* **297**, 428–430.
Dalla-Favera, R., Wong-Staal, F., and Gallo, R. C. (1982a). *Nature (London)* **299**, 61–63.
Dalla-Favera, R., Franchini, G., Martinotti, S., Wong-Staal, F., Gallo, R. C., and Croce, C. M. (1982b). *Proc. Natl. Acad. Sci. U.S.A.* **79**, 4714–4717.
De Klein, A., Van Kessel, A. G., Grosveld, G., Bartram, C. R., Hagemeijer, A., Bootsma, D., Spurr, N. K., Heisterkamp, N., Groffen, J., and Stephenson, J. R. (1982). *Nature* **300**, 765–767.
Dhar, R., Ellis, R. W., Shih, T. Y., Oroszlan, S., Shapiro, B., Maizel, J., Lowy, D., and Scolnick, E. (1982). *Science* **217**, 934–937.
de Martinville, B., Giacolone, J., Shih, C., Weinberg, R. A., and Franke, U. (1983). *Science* **219**, 498–501.
Erikson, J., Martinis, J., and Croce, C. M. (1981). *Nature (London)* **294**, 173–175.
Gooderham, K., and Jeppesen, P. (1983). *Exp. Cell Res.* (in press).
Hamada, H., and Kakunaga, T. (1982). *Nature (London)* **298**, 396–398.
Harper, M. E., Simon, M. I., Franchini, G., Gallo, R. C., and Wong Staal, F. (1983). *Proc. Natl. Acad. Sci. U.S.A.* (in press).
Heisterkamp, N., Groffen, J., Stephenson, J. R., Spurr, N. K., Goodfellow, P. N., Solomon, E., Carritt, B., and Bodmer, W. F. (1982). *Nature (London)* **299**, 747–749.
ISCN (1981). "An International System for Human Cytogenetic Nomenclature—High Resolution Banding, 1981". *Birth Defects, Orig. Artic. Ser.* XVII:5. March of Dimes Birth Defects Foundation, New York.
Kirsch, I. R., Morton, C. C., Nakahara, K., and Leder, P. (1982). *Science* **216**, 301–303.
Klein, G. (1981). *Nature (London)* **294**, 313–318.
Klinger, H. P. (1982). *Cytogenet. Cell Genet.* **32**, 68–84.
Krontiris, T. G., and Cooper, G. M. (1981). *Proc. Natl. Acad. Sci. U.S.A.* **78**, 1181–1184.
Lamb, M. M., and Daneholt, B. (1979). *Cell* **17**, 835–848.
Lenoir, G. M., Preudhomme, J. L., Bernheim, A., and Berger, R. (1982). *Nature (London)* **298**, 747–746.

McBride, O. W., Hieter, P. A., Hollis, G. F., Swan, D., Otey, M. C., and Leder, P. (1982a). *J. Exp. Med.* **155**, 1480–1490.

McBride, O. W., Swan, D. C., Santos, E., Barbacid, M., Tronick, S. R., and Aaronson, S. A. (1982b). *Nature (London)* **300**, 773–774.

McCready, S. J., Jackson, D. A., and Cook, P. R. (1982). *In* "Progress in Mutation Research" (A. T. Natarajan, G. Obe, and H. Altmann, eds.), Vol. 4, pp. 113–130. Elsevier, Amsterdam.

McIntosh, R. V., Cohen, B. B., Steel, C. M., Read, H., Moxley, M., and Evans, H. J. (1983). *Int. J. Cancer* **31**, 275–279.

Malcolm, S., Barton, P., Murphy, C., Ferguson-Smith, M. A., Bentley, D. L., and Rabbits, T. H. (1982). *Proc. Natl. Acad. Sci. U.S.A.* **79**, 4957–4961.

Manolov, G., and Manolova, Y. (1972). *Nature (London)* **237**, 33–34.

Marshall, C. J., Hall, A., and Weiss, R. A. (1982). *Nature (London)* **299**, 171–173.

Mayfield, J. E., Serunian, L. A., Silver, L. M., and Elgin, S. C. R. (1978). *Cell* **14**, 539–544.

Miller, D. A., Okamoto, E., Erlanger, B. F., and Miller, O. J. (1982). *Cytogenet. Cell Genet.* **33**, 345–349.

Miller, D. M., Turner, P., Nienhuis, A. W., Axelrod, D. E., and Gopalakrishnan, T. V. (1978). *Cell* **14**, 511–521.

Mohandas, T., Sparkes, R. S., and Shapiro, L. J. (1981). *Science* **211**, 393–396.

Müller, R., Slamon, D. J., Tremblay, J. M., Cline, M. J., and Verma, I. M. (1982). *Nature* **299**, 640–644.

Neel, B. G., Jhanwar, S. C., Chaganti, R. S. K., and Hayward, W. S. (1982). *Proc. Natl. Acad. Sci. U.S.A.* **79**, 7842–7846.

Nomura, T. (1982). *Nature (London)* **296**, 575–577.

Nordheim, A., Pardue, M. L., Lafer, E. M., Möller, A., Stollar, B. D., and Rich, A. (1981). *Nature (London)* **294**, 417–422.

Prakash, K., McBride, O. W., Swan, D. C., Devare, S. G., Tronick, S. R., and Aaronson, S. A. (1982). *Proc. Natl. Acad. Sci. U.S.A.* **79**, 5210–5214.

Rechavi, G., Givol, D., and Canaani, E. (1982). *Nature (London)* **300**, 607–611.

Sakaguchi, A. Y. (1983). *In* "Oncogenes and Retroviruses" Alan Liss Inc., New York (in press).

Sakaguchi, A. Y., Naylor, S. L., and Shows, T. B.(1983). *Prog. Nucleic Acid Res.* (in press).

Santos, E., Tronick, S. R., Aaronson, S. A., Pulciani, S., and Barbacid, M. (1982). *Nature (London)* **298**, 343–347.

Shih, C., Padhy, L. C., Murray, M., and Weinberg, R. A. (1981). *Nature (London)* **290**, 261–264.

Singleton, C. K., Klysik, J., Stirdivant, S. M., and Wells, R. D. (1982). *Nature (London)* **299**, 312–316.

Swan, D. C., McBride, O. W., Robbins, K. C., Keithley, D. A., Reddy, E. P., and Aaronson, S. A. (1982). *Proc. Natl. Acad. Sci. U.S.A.* **79**, 4691–4695.

Taub, R., Kirsch, I., Morton, C., Lenoir, G., Swan, D., Tronick, S., Aaronson, S., and Leder, P. (1982). *Proc. Natl. Acad. Sci. U.S.A.* **79**, 7837–7841.

Tsuchida, N., Ryder, T., and Ohtsubo, E. (1982). *Science* **217**, 937–939.

Venolia, L., Gartler, S. M., Wassman, E. R., Yen, P., Mohandas, T., and Shapiro, L. J. (1982). *Proc. Natl. Acad. Sci. U.S.A.* **79**, 2352–2354.

Wang, A. H. J., Quigley, G. J., Kolpak, F. J., Crawford, J. L., Van Book, J. H., Van Der Marel, G., and Rich, A. (1979). *Nature (London)* **282**, 680–686.

Watson, R., Oskarsson, M., and Vande Woude, G. G. (1982). *Proc. Natl. Acad. Sci. U.S.A.* **79**, 4078–4082.

Westin, E. H., Gallo, R. C., Arya, S. K., Eva, A., Souza, L. M., Baluda, M. A., Aaronson, S. A., and Wong-Staal, F. (1982). *Proc. Natl. Acad. Sci. U.S.A.* **79**, 2194–2198.

Zech, L., Haglund, U., Nilsson, K., and Klein, G. (1976). *Int. J. Cancer* **17**, 47–56.

Zimmerman, F. (1982). *Ann. New York Acad. Sci.* (in press).

Index

A

Abelson leukemia, 347
Abelson virus, 141
Adenoma, pleomorphic, 77, 79
Adenovirus, 248, 259
  type-2 major late promoter, 29–42
  upstream sequence effect, 37–40
Alkaline phosphatase, biotinglation, 276–277
Alloantigen H-2, 141
Anemia, siderblastic, 94
Angioimmunoblastic lymphadenopathy,
  324–325
Aniridia, 107–113
Aniridia–Wilms' tumor, 78, 79, 106–109
Antifolate resistance, 119–123

B

Benzpyrene, leukemia induction, 140
Biotin-labeled probe, colorimetric method,
  273–290
Bladder carcinoma
  cell, EJ, 11
  transforming gene, 47–50
Bombyx mori, 20
Burkitt's lymphoma, 65, 73, 94–95
  chromosome anomaly, 343–346
  c-myc oncogene, 174–178
  immunoglobulin gene translocation,
    167–174
Burkitt tumor, 254

C

Cancer, induced, 140–142
Carcinoma, 65, *see also* specific types
Cervical carcinoma, 77, 79
Chromatin
  alteration
    DNase sensitivity, 303–304
    globin gene domain, 298–304
    methylation, 299–303
  organization, 22–24
Chromosomal scaffold, 18, 20
  breakpoint position, 220
  clone localization, 215–217
  expressed sequence, 217–219
  single copy sequence isolation, 214–215
Chromosome, *see also* specific chromosomal
  numbers
  aberration, external factor effect, 69, 150–156
  anomaly, 341–349
    human oncogene, 342–349
  architecture, 334–336
  deletion, 101–104, 144–148
    11p13 band, 106–112
    13q14 band, 101–104, 109
  Epstein–Barr virus integration, 254–265
  isolation, 197
  nonviral DNA integration, 265–268
  onc gene assignment, 349
  pattern, *see also* Cytogenetics
    clinical significance, 311–331
    Paris nomenclature, 57–60
  Philadelphia, 57, 63, 66–68
  ring, 132